EARTHLY BODIES
&
HEAVENLY HAIR

*Natural and Healthy Personal Care
for Every Body*

BY DINA FALCONI
HERBALIST AND FOUNDER, FALCON FORMULATIONS

ILLUSTRATIONS BY ALAN McKNIGHT
PHOTOGRAPHS BY DAVID GOLDBECK

Ceres Press
Woodstock, New York

Published by Ceres Press, PO Box 87, Dept. EB, Woodstock, New York 12498

Cover design by Mark Larson
Illustrations by Alan McKnight
Photography by David Goldbeck
Book design by Vicki Hickman and David Goldbeck

Printing: 10 9 8 7

First Edition

Library of Congress Cataloging-in-Publication Data

Falconi, Dina
        Earthly bodies & heavenly hair : natural and healthy personal care for every body / by Dina Falconi ; illustrated by Alan McKnight ; photography by David Goldbeck.
        p. cm.
        Includes index.
        ISBN: 1-886101-04-3
        1. Skin—Care and hygiene. 2. Hair—Care and hygiene. 3. Beauty—Personal. 4. Herbal Cosmetics. I. Title. II Title: Earthly bodies and heavenly hair.
        RL87.F35 1997
        646.7'2   97-069510

Printed in Canada

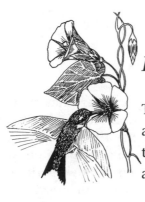

Dedication

This book is dedicated to Sam
and all our Children,
that their world may be safer, healthier
and more enjoyable.

❧ *Acknowledgments* ❧

I want to thank Jennifer Fox for making this book happen. Her support as a friend and her assistance with the actual writing and editing has proved invaluable — without her the book might never have been written. I am also indebted to her and her partner, Lincoln Stoller, for teaching me how to use the computer. They were both there to help me out of computer mayhem. Thanks also to Lincoln for providing the computer this book was written on.

Thanks to all who shared their valuable formulas with me. I am especially grateful to Rosemary Gladstar, who laid the foundation for various formulations. I thank her in particular for the basic cream recipe, basic scrub recipe and Queen of Hungary's Water formula, and for all her inspiration and loving support. Thanks also to Jean Argus, Sage Blue, Ed Smith, Randi Barouch, Ken Landauer, Wendy Weiner, Kate Gilday, Reid, Kim, Rosa Torres, Julie Robbins and Blade.

I am grateful to my first teacher, Mickey Carter, who shared his wisdom and guided me into the world of natural healing. Thanks to Pam Montgomery, who introduced me to wild plants and opened the "green" door to herbalism. I am greatly indebted to William LeSassier, who generously and wholeheartedly shared his herbal expertise, and encouraged me to practice the art of herbal healing.

A special thanks to David Goldbeck for pursuing me to take on this project, and for shepherding it through the transformation from first draft to final publication.

Thanks to Vicki Hickman for designing the book so beautifully and to Alan McKnight for his illustrations that add such grace to the pages. I would also like to thank Meril Schnieder for her generosity in indexing the book.

Thanks to the many people who helped along the way, including Charlie Blumstein, Buzzy Tischler, Motria and Marco.

Finally, my deepest thanks go to Tim Allen, who has endured it all with me.

DINA FALCONI
Kerhonkson, New York
May 1997

❦ *Table of Contents* ❦

❦ *Introduction* ❦

I love introducing people to the art and science of home-crafted body care products. There are so many rewards: Most people rejoice in the new feelings of health and radiance they experience after using formulations made from healing and aromatic herbs. Some simply like the process of creating items for themselves and others that they thought had to be purchased ready-made. Others appreciate the fantastic financial savings. Then there are those who are taken with the minimal impact they are having on the environment. No matter what the motivation, the result is the same — an improvement in individual and planetary health.

I have been teaching and exploring the realm of natural body care for over nine years. My experience has taught me that the physical aspect we present to the world reflects our inner state of being. To me, natural body care is not about masking one's supposed "flaws" with cosmetics, denying the aging process, or living up to some standardized — and unrealistic — concept of beauty. Rather, it involves creating and maintaining inner harmony and outer balance.

Natural body care products, in contrast to commercial ones, are based on the philosophy of working in partnership with nature to support and nurture the body throughout its life cycle. The idea is to start with simple, pure ingredients that are as close to their natural state as possible. These are then combined according to their specific actions into formulas that enable the body to gently soothe, nourish and heal itself.

The shift to natural body care encourages a subtle change in consciousness away from the negative rhetoric of the commercial cosmetic industry. For instance, instead of slathering on "anti-aging" formulas or "fighting" wrinkles, natural body care offers optimum nourishment to the skin to keep it supple and hydrated through all of its cycles and changes. The underlying philosophy of self-acceptance is an acceptance of nature.

Creating and using natural body care products makes good sense for your own well-being and for that of our planet Earth. With a few easy-to-find ingredients, a handful of readily available herbs and some basic kitchen equipment, anyone can produce an array of homemade commodities that will make the common synthetic commercial concoctions superfluous.

When you make your own natural cosmetics you know exactly what you are putting on your body and where the ingredients came from. And you won't sacrifice quality or effectiveness by changing from synthetic, chemically based products to all-natural, nontoxic ones, many of which are actually safe enough to eat. In fact, you will probably find, as I have, that your body thrives on these homemade products.

Earthly Bodies & Heavenly Hair allows you to replace harsh chemicals, dyes and perfumes with pure, simple ingredients that are gentle to your body. Many ingredients used in commercial products are common allergens that can cause such reactions as skin rashes or eye irritations, while strong synthetic scents trigger nausea and headaches in some individuals. Moreover, certain commercial ingredients are suspected carcinogens; others are believed to lead to insidious long-term health effects, such as damage to the liver and central nervous system when they build up in the body over time. The alarming increase in individuals with multiple chemical sensitivities is a testament to the wisdom of replacing commercial, synthetic cosmetics with homemade, natural body care products.

The information and formulas contained in this book will equip you to start creating your own natural body care products. In addition to making these blends for your own consumption, you'll be able to create distinctive gifts that are both personal and economical. Avoiding commercial cosmetic products is also a small gift you can give to the Earth, since the cosmetics industry inevitably spews toxins into the environment and contributes to clogged landfills with its wasteful packaging practices.

Earthly Bodies & Heavenly Hair is about sharing the desire to feel more connected and nurtured physically, emotionally and spiritually. I offer it as an inspirational guide to developing your own natural body care products, and as a resource to help connect you with other people who make and sell products and ingredients in the natural health and beauty arena. I feel that the skin — like the surface of the Earth — is a highly complex and sensitive organ that responds to everything that comes into contact with it. You might say that if it's not good for the environment, it's not good for your skin. An oil slick is no better for your face than for the Alaskan coastline, yet many commercial facial creams rely on petroleum by-products as primary ingredients. Your body is a world unto itself, so it makes sense to treat it with the same basic love, care and respect that you would the Earth.

My own entrée to herbal body care was through natural healing, which continues to be the focus of my work and my heart's true path. I started this journey as a child growing up in New York City's East Village when, at age eleven, I began to be plagued with painful, migrainelike headaches. At that time a friend of my family's, Mickey Carter, an elderly man who had cured himself of a terminal illness, became my mentor and helped guide me back to health. Under his direction I eliminated all processed products from my diet and replaced them with fresh, natural whole foods. This entailed a considerable change of lifestyle, since I was a typical junk food devotee. Within a year of adopting Mickey's health regime, not only did my headaches disappear, but my hair grew glossy and thick and my complexion took on a new vibrancy. The changes related to my new lifestyle affected me at the core of my being — I knew that I was onto something that felt right. I also became sensitive to what I was putting *on* my body. Commercial synthetic skin and hair preparations felt unhealthy to me, so I began to explore the alternatives. At that point in my life, this meant frequent trips to the health food store to buy body care products.

Six years later, when the time came for me to leave home for college, I took the next step and moved away from the city to a rural setting in upstate New York. In 1987, during my final year in college, when I was pregnant with my son Sam, I began to explore the nutritive and healing value of herbs. This is when I was first introduced to the wild plants that literally grew outside my back door. In addition to harvesting these wild "weeds," I eventually began cultivating my own herb and vegetable garden. To a city girl, this new sense of self-sufficiency and awareness of nature's bounty was a profoundly liberating and empowering experience.

In 1988, I began my formal training as a wildcrafter and medicine-maker with the herbalist Pam Montgomery, creator of a line of herbal products known as *Green Terrestrial*. In 1991, I pursued more advanced studies in clinical herbalism with William LeSassier, who draws on both Eastern and Western herbal traditions in his healing practice. When I began to teach herbalism at herbal conferences, in women's groups and in community and continuing education programs, I found my way into natural skin care. This interest was inspired by my students, who, besides wanting to know about herbal health care, were also hungry for information on natural skin and hair care. I eventually developed Falcon Formulations, a well-received line of herbal skin and hair care products.

Although this book is about creating body care products, I have a firm belief in the importance of caring for the body from the inside as well. This means eating a balanced diet of nourishing whole foods, drinking plenty of pure water, getting enough rest and exercise and treating yourself to a daily dose of fresh air and sunshine. These factors contribute to your appearance even more than what you put on your skin and hair. Not surprisingly, many of the food items that form the basis of a wholesome diet are the very ingredients found in the body care formulas presented here.

Earthly Bodies and Heavenly Hair is intended to be a garden of herbal skin and hair care. Writing it provided an opportunity for me to organize and share more widely what I have learned about natural personal care. Other herbalists have enriched the book by generously providing me with their successful and highly prized formulations, and I am very grateful to them for their generosity.

The book is organized to provide ready access according to your needs. There are special chapters for men, teens, babies and elders — people often ignored in a book of this type. To make things as easy as possible, I have specially marked basic and beginner formulations which rely mostly on common household ingredients with the basic bee 🐝. If you find you don't have the time or inclination to produce all of your own body care products, there is a reference section at the end of the book listing individuals and small businesses that offer Earth-conscious products made with the utmost respect for nature. If you decide to buy rather than make your own natural personal care products, you can use this book to discover which herbal products are best for your particular needs. Those who would like more information will find at the back of this book a list of other books on herbalism and nutrition.

Once you have mastered the fundamental techniques and sampled some of the formulations, let your imagination fly — that and Earth's bounty are the only limits to what you can create.

Dina Falconi

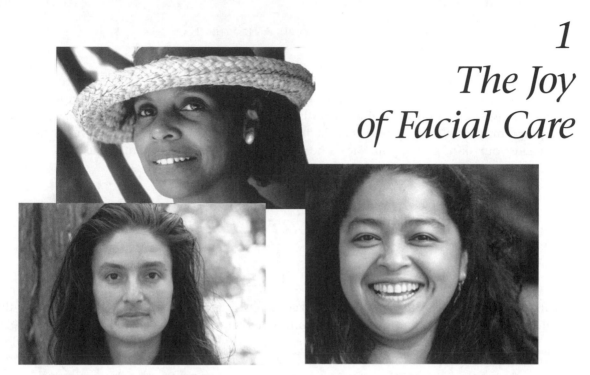

1
The Joy of Facial Care

Your face, perhaps more than any other part of your body, serves as an outer expression of your inner state of being. When you are happy, relaxed and well-nourished, your face glows with health and contentment; when you are upset, stressed or sick, your face may look tense, dull or drawn. While you likely clothe and protect other parts of your body according to social custom and the imperatives of the environment in which you live, your face is most often left exposed to the world. Even if you customarily wear a "mask" of some sort — such as eyeglasses, sunglasses, makeup and the like — your face still communicates your feelings and inner essence to others. Because of its high degree of exposure and its key role in communication, your face deserves a great deal of care and attention. Thus, the perfect place to start a regimen of natural and healthful body care is with the face.

Facial skin is especially sensitive to chemical and environmental influences, because it tends to be thinner and more porous than skin elsewhere on the body. Most people who have experimented with different commercial facial products have probably experienced anything from a mild irritation or reddening of the skin to a full-blown rash at some point. The nose, eyes and mouth are direct openings to the interior of the body, and provide obvious routes of entry for irritating substances; allergic responses, such as headaches, sinus congestion and lung disorders, are some of the possible side effects that can result. Facial preparations and treatments should therefore be as gentle as possible without compromising effectiveness.

A good, basic facial care program is composed of three phases: cleansing, toning and moisturizing. Each of these phases, in turn, may consist of one or more processes, depending on your skin type and special needs. Note that in general, whatever you do for your face can also be extended to your neck region. The most sensitive areas of your face — the eyes and lips — sometimes need a little extra care, no matter what type of skin you have.

This chapter is organized into three sections, corresponding to each of the above-mentioned phases of facial skin care, followed by a section dealing with eye care. Each of the formulas indicates the type of skin or conditions for which it is appropriate. Facial care regimens for different skin types appear at the end of the chapter. These help provide a starting point for creating a customized program that works best for you. As you embark on your natural facial care program, you will likely find that the treatments offered here help to relieve tensions and rejuvenate your skin, giving your face a healthier, more open and inviting aspect.

◊ *Facial Care Phases* ◊

PHASE 1: CLEANSING

For most people the word "cleansing" suggests washing with soap and water. Although this is one way to cleanse your skin, it is certainly not the only, nor even the best way, to begin your skin care routine. Steams, scrubs, masques, cleansing oils and cleansing creams are alternatives that can offer benefits not provided by the traditional soap-and-water method. And sometimes just a gentle rinse with pure spring water is all the cleansing your skin may need.

The first principle to understand about cleansing — despite what the advertisements say — is that you don't necessarily need to cleanse your face every day. If your facial skin looks clear and feels clean, frequent cleansing is not desirable. This is because your skin produces a natural protective oily substance called sebum that helps to keep it healthy by providing a natural antibacterial layer and holding in moisture. Habitually stripping away this protective layer can stress or damage your skin. The goal in cleansing is to gently remove impurities and dead skin cells while encouraging the skin to produce a healthy, protective mantle of sebum. Overcleansing is especially damaging to dry skin, since it leaves it vulnerable to moisture loss. However, too much cleansing — particularly when it involves scrubbing — can also be detrimental to oily skin by stimulating sebum overproduction. The key is to tailor your cleansing process to your skin's particular needs, and to proceed with moderation; remember that more is not necessarily better.

Experiment to find what works best for you, bearing in mind that you will probably want to use a combination of cleansing techniques. For example, in general my face does not require a daily cleaning. However, because the pores around my nostrils tend to get clogged with excess oil, this area benefits from a daily "spot" cleansing. To do this I simply apply oil or astringent to a small piece of cotton cloth and wipe it gently over the appropriate areas. In addition, about once a week I like to cleanse my face by rubbing it all over with olive oil, wiping off the dirt and residue with a soft cotton cloth, then following up with a 20-minute herbal steam treatment. I like to follow the steam treatment with an exfoliating or nourishing masque, and then to tone and moisturize as needed. I am attentive to seasonal changes in my skin as well, and vary my cleansing routine accordingly. For example, I tend to cleanse my face less frequently in the winter, when indoor heating dries out my skin.

Cleansing Oils and Creams

Cleansing oils and creams are lubricating solvents that effectively remove makeup and other oil-soluble dirt from the skin. They provide a gentle and nutritive approach to cleansing dry, damaged and irritated skin. This cleansing approach may not be as suitable for oily or blemished skin types, though I have seen acne clear up with the use of oil-based cleansers.

BASIC CLEANSING TECHNIQUE USING OILS AND CREAMS. To cleanse the face with a cleansing cream or oil, spread a small amount of oil or cream onto the face with your fingers and massage gently into the skin for a couple of minutes to help loosen dirt and grime. Wipe off the oil with a soft cotton cloth. Cleansing creams are especially effective for removing makeup or other greasy grime. For makeup removal, saturate a disposable cotton ball or pad with cleansing oil or cream and wipe the area to be cleaned. Repeat, if necessary, until the area is completely clean. Cleansing oils and creams are often the first step in a cleansing regimen, and may be followed by a deep cleansing treatment such as a scrub, masque or steam.

Choose from among the oils mentioned in the Ingredients chapter that are appropriate for your skin type, or refer to the following table. The table provides a quick review of which oils are appropriate for which skin types based on my experience. Remember that each person is different and will respond uniquely to each oil, so trial and error is your best teacher.

Oils and Corresponding Skin Type

When I teach classes on natural skin care, I like to introduce people to different carrier oils and butters by passing around samples for everyone to apply to their skin. The students note which oils sit on the skin's surface and which ones are absorbed right away, whether they leave the skin softer or drier and whether the aroma is strong or mild. Each person will have a unique response to each oil, learning firsthand which ones are best suited for their skin. Although generalizations can be made about the different types of oil — for example, that grapeseed oil tends to be drying, while olive oil is more lubricating — each individual's skin will respond a little differently. I recommend testing individual carrier oils in this manner, and making notes on your responses. This will provide a good starting point for making your own customized treatments.

Olive oil for normal to dry skin
Coconut oil for normal to dry skin
Grapeseed oil for normal to oily skin
Jojoba oil for most skin types and especially for dry, damaged and mature skin
Almond or **canola oil** for normal skin

🐝 *Basic Cleansing Oil with Essential Oils* ALL

By adding essential oils to the carrier oils you increase the cleansing action of the oil.

To each ounce of carrier oil add 5 drops of essential oil

Pour the carrier oil into a 1-oz. glass jar, add essential oil, cap the jar and shake well. The oil is ready for use. Makes 1 oz. *Variations follow:*

Grapeseed Orange Cleansing Oil OILY

A fresh-smelling cleansing oil for oily skin. Some oily skin responds well to an oil cleanser and some doesn't. The addition of the orange and sage essential oils improves the grapeseed oil's solvent capacity for oil and grease.
Use 1 oz. grapeseed oil, 3 drops orange essential oil, and 2 drops sage essential oil.

Olive Lavender Cleansing Oil DRY

An invigorating and refreshing cleansing oil for dry skin.
Use 1 oz. olive oil, 3 drops lavender, and 2 drops rosemary essential oil.

Almond Delight Cleansing Oil NORMAL

A refreshing cleansing oil for normal skin.
Use 1 oz. almond oil, 2 drops rosemary essential oil, 1 drop orange essential oil, and 2 drops lavender essential oil.

Cleopatra's Cleansing Oil ALL

A good emollient oil for most skin types with antimicrobial and grime-cleansing action.

1 oz. olive oil
2 oz. canola oil
1 oz. coconut oil
7 drops rosemary essential oil

6 drops orange essential oil
4 drops tea tree essential oil
3 drops sage essential oil

Place olive, canola and coconut oils into a heat-proof measuring cup in a hot-water bath and heat till coconut oil has completely melted. Pour oils into a squeeze bottle or wide-mouth jar and drop in essential oils, stirring well. Cap and shake. It is ready to use. Note that as the oil cools, it will thicken due to the presence of the coconut oil. Yields 4 oz.

Basic Cleansing Cream ALL

This cream is excellent for removing makeup and other grime from the skin. It is an emulsion of water and oil using beeswax and borax as the emulsifying agents. The addition of the water makes this cream lighter than the cleansing oils and in some cases more effective for oily and blemished skin.

7 oz. canola oil
10 oz. distilled water
½ oz. beeswax
1 teaspoon borax

optional: 25 drops rosemary essential oil, 15 drops lavender essential oil, 10 drops orange essential oil

Place beeswax and canola oil into a heat-proof measuring cup in a hot-water bath. Stir occasionally until wax is completely melted into the oil. Then remove from heat and let cool to body temperature. Meanwhile dissolve borax into water and warm to body temperature. Pour oil-wax mixture into a bowl and blend with handheld mixer with one beater, add the water borax mixture a little at a time, then beat until creamy and thick, about 5 minutes. Add optional essential oils and stir in thoroughly. Pour into wide-mouth jars. Note that the addition of the essential oils increases the cleansing action of the cream while adding a wonderful aroma. Makes about 17 oz.

Facial Steams

Facial steams are a wonderful way to relax and deeply cleanse the face, open the pores and increase circulation to the skin. Steaming is an excellent cleansing technique for all skin types, offering a recharging and rejuvenating effect. For added benefits you can use the facial steam as a medium for aromatherapy, adding an appropriate essential oil for the desired effect, such as relaxation or invigoration. Steams are also excellent upper respiratory decongestants, with or without the addition of botanical ingredients. Steams are optimally done about once or twice a week, and are often done prior to applying a masque. After steaming the pores are wide open, which allows the masque to penetrate more deeply.

BASIC STEAM TECHNIQUE. Before steaming, it is helpful to remove makeup and surface dirt from face with oil, cleansing cream or other appropriate cleanser. In general, the technique for doing a steam is to begin by placing the desired ingredients into a quart-size, heat-proof bowl. Pour in one pint of boiling water, preferably pure well water or bottled spring water; avoid using water from a treated or municipal supply. Slowly lower your face over the bowl and place a bath towel over both your head and the bowl to form a "tent" that helps to retain the steam. Be very careful not to lower your face too quickly or too close to the steaming liquid, and never leave the bowl over a heat source while you are steaming! Remain in the steam tent for about 20 minutes. In general, you should allow your face to air-dry rather than toweling off after a steam before proceeding to the next step in your skin care routine. If you are following the steam with a scrub, masque, toner or moisturizer, it is ideal to begin any of these treatments while your skin is still slightly moist.

It is perfectly acceptable to begin a facial treatment with a pure water steam to which no additional ingredients have been added. However, the addition of herbs and/or essential oils chosen for your specific needs offers extra therapeutic value. Following are some of my favorite steam treatments:

❧ *"Christmas Tree" Steam*   ALL

A fabulous year-round steam made with fresh tree clippings. This is especially nice in the winter months, and also useful as a decongestant. To make, simply clip off the tips of some white pine, spruce and/or hemlock trees. You can even recycle your Christmas tree or wreaths for steaming, provided they haven't been sprayed or treated. Use 2 large handfuls of plant material to 1 pint of water. Follow directions for Basic Steam Technique.

🐝 Tea Bag Steam   ALL

Look in your cupboard and choose from among the aromatic herbal teas, such as chamomile, mint and the like. Most tea blends that are commonly consumed can also be used for steaming. Use 3–4 herbal tea bags for 1 pint of water. Follow directions for Basic Steam Technique.

Refer to the table below for a quick glance at herbs and their corresponding skin type properties. (See Botanicals section in Ingredients chapter for more detailed herbal information.)

🐝 Culinary Herb and Spice Steams   ALL

Your kitchen cupboard has aromatic spices and culinary herbs for these steams. Stay away from those with irritating effects, such as black pepper, cayenne or mustard. Desirable and likely finds include anise, fennel, coriander, caraway, basil, oregano, sage, thyme, etc. If using seeds, crush them lightly prior to use. Use a palmful of herbs per 1 pint of water. You may need to use more herbs if yours are old. This is a good use for herbs that are a little past their prime. Follow directions for Basic Steam Technique.

Ocimum basilicum
(Basil)

Refer to the following table for a quick glance at some herbs whose properties make them especially good for certain skin types. (See Ingredients chapter for more detailed herbal information.)

Herbs and Their Steaming Virtues

Most herbs can be used for all skin types in steams. Yet some herbs have a special affinity for certain skin types, and can accordingly address particular skin care needs.

Chamomile for irritated skin
Mint (peppermint, spearmint, black mint) for tired and dull skin
Sage for oily skin
Thyme for oily and pimpled skin
Oregano for oily and pimpled skin
Fennel for dry and mature skin
Lemon/Citrus for oily skin
Licorice for dry skin
Spicy tea blends for cold and oily skin

🐝 *Basic Essential Oil Steams* ALL

Place 1–3 drops of essential oil into a bowl that already contains steaming water. Proceed with extra caution when placing your face over the bowl, as the essential oil vapors could irritate your eyes. Note that the steam will carry the essential oils out into the air and dissipate rapidly, so you may need to add a few more drops in the middle of your steam treatment. Some good essential oil choices are lavender, melissa, rosemary, chamomile, eucalyptus and mint. Follow directions for Basic Steam Technique.

Comptonia peregrina

Sweet Fern Citrus Blend OILY

This delightful-smelling blend contains astringent herbs to help balance oil production.

1 handful each of these dried herbs: oak bark, sweet fern,   mugwort, calendula blossoms, citrus peel, lemon balm

Combine herbs; use a handful of herbal mixture for each steaming. Follow directions for Basic Steam Technique. Store herbal mixture in a dry, cool place. Makes enough for 6 steamings.

Comfrey Fennel Blend DRY

This blend is good for irritated, dry, damaged and mature skin. It smells strongly of fennel.

1 handful each of these dried herbs: elder flower, comfrey leaf,   calendula blossoms, chamomile, crushed fennel seeds

Combine herbs; use a handful of herbal mixture for each steaming. Follow directions for Basic Steam Technique. Store herbal mixture in a dry, cool place. Makes enough for 5 steamings.

Facial Hot Packs

A facial hot pack is essentially a hot compress that is applied to the face. This treatment uses hot liquid, preferably an herbal infusion, in which a cloth is soaked and then applied to the face. It offers another way to deeply clean and tone the skin, clearing away dead cells and debris by opening the pores while increasing circulation. This treatment is extremely relaxing, and can ease tension held in the face. It is especially pleasurable to have someone else apply the compress to your face and neck while you relax in a reclining position. A hot pack is also a good treatment to use for skin affected by acne, especially when herbs such as thyme and echinacea are used. Plain hot water can be used, but an herbal infusion will increase the cleansing and therapeutic effects of the treatment. You might try an infusion of one of the formulas listed in the Facial Steams section above: Choose the Sweet Fern Citrus Blend for oily skin or the Comfrey Fennel Blend for dry, damaged skin. You might also want to try an infusion of chamomile for irritated skin, or sage, thyme or oregano for oily or pimply skin. You can also experiment by adding other ingredients, such as vinegar, carrier oils, essential oils and herbal tinctures, to produce different effects.

DIRECTIONS FOR FACIAL HOT PACKS. You will need a cotton cloth or towel (18 inches by 28 inches is a good size) and 32-oz. of herbal infusion (preferred) or pure spring water.

Make the herbal infusion with 2 handfuls of herbs and 32 oz. of boiling water, allowing it to steep for a minimum of 1 hour. You don't have to strain the infusion unless you think you'll mind the bits of herb that will temporarily adhere to your face.

Pour the infusion or water into a pot and place over very gentle heat. When the liquid is almost too hot to touch, place the cloth in until completely saturated, then wring it out and gently press it onto your face while maneuvering yourself into a reclining position. I find it best to hold the cloth by the two ends in a U shape, placing it with the ends overlapping on my forehead; that way I can create a small opening over my nostrils for breathing. The compress should be as hot as tolerable, but please exercise caution so as not to scald your hands or face. Each time the cloth cools, repeat the procedure. You should allow between 10 and 20 minutes for the entire treatment. Keep the pot covered between cloth dippings to prevent heat loss — you may even want to use an electric cooking pot or hot plate set on low heat to keep the liquid hot. You can also use two cloths alternately, leaving one soaking in the liquid while the other one is on your face. This procedure can be extended to the neck and chest region, in which case you will probably need to use more than one cloth at a time.

Facial Scrubs

Facial scrubs are formulated from dry ingredients that are ground together, moistened and then used to scrub the skin. They gently cleanse and polish, providing excellent exfoliation. Scrubs also help to nourish the skin by stimulating circulation. The specific ingredients you use will contribute to the scrub's nutritive and therapeutic effects. A scrub is used like a soap-and-water wash, but tends to leave the skin smoother and less stripped of its protective oils. If you generally use soap on your face, you may want to replace it altogether with a scrub, since the latter contains no harsh detergents or artificial scents.

Scrubs can be moistened with either plain water or a liquid with the properties suited to your skin type, as indicated in the following table or refer to the Ingredients chapter for further information. For instance, if you have oily skin, you might want to use witch hazel or a few drops of an astringent herbal tincture, such as sage, mixed with water. You might also add a drop of orange or grapefruit essential oil. Even oily skin sometimes needs a lubricating element for its emollient and soothing qualities, so you might choose to add a little jojoba or olive oil as well. If you have dry skin, you might moisten the scrub formula with a combination of honey and jojoba oil. For acne-prone skin, water to which a couple of dropperfuls of an antimicrobial tincture such as calendula, goldenseal or echinacea have been added is appropriate.

Liquids for Moistening Scrubs and Masques

The following liquids can be used alone or in combination. Tinctures and essential oils should be added in small amounts — they serve as aromatic and therapeutic accents to the formula rather than as primary moistening agents.

Liquid	Skin Type/Comments
Water	All
Oil	All/Dry/Damaged
Milk	All/Dry
Yogurt	All/Dry
Cream	All/Dry/Mature/Damaged
Honey	All
Vinegar	All/Oily/Acne
Witch Hazel	All/Oily/Acne
Herbal Infusions	All/Use specific herbs to address specific needs
Juice (orange, apple, carrot, etc.)	All/Oily
Maple Syrup	All
Tinctures	All/Oily/Acne: Add 1–2 dropperfuls per scrub
Essential Oils	All/ Add 1 drop per scrub

BASIC SCRUB TECHNIQUE. To moisten a scrub formula for one treatment, place 1–2 teaspoons of the formula into a small bowl and slowly stir in 1–2 teaspoons of the liquid until it reaches a pasty consistency — the amount of liquid you need will vary according to the scrub formula. To avoid adding too much liquid (and then having to add more scrub) add a teaspoon of liquid at a time. You can also moisten up to a week's worth of the scrub by using proportionately more formula and liquid. Be sure to store the moistened scrub in a small jar with a tight-fitting lid in the refrigerator.

Apply the moistened scrub formula to the skin, then thoroughly and gently massage with your fingertips for about a minute. Be gentle: Rubbing too hard or too long will irritate your delicate facial skin. Rinse with warm water and proceed to the next stage of your skin care regimen while your skin is still slightly moist.

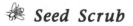 ## Seed Scrub   DRY

Scrubs made from seeds offer exfoliation and lubrication for the skin, and are especially good for dry skin. This scrub and some of the following ones require a seed/coffee grinder or mortar and pestle for proper grinding, and a wire mesh strainer or sieve to sift the scrub through. It is helpful to sift the scrub, remove any large particles and regrind to obtain a uniformly small-grained scrub. The consistency of the scrub is up to you; I personally like it finely ground. The size of the mesh in the strainer will dictate the size of the scrub granules.

**2 tablespoons in total of 1 or all of
these raw unroasted and organic
seeds: sesame, sunflower, pumpkin
and flax**

Grind and sift seeds. To moisten for one application mix 1–2 teaspoon of seeds with desirable liquid such as water, oil or yogurt till pasty consistency is reached. Makes enough for 3-4 applications.

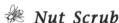 *Nut Scrub*   Dry

Scrubs made from nuts offer exfoliation and lubrication for the skin.

3 tablespoons raw almonds or other nut

Grind and sift nuts as directed in Seed Scrub above. To moisten for one application mix 1–2 teaspoon of scrub with desirable liquid such as water, oil or yogurt till pasty consistency is reached. Makes enough for 3–4 applications.

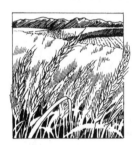

Grain Scrub   Oily

Scrubs made from grains are very exfoliating and absorbent and are good for oily and dirty skin.

2 tablespoons oats, brown rice or other grain

Grind and sift grains as directed in Seed Scrub above. For 1 application moisten 1–2 teaspoons of scrub with witch hazel extract or water till pasty consistency is reached. Makes enough for 3–4 applications.

Bean Scrub   Oily

Beans ground up finely make a good exfoliant for oily and bumpy skin. Ground aduki beans (found in the dry goods sections in health food stores) are a traditional Japanese face cleanser. You may want to dry-roast beans prior to grinding, as this process further dries them and makes them grind better. To dry-roast, place beans in a cast-iron skillet over a low flame for 5–10 minutes, stirring constantly.

2 tablespoons aduki, lentil or other bean

Grind and sift beans as directed in Seed Scrub. For one application wet 1–2 teaspoons of scrub with water and add a few drops of jojoba or olive oil. Makes enough for 3–4 applications.

Sage Scrub   All

A cleansing, astringent, soothing scrub for all skin types.

**2 tablespoons dried sage leaf
1 tablespoon sunflower seeds**

Finely grind the sage and seeds as directed in Seed Scrub. For 1 application wet 1–2 teaspoons scrub with water or yogurt till pasty consistency is reached. Makes enough for 3–4 applications.

Variations: You can substitute the sage for other herbs such as mint for a more refreshing, stimulating scrub, or calendula flowers for a more skin-reparative scrub. And you can also substitute sesame or green pumpkin seeds for the sunflower seeds.

Queen of Leaves Face Cleanser   DRY/NORMAL

A premoistened moisturizing and stimulating exfoliant for tired and dry skin.

2 tablespoons seeds (choose from any or all of the following: sunflower, sesame, green pumpkin, flax)	1 tablespoons honey
	1 tablespoon olive oil
	10 drops peppermint essential oil
2 tablespoons black beans	5 drops lavender essential oil

Grind and sift the seeds and beans as directed in Seed Scrub. Place ground seeds and beans in a small bowl and stir in the honey and then the olive oil until a smooth paste results. Add the essential oils, stirring them in thoroughly; transfer to a small 3- or 4-oz. jar and cap with a tight-fitting lid. This recipe makes about 3 ounces of cleanser, enough for several applications. It is fairly stable, lasting a few weeks out of refrigeration; place in refrigeration for longer storage. This is a premoistened cleanser and ready for use. After massaging cleanser into skin, allow it to stay for a few minutes to further the moisturizing effects before rinsing off with warm water.

Gladstar's Basic Mixed Scrub   ALL

This is a more complex recipe that combines the properties of clay, seeds, nuts, herbs and grains. There is a lot of room to improvise, and it is not necessary to be exact in your measurements, since they serve only as basic guidelines. In some formulas for oily and acne-prone skin, the nuts and seeds are omitted while the herbal component is increased for more healing and cleansing effects. This basic formula provides the basis for the other scrubs that follow.

Mixed Scrub (Small Batch)

4 teaspoons grains	1 teaspoon nuts/seeds
2 teaspoons herbs	3 tablespoons clay

Use a coffee/seed grinder to grind all the ingredients except the clay into a powder. The coarser the powder, the more abrasive and exfoliating the resulting grains will be. You may wish to sift through a fine strainer for a uniform consistency and to ensure that all the ingredients have been properly pulverized. Add the clay and mix thoroughly. Store in an airtight container in the refrigerator. Yields about 5 tablespoons of scrub, enough for several scrub applications and 5 masque applications.

Mixed Scrub (Large Batch)   ALL

1 cup grains	¼ cup seeds/nuts
½ cup herbs	2 cups clay

Using a blender, grind all ingredients except the clay into a powder. The coarser the powder, the more abrasive and exfoliating the resulting grains will be. You may wish to sift through a fine strainer for a uniform consistency and to ensure that all the ingredients have been properly pulverized. Add the clay and mix thoroughly. Store in an airtight container in the refrigerator. Yields 3½ cups of scrub, enough for many applications.

The following scrubs are variations of Gladstar's Basic Mixed Scrub Formula and they are made as directed above. In a couple of the following scrubs the proportions of ingredients differ and certain ingredients are omitted to suit the purpose of the scrub. *Variations follow:*

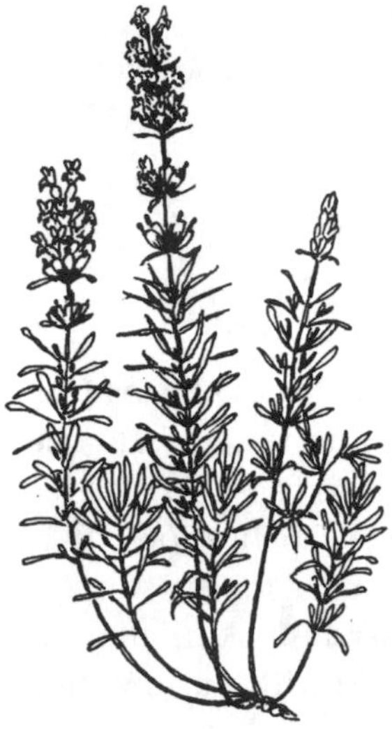

Lavender Calendula Scrub   ALL

Use ¾ cup oats, ¼ cup cornmeal, ¼ cup hazelnuts, ⅛ cup lavender flowers, ⅛ cup calendula flowers, ⅛ cup fennel seeds and 2 cups clay. Follow directions for Mixed Scrub (Large Batch); reserve the cornmeal and add along with the clay after all ingredients have been ground and sifted. Yields 3½ cups, enough for many applications.

Comfrey Fenugreek Scrub   DRY/DAMAGED

A more soothing and lubricating formula for dry, damaged skin.
Use ¾ cup oats, ¼ cup barley, ¼ cup sunflower seeds, 1 teaspoon flax seeds, 1 teaspoon fenugreek seeds, 1 teaspoon powdered comfrey root, ¼ cup chamomile flowers and 2 cups clay. Add the comfrey powder along with the clay after all the ingredients are ground as directed in Mixed Scrub (Large Batch). Yields 3½ cups, enough for many applications.
Variation: Wet the scrub with cream, oil or yogurt to further its soothing action.

Comfrey Fenugreek Scrub (Small Batch)

Use 3 teaspoons oats, 1 teaspoon barley, 2 teaspoons sunflower seeds, ⅛ teaspoon flax seeds, ⅛ teaspoon fenugreek seeds, ⅛ teaspoon comfrey root powder, 2 teaspoons chamomile flowers and 3 tablespoons clay. Add comfrey powder along with the clay after all ingredients are ground as directed in Mixed Scrub (Small Batch). Makes 5 tablespoons of scrub, enough for 5 masque applications and several scrub applications.

Lavandula angustifolia

Rose Blossom Sage Scrub   OILY/ACNE

A more astringent, drying and antiseptic formula that omits the nuts/seeds and increases the quantity of herbal ingredients.
Use ½ cup oats, ½ cup brown rice, ⅛ cup rose blossoms, ⅛ cup citrus peel, ⅛ cup burdock seeds, ⅛ cup sage, ⅛ cup cloves and 2 cups clay. Follow directions for Mixed Scrub (Large Batch). Makes about 3½ cups of scrub, enough for many applications.
Wet the scrub with witch hazel and floral waters and add small amounts of herbal tinctures (a dropperful per scrub application) such as sage, rose or lemon balm to enhance the astringent and cleansing effects. *Variation:* You may also want to add 2 drops of grapefruit and 1 drop of lavender essential oils to each scrub application, giving it a delicious aroma and adding to the therapeutic properties of the scrub.

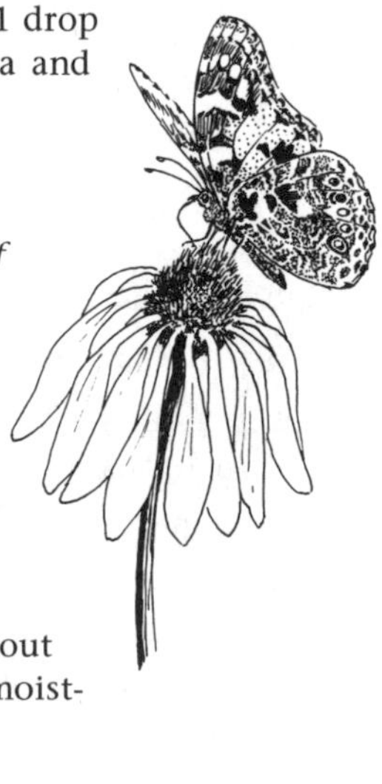

Echinacea Clove Scrub

ACNE/OILY

An antiseptic scrub for erupting, acne-prone skin. It contains a larger quantity of herbs while reducing the clay and omitting the nuts/seeds for stronger action. This is a very strong scrub that can tingle and even irritate sensitive skin. Increase the clay to make a milder scrub.
Use ½ cup oats, ½ cup brown rice, ¼ cup echinacea root, ⅛ cup clove, ½ cup calendula, ¼ cup myrrh and 1½ cups clay; *optional:* tea tree essential oil, lavender essential oil. Add the myrrh powder along with the clay after all the ingredients are ground as directed in Mixed Scrub (Large Batch). Yields 3 cups, enough for many applications.
Wet with witch hazel and tinctures of echinacea, sage and thyme, and also add about 2 drops of tea tree essential oil and about 1 drop of lavender to a 1-oz. batch of moistened grains in order to enhance the cleansing and therapeutic action.

Facial Masques

Facial masques are preparations made from various dried, ground, mashed or powdered ingredients that are moistened to form a thick paste. The paste is spread over the skin and left on for 20 minutes or longer for a sustained cleansing, nourishing and tonic effect. Any scrub formula can be moistened for use as a masque, or you can use fresh plant material, foodstuffs or other ingredients. Because masques penetrate the skin more deeply than scrubs, their use should generally be limited to once or twice a week — otherwise, they can end up stripping the skin of its natural protective oils. However, certain masques are predominantly nourishing, moisturizing and so gentle that they will not dry out the skin; thus they can be used more frequently. Ideally masques should be applied following a steam treatment because the pores are open, which allows the masque formula to penetrate more deeply.

BASIC MASQUE TECHNIQUE. When applying a masque, tie the hair back away from the face. Some of the masques are quite messy, so you might want to wear an old shirt or drape an apron or towel over your chest to protect your clothing. Moisten the formula as for a scrub, gently spread the mixture over your face, then rest quietly for 20 minutes while the masque goes to work. It is best to remain in a reclining posture to aid circulation to your face. You might want to place a towel under your head while reclining to catch any drips. Rinse well with warm water and allow your skin to air-dry rather than toweling it off. While the skin is still slightly moist, proceed to the next step of your skin care program. I find it helpful to use a soft cotton cloth for rinsing off some of the masques.

Symphytum officinale

FACIAL SCRUB MASQUES. The scrubs used for daily cleansing can also be used as masques if applied thickly and left on for 20 minutes or longer. Choose a facial scrub appropriate for your skin type from the Facial Scrubs section using 1–2 tablespoons of scrub per masque application. Moisten with 1–2 tablespoons of an appropriate liquid, such as water, honey, cream, oil, distilled witch hazel, herbal infusion, tincture, etc., until a spreadable paste results. If needed, add more liquid or scrub a half teaspoon at a time, until the desired consistency is reached.

Comfrey Fenugreek Masque   DRY/DAMAGED/AGED

A very emollient-nourishing masque for dry, aged or damaged skin that can be used daily if desired.

1 tablespoon Comfrey Fenugreek Scrub
(see formula page 12)
3 teaspoons dairy cream
(organic preferred)

1 teaspoon honey
a few drops jojoba oil

Mix scrub with liquids until a spreadable paste is formed, adding more liquid or scrub half a teaspoon at a time if needed. Makes enough for 1–2 masque applications.

Echinacea Clove Masque

ACNE/OILY

An antimicrobial masque for oily, pimply or infected skin. You may use this mixture to dry out pimples by putting directly on pimple, leaving it on and repeating throughout the day. In addition, apply before going to bed and leave on throughout the night.

1 tablespoon Echinacea Clove Scrub
   (see formula page 12)
1 tablespoon witch hazel extract

⅛ teaspoon echinacea tincture
2 drops tea tree essential oil

Mix scrub with liquids until a spreadable paste is formed, adding more liquid or scrub by half a teaspoon at a time if needed, and stir in essential oil. Makes enough for 1–2 masque applications. *Variation follows:*

Echinacea Clove with Honey Masque

ACNE/DRY

For sensitive or dry skin use 2 teaspoons of honey and 1 teaspoon of witch hazel and proceed as directed in above formula.

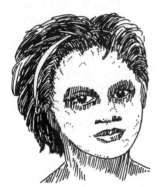

CLAY MASQUES. These masques are absorbent, drawing, cleansing and tightening. They are especially good for oily and large-pored skin, but can sometimes make dry skin uncomfortably taut. Mixing clay with various liquids helps moderate the drying effects, and can make the masque more suitable for dry skin. The longer the clay is left on, the more drawing and tightening the effect. Again, this may be desirable for oily and large-pored skin, but is not necessarily beneficial for dry or depleted skin unless more nourishing substances have been added to the clay. There are many different types of clay available, often identified by color — you can experiment to see which clay feels most appropriate for your skin type. You may want to keep in mind that kaolin clay, which is white, is considered less drying than the colored clays. (For more information about clay see page 198.)

🐝 Basic Clay Masque

ALL/OILY

Good for oily, wide-pored skin, and can also be used to dry out pimples.

1–2 tablespoons clay
approximately 1–2 tablespoons water

Mix the clay and water to create a smooth paste. Add more water if too thick, or more clay if too loose. Apply the paste thickly to your face and leave it on for 5–20 minutes. Makes 1 masque application. The following are variations to the Basic Clay Masque.

🐝 Clay and Oil Masque

DRY

For dry skin, use a carrier oil, such as olive or jojoba oil, or a combination of water and oil to moisten the clay.

🐝 Clay and Cream Masque

ALL/DRY

Even with normal skin, clay masques may be too drying. Moistening the clay with yogurt or cream can balance the drying effect.

🐝 Clay and Vinegar

ACNE

Moisten clay with vinegar, or part vinegar and part water, and put on pimple to dry it out.

All-in-One Clay Masque

ALL

This gently toning masque can be used by most skin types. The clay's drying qualities are balanced by the honey, glycerin and oil and make this masque appropriate even for dry and damaged skin. Yet its astringent and cleansing properties, due to the clay, witch hazel and vinegar, make it suitable for oily and large-pored skin as well. However, keep in mind that this formula may not be the best choice for pimpled skin. This masque can be made ahead of time and stored in the refrigerator, where it will keep for several months. It can be used as frequently as desired.

8 tablespoons clay
4 tablespoons honey
2 tablespoons distilled witch hazel
2 teaspoons almond oil

2 teaspoons vinegar
1 teaspoon glycerin
5 drops lavender essential oil
3 drops rosemary essential oil

Mix ingredients to create a smooth paste. Add more distilled witch hazel if too thick, or more clay if too loose. Apply the paste thickly to your face and leave it on for 20 minutes or longer. This masque will not dry, because it contains honey, oil and glycerin. Store in a tightly sealed jar in the refrigerator. Makes approximately 8 masque applications.

HONEY MASQUES. Honey makes an excellent all-purpose masque that is convenient and easy to use. It delicately rejuvenates, adding moisture and color to the skin, making it appropriate for all skin types, and especially dry and damaged skin. It can be used as frequently as desired. Honey can also be mixed with other ingredients, such as herbs and essential oils, to add fragrance and enhance the masque's effectiveness.

🐝 Basic Honey Masque

ALL

A soothing, cooling, humectant masque for all skin types.

½–1 teaspoon honey per facial

Pat and massage honey onto the skin, spreading it evenly over your face. Leave on for 20 minutes, then rinse off with warm water.

🐝 Honey Masque with Essential Oils

ALL

By combining honey with essential oils one can create an aromatically delightful and healthful array of masques.

1 teaspoon honey
1 drop essential oil

Place honey in palm of hand and stir in the essential oil, massage and pat onto face and leave on for 20 minutes, then rinse off with warm water. Makes enough for 1 application.

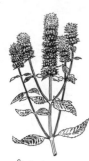

Variations: Following are some masque suggestions. (See Ingredients chapter for more detailed information on essential oils.)
1. Use 1 drop of tea tree, thuja or wintergreen for acned skin.
2. Use 1 drop chamomile, or lavender for irritated and inflamed skin.
3. Use 1 drop peppermint for tired skin.
4. Use 1 drop sandalwood or fennel for dry skin.
5. Use 1 drop orange, lime or lemongrass for oily skin.

🐝 *Honey Masques with Essential Oils (Large Batch)*   ALL

Make larger quantities and store in a tightly capped glass jar away from direct light. Place in attractive antique jars and give away as gifts, labeled with ingredients and instructions.

¼ cup honey
12 drops essential oil

Place honey in jar and stir in essential oils. Apply 1 teaspoon of honey to face, leave on 20 minutes and rinse off with warm water. It will keep outside of refrigeration for many months, although the essential oils may become weaker after a couple of months. If the honey needs to be reinvigorated just add more essential oils. Makes 12 masques.

Variation: You can use a mixture of essential oils to further customize the masque treatment. For example, irritated and acned skin can benefit from 6 drops of chamomile essential oil and 6 drops of tea tree oil. For oily and tired skin you can use 6 drops of peppermint essential oil and 6 drops of lemongrass essential oil.

Using Fruit or Alpha Hydroxy Acids in Masques

Fruits can be very beneficial for helping the skin renew itself, since the naturally occurring acids help to chemically exfoliate the skin in a gentle way. For some people, this natural form of chemical exfoliation is preferable to mechanical scrubbing. Fruit acids have been popularized by the cosmetics industry, and are usually referred to as alpha hydroxy acids. The fruit acids responsible for this gentle stripping action are found in citrus fruits such as grapefruits, limes and oranges; berries such as strawberries and blackberries; and in other fruits, including apples, tomatoes, kiwis, peaches and grapes. Citric, malic, lactic and glycolic acids are the components of the fruits that are believed to be responsible for the exfoliating action. Using fruits in masques is especially well suited for oily, wide-pored and blemished skin. However, fruits can be quite drying and irritating to already dry and damaged skin — especially the citrus fruits. For dry skin, you may want to add a bit of oil or cream to moderate the effects of the fruit. Keep in mind that many people who are allergic to fruits will also have an allergic response to topical fruit preparations.

To use fruits in masques, extract the juice and use it to moisten the masque, or mash or grate the fruit and apply it directly to the face. If using mashed fruit, it may be necessary to add clay or cornstarch to help the fruit adhere to the face. You can also experiment by combining the fruit mash with any of the masque formulas offered here.

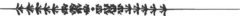

Whole-Wheat Flour Cleansing Masque   OILY/ACNE

An astringent, drawing masque for oily, dirty skin. You may use this masque to dry out pimples by putting directly on pimple, leaving it on and repeating throughout the day. In addition, apply before going to bed.

1 tablespoon organic whole-wheat flour
1 tablespoon clay (any good-quality clay)

1 teaspoon raw apple cider vinegar
1 tablespoon witch hazel extract
¼ teaspoon olive oil
2 drops orange essential oil

Combine ingredients in a small bowl, stirring thoroughly until a smooth paste results. Sprinkle in more witch hazel if the masque consistency is too thick, or more clay if the masque consistency is too thin and watery. When desired consistency is reached, apply masque to face. Note that the apple cider vinegar can make eyes water, so keep masque away from eyes. This masque can be made ahead of time and stored in the refrigerator where it will keep for a few weeks or longer. Makes enough for 1–2 applications.

Vegetable Garden Masque   ALL

This masque gently tones and rejuvenates the skin.

1 large handful fresh leafy greens (some good choices are kale, lettuce, collards and parsley)

½–1 oz. liquid (water, yogurt or milk)
2 tablespoons cornstarch

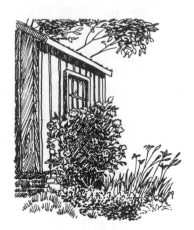

Chop leafy greens and place in food processor (preferred) or blender and process with water, yogurt or milk, pouring liquid in a little at a time until a thick paste results. Add the cornstarch and continue to blend. If the vegetable paste is too loose and won't adhere to your face, sprinkle in small amounts of cornstarch to thicken.

Apply the masque thickly to the face and relax and recline to keep it from dripping off. You can also place gauze or thin cloth over the masque to keep it in place. Leave on for 20 minutes or longer and then rinse off. This masque will not dry. Makes enough for 1 thick masque application.

Herbal Garden Masque

ALL/DAMAGED

Useful on irritated, damaged skin. Choose soothing reparative herbs.

1 large handful fresh herbs (some good choices are violet, comfrey, plantain and calendula; see Botanicals section in About Ingredients)

½–1 oz. of liquid (water, yogurt or milk)
2 tablespoons cornstarch

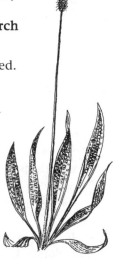

Note: Comfrey leaves may leave the skin feeling tingling and slightly irritated. This sensation only last a few minutes, so don't be alarmed.

Chop herbs and place in food processor (preferred) or blender and process with water, yogurt or milk, pouring liquid in a little at a time until a thick paste results. Add the cornstarch and continue to blend. If the herbal paste is too loose and won't adhere to your face, sprinkle in small amounts of cornstarch to thicken.

Apply the masque thickly to the face and relax and recline to keep it from dripping off. You can also place gauze or thin cloth over the masque to keep it in place. Leave on for 20 minutes or longer and then rinse off. This masque will not dry. Makes enough for 1 thick masque application.

Plantago lanceolata

Avocado Flour Treat

ALL/DRY

A soothing, nutritive, moisturizing, cleansing and toning masque for most skin types. An excellent treatment for the face as well as the body.

1 tablespoon ripe avocado (mashed)
1 tablespoon whole-wheat flour, oat flour or buckwheat flour
½ tablespoon cornmeal

1 tablespoon water
a few drops jojoba oil, peanut oil or other rich oil of choice

Mix flour and cornmeal, add water (a little at a time, until a smooth paste results), add avocado and then oil, stirring both in thoroughly. If the paste is too loose sprinkle in more flour; if it is too thick add water, a little at a time. Massage the skin with the paste and then apply a thick coat of paste over the surface of the skin. Leave on 20 minutes. Rinse off. Makes 1 thick masque application.

Variation: Other masques can be made by substituting the avocado in the above recipe with other fruits such as peaches, strawberries, papaya, etc. and adding them to the flour paste. The flour paste in this recipe provides a basic masque to which other ingredients can be added.

PHASE 2: TONING

The second phase of facial skin care, toning, helps to remove oily residue while refining and tightening the pores after they have been opened during the cleansing process. In general, toners and astringents have a drying effect on the skin; the more alcohol or vinegar used to make a formula, the more astringent and drying it will be. Water-based toners that include glycerin, aloe or other hydrating substances are less astringent and more moisturizing. A toner or astringent can sometimes be used instead of a cleanser. With the addition of an appropriate scent, these formulas can also be used as effective aftershaves.

In general, you should use alcohol- and vinegar-based astringents with moderation, as their overuse can have the opposite of the desired effect. For example, oily skin can become even oilier from too much toning or through use of an overly drying astringent, which can stimulate sebum production. Dry skin, on the other hand, can benefit from an occasional astringent toner, for the same reason. Keep in mind that the floral water toners are very gentle astringents that can be used as often as needed while hardly drying the skin, if at all. The hydrating herbal toners are also moisturizing rather than drying, and can be used throughout the day or as needed. The sebaceous glands, which produce oily sebum, are very responsive to environmental influences, meaning anything that comes into contact with your skin. Overall, the idea in toning is to work with your skin's natural processes, encouraging balance.

BASIC TONING TECHNIQUE. There are two basic methods for applying a toner or astringent to your skin. The first method is simply to moisten a cotton ball or soft cotton or silk cloth (avoid disposable tissues and synthetic cloth, since these can irritate the skin) with the full-strength formula and to wipe it gently over all or part of your face, depending on your skin's needs. In general, this method is appropriate for normal to oily skin types, since it helps remove excess sebum.

The second method is to use an alcohol- or vinegar-based astringent diluted with pure spring or well water, which you splash on your face. Place a bowl of cold water in the sink, add ¼ teaspoon of astringent and splash water onto face, catching the liquid in the bowl. Repeat this for 1–2 minutes.

Alternatively, you can place the diluted formula in a spray bottle and mist your face. The amount of water you add to the astringent will vary depending on the potency of the formula and your skin's needs. However, generally 1 part astringent is diluted with 1 part water for misting. For extra stimulation, try repeatedly patting your face all over with your fingers during the application. In general, this method is appropriate for normal to dry skin types. Proceed to the next stage of your skin care routine while your skin is still slightly moist.

Facial Toners and Astringents

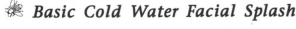 *Basic Cold Water Facial Splash*   ALL

Splashing the face with cold water is a great way to refresh and invigorate the skin and tighten the pores. This is the most commonly used skin toner. Its cleansing and toning action can be improved with the addition of various substances, such as one of the astringent formulas or other simple ingredients.

Bowl filled with about 16 oz. cold water and placed in the sink

Splash face with water, catching the water back in bowl, and repeat for a minute or so. Makes 1 treatment.

Variations: Many different ingredients can be added to the water to modify the splash. Here are a few suggestions. Add a teaspoon of lemon juice to increase the astringency of the splash, especially for oily skin. Add ½ teaspoon of vinegar to increase astringency, especially for oily skin. Add ½ teaspoon of vinegar and ¼ teaspoon of oil for normal to dry skin. This last variation has an astringent, lubricating and moisturizing effect.

Floral Water Toners

Floral waters are gentle, refreshing toners that are often packaged in fancy bottles and sold for a small fortune. Yet they are very quick, easy and inexpensive to make with essential oils and distilled water. You can choose a particular essential oil for its aromatherapy value or for its mild antimicrobial, antiseptic or other therapeutic properties. Floral waters can be used frequently during the day without drying the skin as much as alcohol- or vinegar-based astringents. Since essential oils are not water-soluble, they will separate from the water. The solution should therefore be shaken briefly but vigorously prior to each use. Floral waters are susceptible to bacterial contamination if they contain no alcohol, so these should be made in small batches, stored in the refrigerator and used quickly. By adding a small amount of alcohol you increase the astringent effect and lengthen shelf life. It is best to place floral waters in spray mist bottles in order to minimize bacterial contact. Misting is a pleasurable and effective way to tone and refresh the face.

 ## *Basic Floral Water Formula* ALL/DRY

> **20 drops essential oil**
> **2 oz. distilled water**

Pour water and essential oil into a spray mist bottle, cap and shake. Mist onto face. Makes 2 oz.

Variation: Add 1 teaspoon of vodka per 1 oz. of floral water for increased astringency and shelf life.

Lavender Water ALL

A soothing, reparative skin tonic for all skin types.

> **20 drops lavender essential oil**
> **2 oz. distilled water**

Place water in a 2-oz jar, add lavender essential oil drop by drop, cap and shake. It is ready to use.

Variations: Use chamomile essential oil for irritated skin, fennel and sandalwood essential oil for dry skin, lemongrass, grapefruit and other citrus essential oils for oily skin, and rosemary, tea tree and sage essential oil for acne-prone skin. Refer to the Essential Oils section in the Ingredients chapter for further information.

Facial Splashes with Essential Oils   ALL/DRY

Another simple way to use water and essential oils for toning the face is to add 1–2 drops of desired essential oil into a bowl of cold water and use to splash on face.

1–2 drops essential oil
16 oz. cold water

Place bowl with water and essential oils in sink and splash face over bowl; trying to catch splashed water into bowl, repeat for a few minutes. The cold water and essential oils tone the skin. Makes enough for 1 application.

Herbal-Infused Vinegar Astringents

Herbal-infused vinegars are excellent, easily made astringents that can be highly therapeutic, depending on the herbs used. A little patience is required, however, since they must infuse for 6–8 weeks before being ready to use. But once they are made, they will keep for many months without refrigeration; I have even made herbal-infused vinegars that were still good after 3 years. Use caution when applying these to the face, since a strong vinegar solution can make the eyes burn or water.

The herbs to choose from are endless. Some common favorites are lemon balm, rose, mint, evergreen tips, witch hazel, calendula and oak leaf. You can use any of these alone or in combination.

To use, moisten a cotton cloth or cotton ball with the vinegar and wipe gently over the face. Full-strength vinegar may be too drying for your skin, in which case you can mix 1 or 2 teaspoons of water with 1 teaspoon of vinegar before applying it. You can also use the vinegar as a splash by adding ¼–½ teaspoon vinegar to a pint of cold water in a bowl and splashing it onto your face; this feels especially refreshing. Another technique is to mix 1 part vinegar with 1 part rose water in a spray mist bottle for use as a spritzer. Not surprisingly, many of these herbal vinegars are also delicious on salads or wherever vinegar is called for in recipes. Herbal-infused vinegars are often high in calcium and other minerals, depending on the herbs used, which can help promote health and beauty from within. Keep in mind, however, that certain herbs, such as witch hazel and oak bark, are very astringent and not very tasty.

Queen of Hungary's Water   NORMAL/OILY

My variation on an ancient toner formula and revived for contemporary times by Rosemary Gladstar. This formula requires a 2-month period of steeping before it is ready, but once made will keep for many months outside refrigeration.

Approximately a total of 3 oz. equal quantities fresh lavender, chamomile, comfrey, calendula, lemon balm, roses, sage and thyme (enough to fill an 8-oz. jar)

approximately 5 oz. of raw apple cider vinegar, (enough to cover the herbs in the jar and fill the jar to the top)
about 5 oz. witch hazel extract
about 100 drops lavender essential oil

Fill a jar with the just-mentioned garden-fresh herbs; if you do not have equal quantities of the herbs or are missing some of them fill the jar with the herbs that you do have. Pour apple cider vinegar over the herbs, covering them, cap with plastic lid and let steep 2 months. Pour the vinegar through a cloth-lined strainer placed over a bowl. Gather up the cloth ends and squeeze out as much liquid from the plant material as possible. To the strained vinegar add an equal amount of witch hazel. Add 10 drops lavender essential oil to every ounce of vinegar-witch hazel mixture. Makes about 11 oz., enough for many applications.

Shake bottle before use and apply to face with a cotton cloth. Or use as a splash, adding ½ teaspoon to a pint of cold water placed in a bowl and splashing face repeatedly, it's refreshing. Or you can put the astringent diluted with equal parts water or more as needed in a pump spray bottle and spritz onto face. *Variation follows:*

Queen of Hungary's Water with Dried Herbs
You can use dried herbs to make Queen of Hungary's Water in place of the fresh herbs, although I think the resulting product is less potent. To make with dried herb use 2 oz. of herb to 10 oz. of vinegar and proceed as above.

Antimicrobial Astringent   ACNE/INFECTED/OILY

For pimples, acne and infected skin. This formula requires a 6-week period to make, but once made will keep for many months, if not years, outside refrigeration.

> 2 oz. dry herb (or approximately 6 tablespoons freshly powdered herb, or 12 tablespoons cut and sifted herbs)

> 8 oz. vinegar
> 2 drops tea tree essential oil per application

Choose from one or all of the following herbs: goldenseal, echinacea, myrrh, spilanthes, yarrow, calendula. Coarsely grind herbs and follow Directions for Herbal-Infused Vinegar with Dried Herbs.

Dilute prior to use by adding 1 teaspoon of Antimicrobial Astringent to 1–2 tablespoons of water. Add 2 drops of tea tree essential oil to increase the antimicrobial action. Apply directly to problem area with cotton swab and repeat as needed. This preparation is also excellent for cleaning wounds. Makes about 6 oz. of astringent.

Variation: Vodka can be used in place of the vinegar for a stronger cleansing effect.

Spirited Astringents

Astringents can also be made by starting with an alcohol base, such as vodka or brandy, and adding juices or infusions. Note that alcohol can be very drying, so this may not be the ideal toner for already dry and damaged skin. Check to see how your skin responds to these spirited astringents. You can also try reducing the amount of alcohol to make the formula less astringent. If you reduce the alcohol content significantly or replace it altogether with water, then you must refrigerate the astringent and use them up quickly, since they are subject to spoilage.

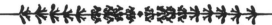

Using Alcohol as a Preservative

When I began to make products for sale in retail shops, I needed to find ways to make them more stable. Although products containing alcohol are not suitable for all skin types, they are often appropriate for oily and large-pored skin. Many of the water based preparations in this section are preserved with alcohol. You can choose to omit the alcohol, but in so doing you reduce the shelf life of the product from many months to just a few days. I am a firm supporter of making the freshest possible products for body care, but when an extended shelf life is desirable, or if you are making products for skin that responds positively to diluted alcohol, this information will prove beneficial.

Using Alcohol as a Preservative Basic Formula

As a general rule, ¼ cup water-based liquid such as juice or an infusion will be preserved by ¼ cup of 80 proof liquor. A product needs to contain 15–20 percent alcohol to stay preserved.

Carrot Parsley Brandy Astringent   ALL

Good for all skin types due to its nutritive and skin-toning effects of the carrot and parsley and the tightening, toning and cleansing effects of the brandy.

¼ cup fresh-pressed carrot juice from
   1 large carrot
a handful of parsley

¼ cup brandy
optional: 1 teaspoon glycerin

Press juice from a large carrot and a handful of parsley in a juicer. Pour juice into a jar with the brandy. Cap tightly and shake vigorously. It is ready for use. You can add the glycerin to the astringent for a more hydrating, humectant effect for very dry skin. If you don't have a juicer and you do have a blender or food processor, place grated carrot with a handful of chopped parsley into food processor, add the brandy and blend till everything is pureed. Pour puree into a cloth-lined strainer placed over a bowl, gather up the cloth ends and squeeze the liquid out. If desired, add glycerin for a more hydrating effect and shake well. It is ready for use. Makes about 4 oz.

Variation: Replace the carrots with apples for a more astringent effect. Repleace ¼ cup of brandy with calendula or other tincture of choice to increase reparative action.

While you are making the carrot parsley juice don't forget to make an extra 6–8 ounces of juice for yourself, as this nutritious juice is excellent for making one healthy and beautiful.

Berry Leaf Skin Toner   ALL/OILY

An excellent skin tonic for oily, large-pored "dirty" skin. Makes enough for a year's supply.

2 large handfuls of any or all of the following: fresh strawberry, raspberry or blackberry leaves (enough to tightly fill an 8-oz. jar)

approximately 5–6 oz. 80 proof vodka (enough to fill the jar and cover the berry leaves)
6 oz. distilled rose water

Follow Directions for Alcohol Tinctures Using Fresh Herbs using the berry leaves and the vodka, strain tincture and combine with the rose water in a 12-oz. glass jar, cap and shake well. Can be used immediately. Put in a mister bottle or apply to a cotton cloth and wipe onto skin. Makes 12 oz.

HERBAL-INFUSION ASTRINGENTS. These formulations combine the therapeutic action of water-based herbal infusions with the toning, tightening and cleansing properties of alcohol. If your skin is sensitive to alcohol you may want to omit it and simply use the fresh infusion. In this case, the formula will have to be stored in the refrigerator and used within a few days. The nonalcoholic versions of these formulas are more like gentle hydrating skin toners than astringents. You can also reduce the amount of alcohol in these formulas according to your own preference and still obtain the therapeutic effects of the alcohol; however, you will need to use these reduced-alcohol formulas more quickly, as they will have a reduced shelf life. The addition of glycerin helps to counteract the alcohol's drying properties and can offer a mildly preservative effect to low- or no-alcohol formulas.

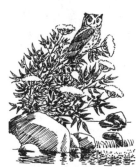

I enjoy making herbal-infusion astringents for classes at herbal conferences, since they are so easy to make and are ready for use within a short time. When making them, just be sure to allow the herbs to steep fully before straining the infusion and mixing it with alcohol.

Chamomile Blend Astringent   ALL/OILY

A soothing, anti-inflammatory astringent for all skin types. My students and I made this astringent in a class at the Green Nations Gathering, one of the popular annual herbal conferences in the Northeast. We passed the astringent around in a spritzer bottle and enjoyed the refreshing mist. One woman with sensitive and oily skin was extremely impressed to finally find an astringent that felt just right for her.

Combine the following freshly dried herbs to equal a large handful (total 1 oz.): chamomile, elder flower, comfrey root (crushed or powdered prior to use), nettle leaf

16 oz. water
8 oz. 80 proof vodka (or other 80 proof liquor)
optional: 2 teaspoons glycerin

Make an infusion of herbs with water and let steep for 4 hours. Pour 8 oz. strained herbal infusion into 16-oz. jar, add vodka and if you desire, glycerin. Cap and shake well. It is ready to use. Makes 16 oz.

Basil Blend Astringent   ALL/OILY

A sweet-smelling, cleansing and invigorating astringent for all skin types.

Combine the following freshly dried herbs to equal a large handful (total 1 oz.): basil, thyme, fennel seeds (crushed with a mortar and pestle prior to use)

16 oz. water
8 oz. 80 proof vodka (or other 80 proof liquor)
optional: 2 teaspoons glycerin

Make an infusion of herbs with water and let steep for 2 hours. Pour 8 oz. of strained herbal infusion into 16-oz. jar, add vodka, and if you desire glycerin. Cap and shake well. It is ready to use. Makes 16 oz.

Hydrating Herbal Toners

If your skin is dry or damaged, you may want to try one of the following hydrating toners made with herbal infusions, glycerin and aloe. These formulas are really more like moisturizing toners than astringents. They omit the alcohol and contain glycerin, which helps to extract the herbal properties while functioning as a mild preservative. Glycerin, unlike alcohol, also helps attract moisture to the skin. These hydrating toners should be used up within a couple of months and stored in the refrigerator. I prefer to keep them in spray mist bottles. Misting them onto the face feels great, and this method of storage will also help prevent bacteria from contaminating the toner. Many people find these toners especially helpful during the winter months, when indoor heating takes its toll on their skin. They are also nice after overexposure to sun or wind.

One drawback to the use of glycerin in a facial toner is that it can make the skin feel sticky. The amount of glycerin you use in a facial toner will determine how sticky your face feels after the application. I found that 1 part glycerin to 12 parts water or other water-based liquid seems to produce the best results. You may want to increase the glycerin if your skin needs the extra moisture, but note that it will result in increased stickiness.

Luscious Face Toner   ALL/DRY/MATURE

A gentle hydrating toner for all skin types.

2 tablespoons plus 2 teaspoons distilled water or herbal infusion of choice
3 teaspoons aloe vera gel

1 teaspoon glycerin
5 drops lavender essential oil
3 drops ylang-ylang essential oil
2 drops lemongrass essential oil

Pour all ingredients into a spray mist bottle, cap and shake well. It is ready to use. Use up within a couple of months, keep refrigerated and check for bacterial contamination periodically. Yields 2 oz.

Variation: You can use lavender, chamomile, rose, comfrey or other infusion of choice in place of the distilled water to create an even more effective preparation.

Rose Lavender Marshmallow and Nettle Toner

ALL/DRY/MATURE

Another excellent toner for dry to normal skin.

Use these dried herbs: 1 tablespoon lavender blossoms, 1 tablespoon marshmallow root freshly crushed, 2 tablespoons rose flowers, 2 tablespoons nettle leaf

8 oz. water
2 oz. plus 1 tablespoon glycerin
1 tablespoon aloe vera gel

Make herbal infusion with herbs, 2 oz. of glycerin and water. Let steep for 4–8 hours. Pour 3 oz. of strained infusion, 1 tablespoon of glycerin, and 1 tablespoon of aloe into a jar (preferably a spray mist bottle) and shake. Use up within a couple of months, keep refrigerated and check for bacterial contamination periodically. Apply after cleansing the face or as needed and especially before night slumber. You will end up with extra infusion, which you can use for hair rinse or soaks. Makes 4 oz.

Variation: Add 14 drops of lavender essential oil and 8 drops of rose geranium essential oil. The essential oils, although not necessary, add an appealing scent to the toner, help to preserve it and amplify skin reparative effects.

Rose Aloe Face Toner

ALL

This is a moisturizing toner for all skin types. It combines rose vinegar's toning properties with the humectant and soothing qualities of glycerin and aloe. The presence of the vinegar makes this toner slightly more drying and less perishable than the previous hydrating toners.

1 oz. rose-infused vinegar (preferred) or plain apple cider vinegar
1 oz. distilled witch hazel (store-bought)
1 tablespoon plus 1 teaspoon aloe gel

2 teaspoons glycerin
1 oz. distilled water
optional: 20 drops rose geranium essential oil

Place ingredients in a spritzer jar, shake and use as needed. Use up within a few months or store in the refrigerator. Makes 4 oz.

PHASE 3: MOISTURIZING

Moisturizing the face with a combination of oil, water, herbs and other natural ingredients is an ideal way to nourish, soothe, lubricate and hydrate the skin. The act of massaging in the moisturizer also helps stimulate circulation, which brings a fresh blood supply to the skin, thereby ensuring a healthy complexion. The best moisturizers leave the skin feeling soft and supple but not clogged or greasy. You should tailor the application of moisturizers to your skin's particular needs. As a rule, dry, damaged or weathered skin benefits from more frequent use of moisturizers than oily or acne-prone skin. But pay close attention to how your skin actually responds to the use of moisturizers — don't simply apply them out of habit. Remember too that dry skin can actually become drier with the overuse of moisturizers. Note that oils and creams can also be used as cleansers for removing makeup and other oil-soluble dirt from the skin while providing a gentle cleansing option for dry, irritated or sensitive skin.

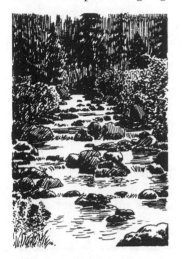

BASIC MOISTURIZER TECHNIQUE. If you choose to use a moisturizer after cleansing and/or toning, be sure to apply it while your skin is still slightly moist; this will work synergistically with the formula to hydrate your skin. Apply the moisturizer with your fingertips and massage it into your face lightly but thoroughly, using small, circular strokes. Be especially gentle when applying the formula to the skin around your eyes, using light, dabbing strokes with your fingertips. Wait several minutes for the moisturizer to soak in before optionally patting off any excess with a soft natural-fiber cloth or cotton ball. Avoid using synthetic "cotton" balls and disposable tissues, since these can clog the pores or irritate the skin. Some of my favorite moisturizing formulas and treatments follow.

Facial Oils

Oils can provide rich nourishment, lubrication and protection for your skin. By themselves oils do not hydrate, so technically they are not moisturizers. Yet at times, when hydration is not an issue or when skin is deficient, thin, damaged or not producing sufficient sebum, all you may need is the application of a little oil. Oils can act as moisture barriers when applied to a damp face that has been cleansed and rinsed. If you opt for an oil treatment in this phase of your skin care routine, you might choose one of the following (see also Botancials Section in the Ingredients chapter):

Olive oil is good for most skin types, with the exception of very oily skin.

Almond oil is good for most skin types.

Grapeseed oil is drying, and is thus good for oily skin.

Jojoba oil is good for most skin types, especially dry, aging or damaged skin.

Golden Oil
ALL/DRY

This is a nourishing, balanced oil for most skin types.

1 oz. jojoba oil
1 oz. peanut oil

2 oz. almond oil

Pour jojoba oil, peanut oil, and almond oil in 4 oz. jar, cap and shake well. It is ready for use. Makes 4 oz.

Variation: Add 5 drops of essential oil of lavender, chamomile or rosewood.

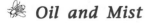 Oil and Mist
ALL

This treatment combines the hydrating effects of water with the lubricating effects of oil. Choose oils and water-based liquids appropriate for your skin type. The water-based liquids — spring or filtered water, floral water, facial astringent or herbal infusions — can either be used individually or in combination, and are generally placed in a spray mist bottle.

Dab the oil onto the forehead, chin and cheeks and mist the liquid onto the face. Massage the face, working the liquid and oil into skin. The following is a favorite variation of oil and mist:

Rose Water and Jojoba Oil ALL

A nourishing, tonic moisturizer for all skin types.

Apply a dab of jojoba oil on forehead, chin and cheeks. Then place rose water in a pump spray bottle and mist on face. Massage face, working oil and water into skin.

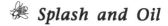 Splash and Oil ALL

The same lubricating and hydrating effect as Oil and Mist can be obtained by this procedure, without the use of spray mist bottles.

Palmful of rose water or other water of choice   **a few drops of jojoba oil or other oil of choice**

Splash rose water onto face and oil fingertips. While face is still damp, massage face with oiled fingertips. By the way, this common technique can be performed as the last phase of the face care program, after rinsing the face with plain water or toner; just apply the oil while the skin is still damp.

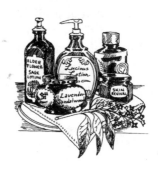

Moisturizing Creams

In the classes I teach, moisturizing creams rank as one of the favorite formulas to both make and use. Students are always thrilled to see the transformation of oil and water into rich, delightfully fragrant emulsions. Creams combine the hydrating effects of water and the nourishing, lubricating effects of oil into one product. The Basic Cream Formula yields about 19 oz., enough to share with family and friends. You can choose to omit the essential oils from the following formulas if you are sensitive to scents. Since these creams are made without chemical stabilizers or preservatives they can be quite perishable, especially if you omit the essential oils. The best solution is to use them up quickly. However, you may want to refrigerate your creams to increase their shelf life. Note that cold temperatures can cause the consistency to change; the water may bead onto the surface of the cream, and slight granulations sometimes appear. Don't worry about such changes in appearance, since they don't alter the effectiveness of the cream. Because creams are made from natural ingredients, they may at times develop a bit of mold on the surface. If this happens, you can simply scrape off the affected portion and use what remains. If at any point your cream gives off a rancid odor, however, be sure to discard it and make a fresh batch, since rancid oil produces toxins. When applying these creams use a little at a time, as they are very concentrated and a little goes a long way. To make the following formulas, please refer to Directions for Creams in Techniques and Definitions chapter.

Lavender Sandalwood Moisturizing Cream
ALL/DRY

An excellent face and body cream for most skin types, with a truly delicious aroma. This is one of my most popular-selling creams, and Greatgrandmother Millie's favorite. I make her jars of it for holiday gifts and she gives it to all of her friends and raves about how it makes her feel young and beautiful. Note that this formula is made with fewer essential oils than the Lavender Sandalwood Cream in the Whole Body Treatments chapter.

6 oz. canola oil (expeller pressed)	60 drops lavender essential oil
3 oz. coconut oil	20 drops sandalwood essential oil
1 oz. beeswax	9 oz. distilled water

Follow Directions for Creams. Makes 19 oz.

Luscious Lotion
ALL/OILY

An excellent face and body moisturizer for normal to oily skin, with the added healing properties of calendula and St. Johnswort. This is a favorite cream of many friends and customers for its moisturizing abilities and its intoxicating aroma. Note that the formula in this section is made with fewer essential oils than the Luscious Lotion in the Whole Body Treatments chapter.

3 oz. canola oil	1 oz. beeswax
1 oz. peanut oil	35 drops ylang-ylang essential oil
1 oz. St. Johnswort-infused olive oil	35 drops lavender essential oil
1 oz. calendula-infused olive oil	10 drops lemongrass essential oil
3 oz. coconut oil	9 oz. distilled water

To make St. Johnswort–infused olive oil, use fresh St. Johnswort flowers and buds, or flowering tops and cold pressed olive oil, and follow Directions for Herbal-Infused Oil with Fresh Herbs. Yield of herbal-infused oil made with fresh herbs varies according to how much you choose to make. To make calendula infused-olive oil, use 2 oz. of freshly dried calendula flowers, coarsely ground, and 10 oz. of cold pressed olive oil and follow Directions for Herbal-Infused Oils with Dried Herbs. You will end up with about 7 oz. of calendula-infused olive oil.

Follow Directions for Cream. Makes 19 oz.

Skin Revival
ALL/DRY /DAMAGED

A nourishing, protective, healing moisturizer for dry, aged and damaged skin and for eczema and dermatitis. It also has some ultraviolet protection, approximately SPF-4, and makes an excellent night cream as well as a winter face cream. (The sun protection factor (SPF) is based on empirical research and not from laboratory testing.)

Liquid oils should total 6 oz.:
   3 tablespoons jojoba oil,
   2 tablespoons avocado oil,
   2 tablespoons peanut oil,
   2 tablespoons calendula-infused
   olive oil (see Lucious Lotion above),
   2 tablespoons wheat germ oil,

1 tablespoon plus 2 teaspoons
burdock root-infused olive oil,
2 teaspoons lecithin
Solid oils should total 3 oz.:
   3 tablespoons shea butter,
   3 tablespoons coconut oil

½ oz. beeswax
9 oz. distilled water
2 teaspoons vegetable glycerin

25 drops lavender essential oil
8 drops geranium egypt essential oil
5 drops cedarwood essential oil

Note: Less beeswax is used in this recipe than in the Basic Cream Formula found in the Techniques and Definitions chapter. This is because the addition of lecithin helps emulsify creams and therefore can be used to replace some of the beeswax within a cream formula.

You can make your own calendula and burdock root-infused oils or you can purchase them (see Resources). To make burdock root-infused olive oil, use 3 oz. of burdock root, freshly dried and coarsely ground, and 12 oz. of cold pressed olive oil and follow Directions for Herbal-Infused Oils with Dried Herbs. Makes about 9 oz. of oil.

Follow Directions for Creams. When making Skin Revival add the lecithin to the liquid oil component and the glycerin to the water component. This cream is very thick and rich and is harder to pour than other creams, so you will need to scoop it out. The more lecithin you add the thicker the cream, as lecithin is an emulsifier. It's messy, but worth it. Skin Revival is also the most perishable of the creams and so should definitely be refrigerated. This cream's consistency is not negatively affected by refrigeration. Makes 19 oz. of cream.

Blue Chamomile Face Cream from Jean's Greens   All/Dry/Mature

Thanks to Jean Argus for sharing her secret formula and technique for making this cream. This is a rich, nourishing, reparative moisturizer for day and night use. Combines the therapeutic properties of herbs with the oils of blue chamomile and rose hip seed oil.

3 teaspoons roses
½ teaspoon dill
2 teaspoons calendula
1 teaspoon passion flower
1 teaspoon comfrey leaf
½ teaspoon lemon balm
2 teaspoons chamomile
½ teaspoon hibiscus
1 teaspoon nettle
½ teaspoon parsley

1 teaspoon lavender
1 teaspoon plantain
1½ cups sweet almond oil
1 oz. beeswax
1 teaspoon blue chamomile essential oil
1 teaspoon rose hip seed oil
1 teaspoon borax
20 drops honeysuckle flower essence

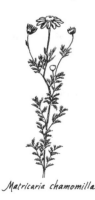

Matricaria chamomilla

Part One: Make herbal infusion with the dried herbs by placing them in a glass jar and pouring boiling water over them, allowing water to be half an inch above the herbs. Cover the jar and let steep overnight. Strain the infusion and use 1 cup per batch of cream. The leftover infusion makes a delightful addition to a warm bath.

Part Two: Warm up the almond oil in a double boiler or hot water bath. Grate the beeswax into the oil and heat until melted. Remove from heat, put in a large mixing bowl and let cool to body temperature. Add the rose hip seed oil and blue chamomile essential oil. Add the borax and the honeysuckle flower essence to the 1 cup of strained herbal infusion and warm to body temperature. Gradually pour herbal-infusion mixture into oil mixture while beating with a handheld electric mixer, (Jean prefers the Braun).

The cream will thicken as it cools and whipping should continue until you can form peaks. Spoon into jars immediately and allow to settle. Let cool completely before capping. Makes about eight 2-oz. jars.

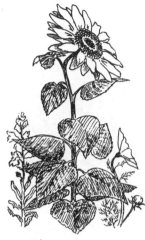

Helianthus annus

Sun Butter Face Cream   ALL/DRY/DAMAGED

A rich, nourishing, protective cream which I would rate at approximately SPF-15. (Note that my SPF ratings are based on empirical research and not on laboratory testing.) The oils used in this cream provide a natural sunscreen factor and are augmented by the PABA. Observe how your skin responds in the sun with this cream. If it burns you need to increase the SPF by adding another teaspoon of PABA per 19-oz. batch. Likewise, if your skin is not tanning reduce or omit the PABA.

3 oz. jojoba oil
3 oz. sesame oil
2 oz. shea butter
1 oz. cocoa butter
½ oz. beeswax
9 oz. green tea-infusion made from 3 tablespoons of green tea
　　and 16 oz. water
1 tablespoon PABA (see Resources)

Make herbal infusion with green tea and water, let steep for 4 hours. Use 9 oz. strained infusion for the water component, add PABA to warmed infusion and then follow Directions for Creams. Note: The PABA is added to the water component, as it is water-soluble. PABA can make the cream slightly granular; if this should happen, don't worry — it is still good. (For more information on PABA see the Ingredients chapter.) In this formula less beeswax is needed than in the Basic Cream Formula found in the Techniques and Definitions chapter because cocoa butter is used. Makes 19 oz.

EYE TREATMENTS

The tissues surrounding the eyes are the finest and most delicate on your face. The eyes themselves are extremely sensitive to environmental factors and vulnerable to strain, irritation or infection. The eyes are also a good indicator of a person's general state of health and well-being — one only needs to think of the clear, sparkling eyes of a healthy, happy person, or the dull, puffy eyes of someone who is sick or fatigued. Of course, eye treatments are no substitute for sleep or good nutrition. However, tired, strained or infected eyes and the tissues surrounding them can be helped immeasurably by herbal eyewashes, poultices, compresses and creams. A simple eye treatment can have wonderfully rejuvenating and healing effects.

Eye Compresses

Eye compresses can be made from a variety of herbs or foodstuffs, which are applied to the closed eyelids and left on for 10–30 minutes. They are very relaxing, soothing treatments that can ease tension, rejuvenate tired, irritated or sore eyes and in some cases help clear up inflammations and infections. It is best to lie down comfortably during the treatment. Herbal tea bags are convenient and popular eye compresses. Try combining an eye compress treatment with a facial masque for an especially rejuvenating effect.

 ## *Cucumber Eyes*   ALL

A soothing, cooling treatment for dry, inflamed eyes. Try this treatment instead of eyedrops. It is also nice to do while applying a facial masque.

2 cucumbers (organic preferred) sliced ⅛-inch thick

Lie down in a comfortable place. Place cucumber slices over closed eyes, leave on at least 20 minutes. Replace after 20–30 minutes if desired. Makes 1 treatment.

 ## *William LeSassier's Apple Eye*   ALL/INFECTED

A traditional remedy that is said to cure pinkeye.

Apple (organic preferred), freshly grated

Lie down with head on towel in a comfortable place, and apply grated apple to closed eyelids. Allow the apple juices to seep into the eyes. Leave on for 20 minutes and repeat a couple of times a day as needed. Makes enough for 1 treatment.

Note: When dealing with infections of any kind, is it wise to pay attention to immune support while also applying external help (see Defense Formula on page 100-101).

Variation: Use potato instead of apple.

 ## *Rose Eyes*   ALL

A refreshing astringent for pussy, oozing eyes.

Roses (unsprayed) either fresh or dried
water

Mash a small handful of fresh roses with a little water, or reconstitute dried ones by soaking them in water and then mashing them. To mash roses pound them in a mortar and pestle or in a bowl with a wood pounder. Lie down in a comfortable place with towel under head and apply mashed roses to closed eyes. Leave on at least 20 minutes. Makes enough for 1 treatment. *Variation follows:*

Calendula Eyes   ALL/INFECTED
A healing, antimicrobial treatment for inflamed, sore eyes where infection is present.
Replace roses with calendula flowers.
Leave on at least 20 minutes, allowing the flower juices to seep into the eye. Repeat as needed.

Note: When dealing with infections of any kind, it is wise to do some internal immune support while also applying external help (see Defense Formula page 100–101).

 ## Chamomile Eyes ALL

For tense, strained eyes, and very relaxing to do while applying a face masque.

> **2 chamomile tea bags**
> **very hot water**

Place the tea bags in a cup and cover with very hot water, just enough to saturate them. Place a saucer on top of the cup to prevent the evaporation of the herb's volatile oils. Let tea bags cool to body temperature. Lie down in a comfortable place with a towel under your head and apply a tea bag to each closed eye. Leave on at least 20 minutes, allowing the herbal juices to seep into the eyes. Repeat as needed. Makes enough for 1 treatment. *Variation follows.*

Mint Eyes ALL

A refreshing, cooling treatment for tired, dry and hot eyes, and very nice to do while applying a face masque. Replace chamomile tea bags with mint tea bags

Eyewashes

Eyewashes moisten the eyes and can also soothe irritations and heal inflammations. Distilled water is the most basic eyewash, but well-strained herbal infusions can also be used for added therapeutic value. Herbal tinctures can be used as well, as long as they are sufficiently diluted. Eye cups and eye droppers, available from any pharmacy, are very helpful in administering the following eye preparations.

 ## Rose Water Eyes ALL

The astringent, healing properties of the rose is also found in distilled rose water. Make sure you use pure distilled rose water. A refreshing cleansing eye treatment.

> **Rose water**
> **eye cup or eye dropper**

Place rose water into a very clean eye cup and wash out the eyes. Or drop rose water into the eyes using an eye dropper. Repeat as needed.

"For Your Eyes Only" ALL

"For Your Eyes Only" was developed by Jean Argus' Herbal Tea Works, which makes it available in tea bags or loose tea through Jean's Greens (see Resources).

This herbal blend provides an excellent treatment for eye irritation. It can also be taken internally, 1–2 cups of tea a day, to promote eye health.

> **Use these dried herbs: 1 part eye bright, 1 part chickweed, 1 part calendula, 1 part lavender, ½ part goldenseal leaf**

Herbs can be measured either by weight, tablespoon or cup depending on how much you want to make.

Combine herbs and make a strong infusion using 1 large handful of herbs (1 oz.) and 16 oz. water, and let steep for 3 hours. You can make more or less infusions as needed. Be sure to strain infusion through a tightly woven cloth. Apply to eyes with eye dropper or eye cup, along with drinking it. Store unused portion in the refrigerator and use up within 2–3 days. Makes about 13 oz.

To use tea bag method, coarsely grind herbs together and put them in tea bags. Place two tea bags in a cup and cover with very hot water. Place a saucer on top of the cup to prevent the evaporation of the herb's volatile oils. Let tea bags cool to body temperature. Lie down in a comfortable place with a towel under your head and apply a tea bag to each closed eye. Leave on at least 20 minutes, allowing the herbal juices to seep into the eyes. Repeat as needed. Makes enough for 1 treatment.

Ed Smith's Rue Fennel Compound ALL

This refreshing tonic for the eyes was provided to me by herbalist Ed Smith. It is mildly soothing, cleansing and astringent. Especially indicated for "tired eyes" and for burning and inflamed eyes and conjuctivia: allergies, conjunctivitus (pinkeye) and bloodshot eyes. The following formula is made from herbal tinctures, but Ed Smith has told me that it can also be brewed into a strong infusion using equal parts of each herb dried. For simplicity's sake I am omitting the 1 percent boric acid from the original formula. Ed Smith is a highly respected formulator and extract maker and is the proprietor of HerbPharm, one of the most successful and highly acclaimed tincture companies in the United States. This compound tincture is available ready-made from HerbPharm (see Resources).

1 teaspoon rue tincture made from
  fresh rue tops with immature seeds
1 teaspoon dried fennel seed tincture
1 teaspoon fresh eyebright flowering
  herb tincture
1 teaspoon dried goldenseal rhizome
  and root tincture

1 teaspoon fresh mullein flower with
  leaf tincture
small amber glass jar with an eye
  dropper top or tight-fitting lid

Make tinctures with herbs following the directions in the Techniques and Definitions chapter. You can make simple tinctures with each herb separately and combine them after they are strained. Then measure out teaspoons of strained tincture into a small measuring cup with a spout and pour into jar. Makes about ¾ oz.

You can also make this formula as a compound tincture using equal parts of each herb and tincture them together, in which case they are premixed and ready to use after they are strained.

Place 3–15 drops in an eye cup with saline solution (available at pharmacy) and stir with the glass dropper until well mixed. The number of drops that can be tolerated will vary with the individual and his or her situation. If the wash seems too strong, lower the number of drops until it feels comfortable. Do an eyewash with this mixture (approximately 1 or 2 minutes for each eye) 1–3 times per day. While doing the wash make sure to keep the eye opened widely and to rotate it in all directions.

Wild & Weedy Eye Pillows From Randi Barouch

Eye pillows are aromatic pillows for your eyes. Through the centuries and across cultures aromatic herbs, seeds and grains have been tucked into small sacks or bags and placed on closed eyes to promote sleep and relaxation. Eye pillows gently caress the eyes with the gentle, cool pressure of the seeds and grains while offering the soothing aroma of herbs. If your eyes are photosensitive, or if you are trying to go to sleep in a room that is not completely dark, eye pillows can also help block out the light. Randi recalls that Granny Barb used old socks that had lost their mates for eye pillows. For those of us who want something a little more "appealing to the eye," Randi offers the following instructions:

Materials:
> 2 pieces of 4½-by-9-inch natural fiber cloth, such as cotton, silk, linen, etc. thread, needle, straight pins
> 1 cup flaxseeds
> 1 cup dried herbs, (lavender, chamomile, lemon balm, peppermint, or any other aromatic herb of your liking)
> paper rolled into a funnel
> chopstick or pencil
> plastic container with lid

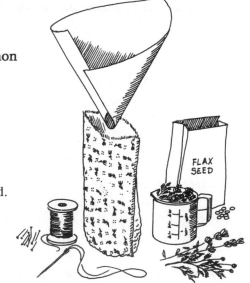

To assemble:
1. Place 2 cloths together, right side facing in, and pin, leaving a 2-inch opening on one end.
2. Sew cloths together, leaving the 2-inch opening for filling.
3. Turn inside out so that right side is facing out; push corners out with pencil or chopstick.
4. Mix 1 cup of flaxseeds with 1 cup of herbs of choice in plastic container.
5. Mix flaxseed herb mixture and pour through funnel into pillow. Use pencil or chopstick to push contents through funnel.
6. Sew up opening to complete the pillow.
   Your herb pillow will last for about a year, at which point it should be re-opened and refilled with fresh seeds and herbs. It makes an excellent gift, especially for elders.

Eye Creams and Emollients for the Skin Around the Eyes

The skin around the eyes is so thin and delicate that it often benefits from a little extra pampering with rich creams gently applied. While mature skin often benefits greatly from the use of special emollient eye creams, using these preparations while your skin is still young and supple can help prevent the area around your eyes from drying out prematurely.

Sandalwood Jojoba Eye Oil All/Dry/Mature

Jojoba's rich, emollient, and protective properties, combined with sandalwood's hydrating and anti-inflammatory effects, are helpful around the eyes.

>   1 oz. jojoba oil
>   5 drops sandalwood essential oil

Pour jojoba oil into 1-oz. jar, leaving about ⅛ of an inch of space at the top, drop in the sandalwood essential oil, cap and shake well. It is ready for use.

Apply jojoba oil to index and middle fingertips and gently massage the skin around the eyes and the eyelids. Allow oil to soak in for 10–20 minutes and then wipe off any excess if desired. Makes 1 oz.

🐝 *Bennay's Beauty Oil* Dry/Mature

This wrinkle-preventing and -rejuvenating skin treatment has been practiced by a friend for the past 20 years. She claims that her youthful and vibrant complexion is the result of this daily castor oil ritual. Its origins are from Native American skin care.

>   ⅛ to ¼ teaspoon castor oil; use more or less as needed

Massage castor oil into the skin after the face has been washed but is still slightly moist and warm. The warmth and moisture allow the thick viscous consistency of the castor oil to spread easily over the skin and contribute to the success of this treatment. Pat off excess oil if desired. Makes enough for 1 treatment.

Comfrey Salve (Loose Version) All/Dry

Apply salve lightly around the eyes and gently massage, especially before sleep, to help reduce swelling and irritation. This is a looser salve than others and will spread more easily around the delicate eye area.

>   4 oz. comfrey-infused olive oil
>   1 oz. beeswax

Make a salve with infused oil and beeswax (See Techniques and Definitions pp. 223–224). Note: To make comfrey-infused oil use 1 oz. of freshly dried and ground comfrey leaf, 1 oz. of dried and ground comfrey root, and 8 oz. of cold pressed olive oil. Then follow Directions for Herbal-Infused Oils with Dried Herbs. You can also purchase excellent ready-made comfrey salve (see Resources). Makes 5 oz. of salve.

Fennel Shea Eye Cream
ALL/DRY/MATURE

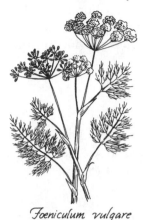

A rich, hydrating and gentle cream for the skin around the eyes.

9 oz. fennel infusion (preferred) or distilled water
3 oz. almond oil
2 oz. avocado oil
1 oz. jojoba oil
2 oz. coconut oil
1 oz. shea butter
1 oz. beeswax
20 drops fennel essential oil

Note: To make fennel infusion use 3 tablespoons fennel seeds (freshly crushed) and 16 oz. water and let steep for 4 hours and strain.

Follow Directions for Creams. Makes 19 oz. of cream.

Foeniculum vulgare

Blue Chamomile Face Cream from Jean's Greens
ALL/DRY/MATURE

This cream's rich, nourishing, reparative and moisturizing capabilities make it an excellent cream for around the eyes. It combines the therapeutic properties of herbs with the oils of blue chamomile and rose hip seed oil. To make, see formula pp. 30–31 or order it from Jean's Greens (see Resources).

Skin Revival
ALL/DRY/MATURE

A nourishing, protective and healing moisturizer for dry, aged and damaged skin, eczema and dermatitis. It has some ultraviolet protection: SPF-4. This concentrated cream can be used sparingly around the eyes; however, omit the essential oils when making it for the eye area. See formula pp. 29–30 for how to make it or order it from Falcon Formulations (see Resources).

FACIAL CARE MENUS

The following menus are facial care regimens based on skin type. I would like to emphasize that these are just a few of the choices among infinite possibilities. Don't feel constrained to follow one of these routines to the letter in order to have healthy skin. The best guide is your own experience — through experimentation you will learn which treatments and formulas work best for your skin, and how often to use them. To get you started, I've assembled some of the formulas and techniques from this chapter into daily and weekly step-by-step facial care programs.

Daily Facial Care

For some of us, daily facial care may require little more than an occasional splashing of cold water on the face to wake up in the morning. For others, a more elaborate program may be necessary to maintain a healthy, glowing complexion. Some people find that their skin feels best if they vary formulas and techniques. Some may benefit from a regimented facial care routine, and others do fine tending to their facial skin on an as-needed basis. As you put together your own facial care routine — whether you follow one of the plans below or create your own customized regimen — be sure to refer to the instructions on basic techniques provided in this chapter.

DAILY FACIAL CARE FOR NORMAL SKIN

Program A for Normal Skin

1. Apply cleansing oil: Almond Delight Cleansing Oil or Cleopatra's Cleansing Oil.
2. Apply a toner: Queen of Hungary's Water, Floral Water Toners or Rose Aloe Face Toner.
3. Apply a moisturizer: Rose Water and Jojoba Oil, or Lavender Sandalwood Cream.

Program B for Normal Skin

1. Apply cleansing oil: Almond or Canola Oil.
2. Scrub with: Lavender Calendula Scrub or Sage Scrub.
3. Apply a toner: Luscious Face Toner or Lavender Water.
4. Apply a moisturizer: Luscious Lotion or Golden Oil.

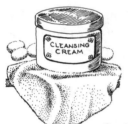

DAILY FACIAL CARE FOR DRY SKIN

Program A for Dry Skin

1. Apply cleansing oil: Jojoba Oil or Basic Cleansing Cream.
2. Apply a toner: Floral Water Toners or Rose Lavender, Marshmallow and Nettle Toner.
3. Apply a moisturizer: Blue Chamomile Face Cream or Skin Revival.

Program B for Dry Skin

1. Apply cleansing oil: Olive Oil or Coconut Oil.
2. Scrub with: Comfrey Fenugreek Scrub or Seed Scrub.
3. Apply a toner: Sandalwood Water.
4. Apply a moisturizer: Lavender Sandalwood Moisturizing Cream for normal to dry skin or Skin Revival for very dry skin.

DAILY FACIAL CARE FOR OILY SKIN

Program A for Oily Skin

1. Apply cleansing oil: Grapeseed Oil or Basic Cleansing Cream. Omit this step if no makeup is worn or if it makes your skin feel oilier.
2. Apply a toner: Berry Leaf Toner or Basil Blend Astringent.
3. Apply a moisturizer: Oil and Mist using Grapefruit Water Toner and Grapeseed Oil. Omit this step if skin feels moist and lubricated.

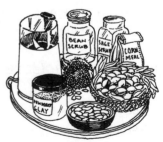

Program B for Oily Skin

1. Apply cleansing oil: Canola Oil. Omit this step if no makeup is worn or if it makes your skin feel oilier.
2. Scrub with: Grain Scrub or Rose Blossom Sage Scrub.
3. Apply a toner: Chamomile Blend Astringent or Lemon Balm Vinegar.
4. Apply a moisturizer: Oil and Mist using Lavender Water and Sesame Oil. Omit this step if skin feels moist and lubricated.

Weekly Facial Care

WEEKLY FACIAL CARE FOR NORMAL SKIN

1. Apply a cleansing oil: Almond Delight Cleansing Oil or Cleopatra's Cleansing Oil.
2. Scrub with: Lavender Calendula Scrub or Sage Scrub.
3. Steam or facial hot pack: Christmas Tree Steam or Lavender Steam.
4. Apply a masque: Vegetable Garden Masque.
5. Apply a toner: Queen of Hungary's Water, Floral Water Toners or Rose Aloe Face Toner.
6. Apply a moisturizer: Rose Water Jojoba Oil or Lavender Sandalwood Cream.

WEEKLY FACIAL CARE FOR DRY SKIN

1. Apply a cleansing oil: Jojoba Oil or Basic Cleansing Cream.
2. Scrub with: Comfrey Fenugreek Scrub or Seed Scrub.
3. Steam or facial hot pack: Comfrey Fennel Blend.
4. Apply a masque: Avocado Flour Treat.
5. Apply a toner: Rose Lavender Marshmallow and Nettle Toner.
6. Apply a moisturizer: Skin Revival.

WEEKLY FACIAL CARE FOR OILY SKIN

1. Apply a cleansing oil: Grapeseed Oil or Basic Cleansing Cream.
2. Scrub with: Rose Blossom Sage Scrub.
3. Steam or facial hot pack: Sweet Fern Citrus Blend.
4. Apply a masque: Whole-Wheat Flour Cleansing Masque.
5. Apply a toner: Berry Leaf Toner.
6. Apply a moisturizer: Oil and mist using Grapefruit Water Toner and Grapeseed Oil. Omit this step if skin feels moist and lubricated.

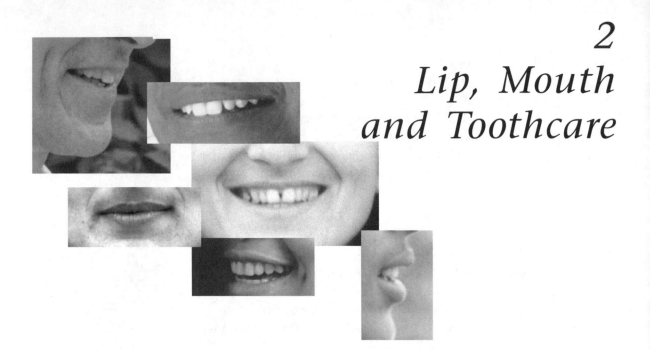

2
Lip, Mouth and Toothcare

Like the eyes, the tissues of the lips and mouth are especially sensitive to environmental influences. And as with the eyes, the appearance of the lips and mouth can be good indi cators of an individual's overall health. We all know how annoying and uncomfortable chapped lips can be, and how self-conscious a cold sore can make you feel. At some point we have all been embarrassed by bad breath or plagued with a toothache. Following are some natural treatments and remedies to prevent or heal chapped or blistered lips, and some pure and simple solutions you can use to rinse your mouth, brush your teeth and even soothe a toothache. Also included are lip gloss formulas made from natural ingredients that are good for your lips.

LIPS AND MOUTH

Lip Balms

Lip balms are made the same way as salves, using 1 part beeswax to 2.5 parts oil. These proportions will yield a fairly hard lip balm. To adjust the consistency, you can increase the beeswax-to-oil ratio for a harder balm or decrease it for a softer one. You can choose oils possessing the desired effects and include appropriate herbal-infused oils and essential oils for a custom formula. The Ingredients chapter offers guidelines for choosing the appropriate herbs and oils. Many of my customers favor the scent of citrus essential oils in lip balms, but it is important to remember that these tend to be drying and may cause the lips to dehydrate if too much is added. The amount of essential oil used in the following recipes shouldn't cause a problem, but pay attention to how they affect your lips and make adjustments in the formulas as you see fit. When making lip balms it is helpful to use heat-proof measuring cups with ounce or half-ounce gradations to help you measure accurately. To make the following formulas, please refer to Directions for Salves and Balms on p. 224.

I find that coating the lips thoroughly with lip balm prior to sleep helps to heal damaged lips. If your lips are dry and chapped, it is also helpful to drink plenty of water and to avoid spicy, salty foods.

All-Purpose Lip Balm   ALL

A light, nourishing, healing lip balm for any time of year.

> 3 oz. expeller canola pressed oil
> 1 oz. calendula-infused olive oil
>   (preferred) or plain olive oil
> 1 oz. wheat germ oil
>
> 2 oz. beeswax
> 56 drops anise, fennel, mint, grape-
>   fruit or other essential oil

Follow Directions for Salves and Balms. When pouring the melted beeswax-and-oil combination into containers, add 2 drops of essential oil per ¼ oz. lip balm, and place lid immediately on the container to prevent the evaporation of the essential oils. Note: ¼-oz. lip balm containers are available by mail order (see Resources). Makes 7 oz. of lip balm or enough to fill twenty-eight ¼-oz. containers if you want to make gifts.

Note: To make calendula-infused olive oil, see Luscious Lotion p. 29.

Superhealing Lip Balm   ALL/DRY/DAMAGED

A therapeutic lip balm with additional nourishing and protective properties for seriously chapped, cracked and damaged lips. Use in summer and winter to protect from harsh weather, sun, wind and dehydration. Apply as needed and especially before night slumber for strongest reparative results.

> 1 oz. coconut oil
> 1 oz. shea butter
> 1 oz. jojoba oil
> ½ oz. wheat germ oil
> ½ oz. calendula-infused olive oil
>   (see Luscious Lotion p. 29)
>
> ½ oz. St. Johnswort-infused olive oil
>   (see p. 29)
> ½ oz. castor oil
> 1 oz. beeswax
> 44 drops lavender essential oil

Follow Directions for Salves and Balms. When pouring the melted beeswax-and-oil combination into containers, add 2 drops of lavender essential oil per ¼ oz. lip balm, and place lid immediately on the container to prevent the evaporation of the essential oils. Note: ¼-oz. lip balm containers are available by mail order (see Resources). Makes 6 oz.

This lip balm uses solid oils as well as liquid oils. The solid oils are solid at room temperature and don't require beeswax to thicken them. So the liquid oils, which add up to 3 oz., will be solidified by 1 oz. beeswax. When following the salve-making directions, measure out the solid oils and add them to the liquid oils and proceed as instructed. Variation follows:

Superhealing Lip Balm with Sunscreen   ALL/DRY/DAMAGED
Add ½ teaspoon PABA per 6-oz. batch of lip balm for an approximate SPF-10 to SPF-15 lip balm. Mix PABA into the melted oil-and-beeswax mixture at the end of the heating process, just prior to pouring the lip balm into containers. The PABA will give the lip balm a slightly grainy consistency.

Echinacea Cold Sore Lip Balm
ALL/DAMAGED

This is an excellent medicated, healing balm with antimicrobial, antiviral and antifungal action. Use on athlete's foot, minor cuts and wounds, bug bites and diaper rash.

1 oz. freshly dried echinacea angustifolia root
1 oz. myrrh powder
1 oz. black walnut hull dried at green stage
1 oz. freshly dried goldenseal root

16 oz. cold pressed olive oil
4 oz. beeswax
3 dropperfuls tea tree essential oil
3 dropperfuls camphor essential oil
3 dropperfuls thuja essential oils

This lip balm requires that you first make an herbal-infused oil with the olive oil and the herbs. Mix and grind echinacea, black walnut hulls, and goldenseal in mortar and pestle or small coffee grinder used exclusively for herbs and seeds. Then mix in the powdered myrrh. Follow Directions for Herbal-Infused Oils with Dried Herbs. Makes about 10–12 oz. oil.

Once you have made and decanted your herbal-infused oil it can be made into a lip balm. Combine 10 oz. infused oil with 4 oz. of beeswax. Follow Directions for Salves and Balms. When pouring the melted beeswax-and-oil combination into containers, add 2 drops of essential oil of tea tree, 2 drops essential oil of camphor and 2 drops essential oil of thuja per ¼ oz. lip balm, and place lid immediately on the container to prevent the evaporation of the essential oils. Note: ¼-oz. lip balm containers are available by mail order (see Resources). Makes 14 oz. balm, enough to use generously on lips and elsewhere on the body as needed.

Lip Gloss

Lip gloss is made by infusing specific dye herbs in oil so that they impart their color to the oil. The quantity of herb used for infusing the oil will affect the intensity of color — the more herb used, the stronger the color. The infused oil is then thickened with beeswax, in the same manner as a salve. For lip gloss, you may want to make a softer, glossier balm by using 1 oz. of beeswax to 3 oz. of oil. Adding a small amount of castor oil will help give the lip gloss a sheen.

Alkanet root and annatto seeds are two commonly used herbs for making lip balms and rouges. Alkanet yields a red color, and annatto yields a yellow-orange shade. Products derived from these oils, even when made with a high concentration of herb, will not be as strongly colored as products made with the synthetic colors used in the cosmetics industry. However, they are often sufficient for adding a subtle touch of color to the face in a completely nontoxic manner. These colored oils can also enhance a product's appearance — for instance, by using the red-infused oil of the alkanet root as the base for an aphrodisiac body oil.

Red Love Lips
ALL

A soothing lip gloss with a red color that can also be applied the cheeks. It is necessary to first make the alkanet-infused oil.

3 oz. dried alkanet root (cut)   1 oz. beeswax
8 oz. olive oil or almond oil   25 drops rose geranium essential oil
1 tablespoon castor oil   or other essential oil of choice

Make infused oil with alkanet root and olive or almond oil (see Directions for Herbal-Infused Oils with Dried Herbs). Once you have made and decanted the alkanet-infused oil make lip gloss by combining 3 oz. of alkanet-infused oil, castor oil and beeswax and follow Directions for Salves and Balms. When pouring the melted beeswax-and-oil combination into containers, add 2 drops of essential oil per ¼ oz. lip gloss and place lid immediately on the container to prevent the evaporation of the essential oils. Makes 4 ½-oz. or eighteen ¼-oz. containers. *Variation follows:*

Orange Love Lips   ALL

This is made with annatto seeds in place of the alkanet root in the Red Love Lips formula and makes an orange- to amber-tinted oil and lip gloss.

Mouthwashes and Breath Fresheners

It is very easy to make effective homemade alternatives to commercial mouthwashes. The formulas offered here reduce bacteria in the mouth while freshening and deodorizing the breath. They are made with essential oils, herbal infusions, tinctures and other natural ingredients. The essential oils, though not used in large proportions, are key ingredients that add antimicrobial action and flavor to the formulas.

Essential Oil Mouthwash   ALL

This simple mouthwash is meant to be used as it is made. You can add more essential oil drops to strengthen the deodorizing effect, but watch for irritating effects from too much essential oil.

2 oz. water   1 drop peppermint essential oil
1 drop tea tree oil   ¼ teaspoon baking soda or salt

Pour water into a cup, add the salt or baking soda, drop in the essential oils and stir well. It is ready to use. Store in a tightly sealed jar to keep the essential oils from dissipating and use up within 1–2 days. Makes 2 oz.

Variation: The peppermint in the previous formula can be replaced by cinnamon, fennel, anise, spearmint, grapefruit or other essential oil of choice.

Essential Oil Mouthwash with Vodka   ALL

The addition of 80 proof vodka (or other 80 proof liquor) to the Essential Oil Mouthwash formula will increase the cleansing action and preserve the mouthwash so you can bottle and travel with it or store it for future use. More essential oil is used in this formula as well. If you like the results, make a larger batch by multiplying the ingredients.

2 oz. water   ½ teaspoon baking soda or salt
6 drops tea tree oil   2 oz. 80 proof vodka
6 drops peppermint essential oil

Place ingredients in a jar and cap with a tight-fitting lid. Shake well before each use. Makes 4 oz.

Variation: The peppermint in the previous formula can be replaced by cinnamon, fennel, anise, spearmint, grapefruit or other essential oil of choice.

Peppermint Breath Freshener I

ALL

This potent formula uses alcohol and essential oil of peppermint to create a very concentrated mouthwash. It will cleanse and deodorize with only 1–2 drops, making it very convenient to travel with.

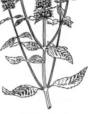

40 drops peppermint essential oil
1 oz. vodka

Pour vodka and essential oil into a small glass jar with a tight-fitting lid. Cap and shake the jar. Place 1–2 drops into mouth and swish around for 10–20 seconds, then spit out. Shake prior to each use. You can also dilute a few drops of Peppermint Breath Freshener into a glass of water for a deodorizing mouth rinse. Yields 1 oz., enough for 50 or more applications.

Mentha piperita

Variations: For a more antimicrobial product, replace the vodka with myrrh, echinacea, spilanthes or other immune-supporting tincture of choice.

Peppermint Breath Freshener II

ALL

This formula is very concentrated. Essential oils are diluted in a honey base and only 1–2 drops are needed to deodorize the mouth.

¼ teaspoon sage essential oil   **1 teaspoon peppermint essential oil**
¼ teaspoon tea tree essential oil   **1 tablespoon plus 1½ teaspoons honey**

Combine ingredients in a small vessel and then pour into a 1-oz. bottle (preferably a small squeeze dropper bottle, like what eyedrops come in) and cap. A funnel may be necessary to get ingredients inside the very small-mouth bottles. You may also need to warm the honey in a hot-water bath if it is too thick to pour. To use breath freshener, place 1–2 drops in mouth as needed. Makes 1 oz., enough for 250 or more applications.

Note: If the honey is too thick to come out of the small opening of the squeeze bottle, enlarge the hole.

Variation: Replace honey with glycerin in the above formula and shake before each use, as the glycerin and essential oils tend to separate.

Clove Prickly Ash Mouth Rinse

ALL

This mouth rinse combines clove's and prickly ash bark's antiseptic, pain-relieving and deodorizing properties with the cleansing action of alcohol. The addition of the alcohol also preserves the product for several months or longer. The formula can be made without alcohol but will not be as cleansing or last as long. It is interesting to note that unlike other water-based infusions, which only last a few days in the refrigerator, clove infusion seems to last for a few weeks or more outside of refrigeration; clove's strong antimicrobial action seems to inhibit the spoilage process. But to err on the side of safety I would store the formulation made without alcohol in the refrigerator and use it up within a week.

1 tablespoon whole cloves	5 oz. 80 proof vodka
1 tablespoon prickly ash bark (cut)	25 drops peppermint essential oil
1 cup water	

Make herbal infusion with herbs and water and let steep for 8 hours or longer. Pour 5 oz. strained infusion into a glass jar, add the vodka and essential oil, cap and shake. It is ready for use. Makes 10 oz. of mouthwash.

Variation: Replace the tablespoon of prickly ash bark with 1 tablespoon echinacea root (coarsely ground) or 1 tablespoon goldenseal root powder.

Grapefruit Seed Extract Mouthwash   ALL

Grapefruit seed extract's antimicrobial action is an aid to cleansing and disinfecting the mouth. Makes enough for 1 mouth application.

3–6 drops of grapefruit seed extract
1 oz. water

Rinse mouth with this combination, swishing it around and keeping it in mouth for as long as desired (at least 1 minute).

Earthly Extract's Herbal Mouth Rinse   ALL

Cleanses and tones the gums. Fights bacterial, fungal and viral infections such as cold sores, gingivitis and irritated gums. Good as a gargle for sore throats. This concentrated mouth rinse can be used straight or diluted in a small amount of water. Available ready-made (see Resources).

1 tablespoon echinacea angustifolia root tincture	1 tablespoon licorice root tincture
1 tablespoon calendula flower tincture	1 tablespoon horsetail tincture
1 tablespoon fresh St. Johnswort flower tincture	2 oz. vegetable glycerin
1 tablespoon sage leaf tincture	10 oz. distilled water
2 teaspoons myrrh powder tincture	12 drops tea tree essential oil
2 teaspoons goldenseal root tincture	60 drops spearmint or fennel essential oil

Make or purchase tinctures of the herbs listed above. Measure and pour the tinctures, glycerin, water and essential oils into a glass bottle, cap and shake. It is ready for use. This mouth rinse can be preserved for a year or more unrefrigerated. Makes about 15 oz.

Garden Mouth Juice   DAMAGED

A mixture of antimicrobial, cell-healing herbs for mouth sores and gum infections. My partner, Tim, who since childhood has periodically suffered from mouth sores, uses this formulation with great success.

> 2 large handfuls of the following
>   mixture of fresh herbs in equal
>   quantities, chopped: Comfrey leaf,
>   violet leaf, spilanthes flowers,
> plantain leaf, echinacea purpurea
>   leaf (when chopped the herbs
>   should equal 2 cups packed)
> 1 cup water

Chop up herbs and place in blender or food processor, add the water slowly to create a slurry with the consistency of very loose pesto or a thick liquid, pour into a jar, cap and store in the refrigerator. Will keep in the refrigerator for 4–5 days.

To use, sip a mouthful and retain inside mouth for as long as tolerable, spit out and repeat several times a day or as needed. These herbs are not only safe but beneficial when ingested, so don't worry about swallowing them.

TOOTHCARE

The Wild Toothbrush

Sumac (*Rhus Glabra, R. typhina*) is a prolific nonpoisonous, red-berried weed shrub or small tree. Do not confuse this with the white-berried sumac, which is poisonous. Look for red berries and you will be safe. You can use a twig from the tree as an improvised toothbrush with superior astringent and cleansing properties. It is excellent for removing plaque and acts as a good gum stimulant. To make a sumac toothbrush break off a twig 4–6 inches long and ½ inch in diameter and peel back the outer skin or thin bark, then scrub the twig tip along the tooth surface and gently massage the gums. Other trees, such as pine and oak, can be used similarly. This is a good thing to know when you've forgotten your toothbrush while traveling.

Tooth Powders

Homemade tooth powders provide a natural alternative to commercial toothpastes. They may take a little getting used to if you've been using sweetened toothpaste all your life, but they are so easy and inexpensive to make, and so effective in cleaning the teeth, that they are worth a try. They are also free of all the chemicals added to commercial toothpastes. Since toxins are easily absorbed through the lining of the mouth, it makes sense to switch to a nontoxic formula. Although my husband initially resisted using these unsweetened preparations, he can no longer stand the taste of commercial toothpaste. He says that his mouth feels fresher and cleaner when he uses an herbal tooth powder. Wet your toothbrush prior to sprinkling on the powder to help it adhere. Salt or spice shakers are a good way to apply tooth powders to a moistened brush. They are convenient for travel and excellent to take camping.

You can make tooth powders with baking soda, sea salt, finely ground herbs, clay and other ingredients. When using baking soda or salt for brushing the teeth, you can add essential oils to increase the antimicrobial action or to flavor the powder and make it more palatable. For example, add 1 drop of tea tree oil per brushing for increased antiseptic properties, or 1 drop of fennel, mint, orange or cinnamon oil per brushing for increased cleansing properties and enhanced flavor. It is best not to swallow the powder when essential oil has been added, since it may be too concentrated. I recommend using finely ground, unrefined sea salt. If you are using coarse, unrefined sea salt, you will need to grind it before using it in a tooth powder.

 ### Baking Soda Tooth Powder ALL

Cleans and deodorizes the mouth and teeth.

Sprinkle baking soda onto moistened toothbrush and proceed to brush. Optional: Add 1 drop of tea tree oil to powdered toothbrush for added cleansing, or other oil for taste. Makes enough for 1 brushing.

 ### Salt Tooth Powder ALL

Gentle abrasive for cleaning the teeth and reducing bacteria in the mouth.

Sprinkle sea salt onto moistened toothbrush and proceed to brush. Optional: Add 1 drop of sage essential oil to powdered toothbrush. Makes enough for 1 brushing.

 ### Salt & Soda Powder ALL

Combines the cleansing and deodorizing effects of salt, baking soda and essential oils.

1 oz. sea salt	5 drops sage essential oil
1 oz. baking soda	10 drops peppermint essential oil
10 drops tea tree essential oil	

Mix salt and baking soda in a glass jar with a tight-fitting lid and add essential oils drop by drop, stirring thoroughly after each addition. To use, sprinkle powder lightly onto moistened toothbrush. Makes 2 oz., enough for 50–60 brushings.

Variation: Replace the peppermint essential oil with cassia cinnamon or fennel essential oils.

Sage Horsetail Tooth Powder ALL

A cleansing, refreshing powder that brightens teeth.

1 teaspoon freshly dried sage	4 drops tea tree essential oil
1 teaspoon dried horsetail	6 drops mint or other oil of choice for
1 teaspoon baking soda	flavor and cleansing purposes
1 teaspoon sea salt	

Grind sage and horsetail in coffee grinder used exclusively for herbs and seeds, sift through fine mesh strainer to get a very fine powder, add baking soda and salt and mix well, drop in the essential oils (stirring after each addition) and store in a glass jar with a tight-fitting lid. To use, sprinkle powder lightly onto moistened toothbrush. Makes enough for 20 or more brushings.

Variation: Instead of sage and horsetail substitute an equal amount of other herbs; some good choices are cinnamon, echinacea, clove, oregano, citrus peel, myrrh, prickly ash bark and oak bark.

Echinacea Prickly Ash Tooth Powder ALL

A strong antimicrobial cleanser.

Use the following dried herbs: 1 teaspoon echinacea root, 1 teaspoon prickly ash bark (cut)
1 teaspoon whole cloves
½ teaspoon myrrh powder

2 teaspoons baking soda
2 teaspoons sea salt
9 drops tea tree essential oil
15 drops mint or other oil of choice for flavor and cleansing purposes

With the exception of myrrh, it is best to buy the herbs as whole as possible and to then cut and grind them prior to use. Grind cut herbs in coffee grinder used exclusively for herbs and seeds, sift through fine-mesh strainer to get a very fine powder, add myrrh powder, baking soda and salt and mix well, drop in the essential oils (stirring after each addition), and store in a glass jar with a tight-fitting lid. To use, sprinkle powder lightly onto moistened toothbrush. Makes enough for 40 or more brushings.

Kim's Herbal Toothpicks

Make your own deliciously flavored toothpicks to cleanse and stimulate your gums. You can create a variety of flavored picks by choosing different essential oils. These toothpicks also make terrific breath fresheners.

This recipe comes from Kim, a childhood friend and the proprietor of Penny's General Store, a wonderful and exotic herbal apothecary in New York City's East Village. When we go to New York City we often visit Kim in his shop. My son Sam is always excited to receive one of Kim's cinnamon toothpicks, which he carries around and enjoys tasting for the next few days.

You will need some good-quality wooden toothpicks and enough essential oil of your choice (cassia cinnamon, fennel, peppermint, orange, anise, nutmeg, and tea tree are favorites) to cover them.

Place the toothpicks inside a jar filled with essential oil and soak overnight. Remove the picks from the oil (you may want to use tweezers) and set them on a platter to air-dry. When completely dry, they are ready to use. Store the flavored picks in an airtight glass or tin jar. Use the herbal toothpicks to clean your teeth and stimulate your gums. You can also suck on them to freshen your breath. The leftover essential oil is still good, and can be used to make other formulas.

Tooth and Gum Pain Remedies

Many herbs, such as clove, yarrow, spilanthes and prickly ash bark, possess pain-relieving and disinfectant properties that are appropriate for pain associated with inflamed gums and tooth-aches. Although these preparations may not address the causes of dental problems, their numb-ing and immune-enhancing properties can be extremely helpful in alleviating pain while re-ducing inflammation and infection.

St. Johnswort Tincture for Pain

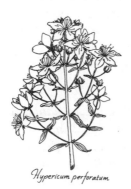

Hypericum perforatum

St. Johnswort's astringent, anti-inflammatory and pain-relieving properties make it very useful for gum and tooth pain, especially if caused by an exposed nerve or cavity. It will not cure the problem but will make the pain tolerable until you can take care of the underlying cause. St. Johnswort tincture has been very helpful in alleviating pain for many people who found no relief from other medicines.

Fresh St. Johnswort buds and flowers, or flowering tops, enough to tightly fill an 8-oz. jar
the highest-proof alcohol available to you, preferably 190 proof, enough to fill and cover the herbs in the jar
water

The higher the percent of alcohol is used to tincture St. Johnswort, the more hypericin is ex-tracted out of the herb. (Hypericin is responsible for its therapeutic action.)

Make tincture with St. Johnswort following Directions for Alcohol Tinctures Using Fresh Herbs. When St. Johnswort tincture has been decanted, store without any additional water. Prior to use, dilute St. Johnswort, tincture with half the amount of water. So for every 1 oz. of St. Johnswort tincture, add ½ oz. of water and drop directly onto problem area as often as needed. Note: Excellent-quality St. Johnswort tincture can also be purchased ready-made (see Resources).

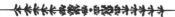

Searching for St. Johnswort

Take a "weed walk" any time from the end of June through mid-July in many parts of North America and you will find blooming St. Johnswort (*Hypericum perforatum*). Put some up in oil and alcohol so that you can benefit from the healing virtues of this powerful medicinal. Wandering through the fields and meadows to gather St. Johnswort is a special ritual I look forward to every year, and a wonderful way to welcome the summer. The plant's name reveals its traditional role as a herald of summer, since it blooms around the time of the Feast of St. John, near the summer solstice.

Myrrh Tincture

Myrrh's antimicrobial and immune-supporting actions are useful for gums, teeth and mouth sores and inflammations.

2 oz. myrrh powder   **1 tablespoon water**
8 oz. 190 proof alcohol*

*The high alcohol content is necessary for extracting medicinal properties from resins and gums like myrrh.

Make a tincture with myrrh, alcohol and water. Follow Directions for Alcohol Tinctures Using Dried Herbs. Apply myrrh tincture directly onto problem area. If myrrh tincture feels too strong dilute with half water prior to use. Note: Myrrh tincture is available in pharmacies, health food stores and by mail order (see Resources). Makes 5–6 oz. myrrh tincture.

Spilanthes Flower Power Chews

Spilanthes is a medicinal plant from South America, where it is referred to as "toothache plant"; it is very helpful in alleviating the pain of mouth sores and gum infections. It is analgesic and antimicrobial, helping to numb and clean sores and to reduce infection or inflammation. By the way, this herb is easy to grow as an annual in the Northeast. Seeds are available via mail order (see Resources).

Fresh spilanthes flower

Chew flower and pack onto the problem area, leaving on for as long as possible. Repeat throughout the day as needed. Note: The flowers will create a tingling sensation in the inner surfaces of the mouth.

Yarrow Chews for Pain

Yarrow's strong antiseptic, analgesic and astringent effects are useful in cleansing and healing mouth sores and gum and tooth problems. It's also used to clean the teeth.

Fresh yarrow flowers and leaves

Chew flower and/or leaf and pack onto the problem area, leaving on for as long as possible. Repeat throughout the day as needed. Note: Yarrow will create a tingling sensation in the inner surfaces of the mouth. To use as a tooth cleaner, rub yarrow leaf or flower thoroughly onto teeth and into gum surfaces.

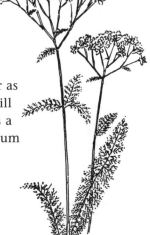

Achillea millefolium

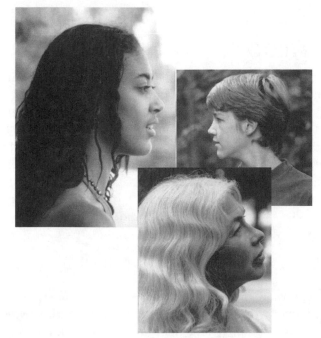

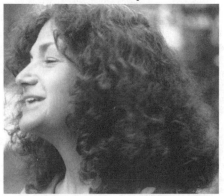

3
Beautiful Hair
Healthy Scalp

Hair care begins with the understanding that hair is essentially an extension of the skin, so many of the principles that apply to skin care also apply to care of the hair and scalp. As a general rule, your hair type will correspond to your skin type, whether it tends to be dry, oily, normal or some combination thereof. For this reason, many of the basic ingredients that are beneficial to your skin can also help your hair and scalp. Commercial hair preparations — shampoos, styling gels, sprays and even conditioners — can be among the most damaging and drying body care products on the market. Combine these harsh preparations with the tendency that many people have to overuse them, and the result can be hair that is lifeless, depleted, frazzled, stripped of its natural oils or coated with artificial ingredients.

The two basic steps in a good hair care program are cleansing and conditioning, which may be accomplished either separately or in a single treatment. This chapter offers an array of formulas that address the cleansing and conditioning needs of various hair types, some of them specially formulated for either light or dark hair. For cleansing you will find a number of shampoos and non-soap cleansers. For conditioning you can either choose one of the conditioning shampoos or follow up with a hair rinse or hair and scalp emollient, according to your specific needs. You will probably want to experiment to see what works best for your hair.

I personally prefer to avoid shampoos, which strip away the protective oils from the scalp and hair. (Note that my hair is long, thick, black and on the dry side. People with thin, limp, light or oily hair may do better with one of the other cleansing methods listed below.) Instead, about once or twice a week I apply a rich oil or pomade containing antimicrobial essential oils, such as the ones found in the Hair and Scalp Emollients section, and massage it into my hair and scalp with a brush. The act of brushing distributes the oil evenly and removes lint and other debris from the hair. I leave this preparation in my hair so that it can thoroughly penetrate the hair shafts and scalp. My hair looks shiny and damp for about a day until the oil has been absorbed. The carrier oil provides excellent conditioning, while the essential oils help to eliminate odor and funk. I only rinse my hair with water on an as-needed basis.

SHAMPOOS

The following shampoos are gentle and free of the synthetic ingredients used in commercial shampoos, including many of the "natural" ones. The only synthetic ingredient found here is the chemical alkali contained in the castile soap that serves as the base of these shampoos (see following explanatory box). The shampoos are formulated to protect to your hair and scalp while offering a mild cleansing action. Unlike commercial shampoos, they are not meant to leave your hair squeaky clean, a result of stripping away all of the protective oils. Rather, they will cleanse your hair of dirt and excess oil, leaving it feeling soft and conditioned. They can also be used as gentle soaps for the face or body.

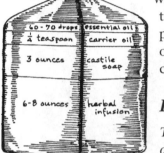

60 - 70 drops | essential oil
¼ teaspoon | carrier oil
3 ounces | castile soap
6-8 ounces | herbal infusion

Basic Shampoo Formula

Basic Shampoo Formula

ALL

This basic formula provides the framework upon which to devise your own customized shampoo. Note that if you would like to increase the detergent effect of a shampoo, simply add more castile soap. And keep in mind that if you do not use up a batch of shampoo within a couple of weeks, it is best to store it in the refrigerator. The shampoos that follow are based on this basic formula.

6–8 oz. herbal infusion of choice
3 oz. of liquid castile soap
¼ teaspoon carrier oil of choice

up to 60–70 drops essential oils of choice

Pour strained infusion, liquid castile soap, carrier oil and essential oils into a jar or squeeze bottle, cap and shake. It is ready for use. Always shake these shampoos before use. Makes about 9–11 oz. of shampoo.

Variations: The amount of essential oil you use will depend on which ones you choose and the effect you are trying to obtain. You can omit the carrier oil if your hair is very oily, or add more if your hair is very dry. Additional ingredients, such as aloe, tinctures, etc., may be added to this basic shampoo recipe to adapt it for various hair and scalp needs.

❦❦❦❦❦❦❧❧•♗♗♗♙♙♙♙♙

A Word About Soap

Soap is made with fats — either of animal or vegetable origin — combined with harsh chemical alkalis such as sodium hydroxide or potassium hydroxide. The fat is combined with the alkali to create a chemical reaction known as saponification; in plain language, the alkali helps turn the fat into soap. All soaps, no matter how gentle or "natural," are made with some form of alkali. This inevitably means that you are using a harsh chemical when using soap. A truly natural soap may have been made many years ago using wood ash as the alkali, but I know of no contemporary soap companies that use this ancient and crude method, since it does not offer the same control as using the new chemical alkalis. While today's soaps are not truly natural products, one can still make the best choices among those available commercially. Choose soaps that have been made with good-quality oils and fats and that have been produced with the least amount of synthetic chemicals, stabilizers, preservatives, coloring agents and artificial scents. Liquid castile soap, such as Dr. Bronner's, is a good-quality basic soap made without the use of additional chemicals. When you do use soap, use only as much as necessary to accomplish the job. Remember that soap acts as a solvent, removing oil and grime from the hair and scalp. This means that it will also remove the natural protective coating your body secretes, leaving the skin and hair dry and unprotected.

Golden Shampoo

LIGHT HAIR

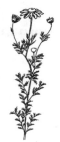

Use the following freshly dried herbs:
  1 teaspoon chamomile, 1 teaspoon calendula, 1 teaspoon marshmallow root (cut)
1 cup water
¼ teaspoon olive oil (use sesame oil for oily hair and jojoba oil for dry hair)

3 oz. castile soap
10 drops lemongrass essential oil
15 drops grapefruit essential oil
10 drops tea tree essential oil

Make herbal infusions with herbs and water, let steep for 4 hours and strain. Pour strained infusion, liquid castile soap, olive oil or other oil of choice and essential oils into a jar or squeeze bottle, cap and shake. It is ready to use. Always shake before use. Makes about 9 oz.

Midnight Beauty

DARK HAIR

Use the following freshly dried herbs:
  1 teaspoon black walnut hull, 1 teaspoon sage, 1 teaspoon comfrey root (cut), 1 teaspoon rosemary
10 oz. of water
3 oz. castile soap

¼ teaspoon olive oil (use sesame oil for oily hair and jojoba oil for dry hair)
45 drops tangerine essential oil
15 drops nutmeg essential oil

Make herbal infusion with herbs and water, let steep for 8 hours and strain. Pour strained infusion, liquid castile soap, olive oil or other oil of choice and essential oils into a jar or squeeze bottle, cap and shake. It is ready to use. Always shake before use. Makes about 11 oz.

Garden Blend

ALL HAIR COLORS

Use the following freshly dried herbs:
  1 teaspoon nettle leaf, 1 teaspoon comfrey root (cut), 1 teaspoon basil
10 oz. water

¼ teaspoon almond oil
3 oz. castile soap
20 drops sweet basil essential oil
30 drops lavender essential oil

Make herbal infusion with herbs and water, let steep for 8 hours and strain. Pour strained infusion, liquid castile soap, almond oil, and essential oils into a jar or squeeze bottle, cap and shake. It is ready for use. Always shake before use. Makes about 11 oz.

Defunk Shampoo
ITCHY/FUNGAL SCALP

Use the following freshly dried herbs:
1 teaspoon mugwort, 1 teaspoon oregano, 1 teaspoon thyme, 1 teaspoon calendula, 1 teaspoon burdock root (cut)
10 oz. water

¼ teaspoon olive oil
3 oz. castile soap
20 drops tea tree essential oil
20 drops rosemary essential oil
20 drops lavender essential oil

Make herbal infusions with herbs and water, let steep for 8 hours and strain. Pour strained infusion, liquid castile soap, olive oil and essential oils into a jar or squeeze bottle, cap and shake. It is ready for use. Always shake before use. Makes about 11 oz.

Luxurious Shampoo
DRY/DAMAGED

For dry, damaged hair and irritated scalp.

Use the following freshly dried herbs:
1 teaspoon comfrey root, 1 teaspoon violet leaf, 1 teaspoon marshmallow root (cut), 1 teaspoon plantain leaf

10 oz. water
½ teaspoon shea butter
¼ teaspoon jojoba oil
3 oz. castile soap
60 drops lavender essential oil

Make infusion with herbs and water, let steep for 8 or more hours and strain. Gently reheat strained infusion until it becomes quite warm but not boiling and add shea butter, stirring it in until thoroughly melted, then add liquid castile soap and jojoba oil. Pour into jar or squeeze bottle, add essential oil, cap and shake. It is ready for use. Always shake before use. Makes about 11 oz.

Citrus Shampoo
OILY HAIR

Use the following freshly dried herbs:
1 teaspoon nettle leaf, 1 teaspoon citrus peel, 1 teaspoon lemongrass, 1 teaspoon Irish moss
9 oz. water

4 oz. castile soap
20 drops lime essential oil
25 drops orange essential oil
10 drops cassia cinnamon
3 tablespoons aloe vera gel

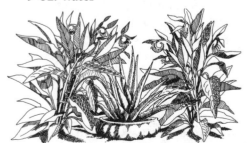

Make herbal infusion with herbs and water, let steep for 8 hours and strain. Pour strained infusion, liquid castile soap, aloe and essential oils into a jar or squeeze bottle, cap and shake. It is ready for use. Always shake before use. Makes about 11 oz.

CLEANSERS FOR NORMAL TO OILY HAIR

You can easily clean the hair and scalp without the use of soap. Essential oils, either used alone or diluted in a base such as alcohol and water, are excellent for this purpose. Certain tinctures made with antifungal and antiseptic herbs also make good scalp cleansers. These cleansers help to disinfect and deodorize the hair and scalp while cutting through excess oil. Note that these formulas may be too drying for dry hair, and if used too frequently can even dry out oily hair. They are used without water and are convenient and easy to use when camping or traveling.

 ## *Essential Oil Drops* ALL/OILY

Use essential oils to disinfect and deodorize the hair and scalp.

Choose from this list: rosemary, lavender, chamomile, sage, tea tree

Apply 1–2 drops of essential oil of choice onto comb or brush and pass through hair. Or drop 1–2 drops of essential oil with eye dropper directly onto hair and massage or brush through hair and into scalp. Be careful not to use more than 1–2 drops, as the essential oils are very concentrated and can easily burn and irritate the skin. For more information on essential oils, see Ingredients chapter.

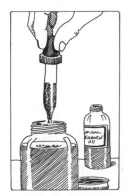

Vodka Tea Tree Hair Cleanser ALL/OILY

A cleanser for oily hair with antimicrobial and deodorizing properties.

1 oz. vodka	5 drops tea tree essential oil
7 drops lavender essential oil	8 drops grapefruit essential oil

Pour vodka into a jar or spray mist bottle, drop in essential oils, cap and shake. Spray into hair or with an eye dropper dispense 10–20 drops of liquid onto scalp and brush through hair. Can be diluted with equal parts distilled water and used as an underarm deodorant. *Variation follows:*

Rosemary Sage and Sandalwood ALL/OILY

Replace the essential oils in the above formula with 7 drops rosemary essential oil, 5 drops sage essential oil, 8 drops sandalwood essential oil.

Nettle Seed Cleanser and Conditioner ALL/OILY

Nettle seed tincture for cleansing and deodorizing oily scalp and hair is used to balance sebaceous gland secretions.

Make nettle seed tincture with fresh nettle seeds and vodka. Follow Directions for Alcohol Tinctures Using Fresh Herbs. Dispense nettle seed tincture with an eye dropper onto the scalp. Use about ½–1 full dropperful of tincture, or more as needed. Massage into scalp and brush through hair.

Variations: Try using calendula, sage, lavender and thyme tinctures for cleaning the hair and scalp.

Hair Rinses

Hair rinses are conditioning treatments that soften the hair, encourage shine and body, and make hair more manageable. Rinses can also help to bring out the natural highlights in hair. The hair rinses offered here are made with a base of herbal infusions or herbal-infused vinegars. Some contain emollients and essential oils for additional benefits.

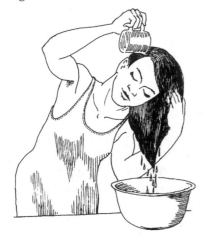

Herbal Infusion Hair Rinses

These formulas are herbal blends made from dry herbs steeped in water to make an herbal infusion, which is then used to rinse the hair. The possibilities for herbal mixtures are infinite, but the following formulas offer some excellent choices. I have included the essential oils as optional ingredients, but bear in mind that they will increase the deodorizing and conditioning effects of the hair rinse. These formulas make enough for 1–2 applications. If you like a particular formula, you might want to increase the amount of dry herb mixture you make by multiplying the ingredients proportionately. Store the mixture in an airtight container away from light and heat, and it will be ready to infuse when needed. Please keep in mind that once you have made the infusion, you should use it within 1–2 days.

Applying Herbal-Infusion Hair Rinses. The best way to apply these hair rinses is to thoroughly massage a few ounces into the scalp and hair. Then hold your head over a bowl or basin, making sure that the ends of your hair are either in or over the container. Pour about a cup of infusion over your head, allowing it to drain into the container. Work the infusion through with your fingers, then repeat the process several times. Make sure that the entire scalp and hair are saturated. Follow with a freshwater rinse if desired.

Golden Rinse
Light Hair

- 1 tablespoon chamomile flowers
- 1 tablespoon calendula flowers
- 1 teaspoon fenugreek seed
- 1 tablespoon marshmallow root (powdered or cut and sifted)

16 oz. water
optional: 1 drop lemongrass essential oil, 1 drop grapefruit essential oil, 1 drop tea tree essential oil

Make herbal infusion with herbs and water, let steep for 3 hours and strain. Gently warm infusion if desired, add essential oils and apply to the hair and scalp, taking the time to massage it in thoroughly. To pour rinse onto head, hold a bowl at the end of the hair strands to catch the liquid and reapply. Repeat this several times. Rinse out if desired. Makes enough for 1–2 treatments.

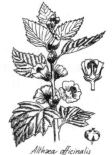

Althæa officinalis

Midnight Beauty Rinse
DARK HAIR

1 tablespoon black walnut hull
1 tablespoon sage
1 tablespoon comfrey root (cut or powdered)

1 tablespoon rosemary
16 oz. water
optional: 1 drop tangerine essential oil, 1 drop nutmeg essential oil

Make herbal infusion with herbs and water, let steep for 8 hours and strain. Gently warm infusion if desired, add the essential oils and apply, taking the time to massage the infusion into the scalp and hair. When pouring rinse onto head, hold a bowl at the end of the hair strands to catch the liquid and reapply. Repeat this several times. Rinse out if desired. Makes enough for 1–2 treatments.

Garden Blend Rinse
ALL HAIR COLORS

1 tablespoon nettle leaf
1 tablespoon comfrey root (cut or powdered)
1 tablespoon basil

16 oz. water
optional: 1 drop sweet basil essential oil, 2 drops lavender essential oil

Make herbal infusion with herbs and water, let steep for 8 hours and strain. Gently warm infusion if desired, add the essential oils and apply to scalp and hair, taking the time to massage the infusion in thoroughly. When pouring rinse onto head, hold a bowl at the end of the hair strands to catch the liquid and reapply. Repeat this several times. Rinse out if desired. Makes enough for 1–2 treatments.

Defunk Rinse
ITCHY/FUNGAL SCALP

1 tablespoon mugwort
1 tablespoon oregano
1 tablespoon calendula
1 tablespoon thyme
1 tablespoon burdock root (cut or powdered)
1 drops tea tree essential oil
1 drop rosemary essential oil
2 drops lavender essential oil
16 oz. water

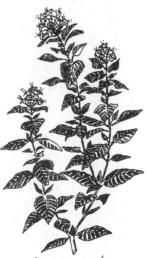

Origanum vulgare

Make herbal infusion with herbs and water, let steep for 8 hours and strain. Gently warm infusion if desired, then add essential oils and apply to scalp and hair, making sure to massage the infusion in thoroughly. When pouring rinse onto head, hold a bowl at the end of the hair strands to catch the liquid and reapply. Repeat this several times. Rinse out if desired. Makes enough for 1–2 treatments.

Note: The essential oils augment the antimicrobial action and are necessary and not optional in this formula.

Luxurious Rinse

DRY, DAMAGED HAIR AND IRRITATED SCALP

1 tablespoon comfrey root (cut or
  powdered)
1 tablespoon violet leaf
1 tablespoon marshmallow root (cut
  or powdered)

1 tablespoon plantain leaf
16 oz. cold water
¼ teaspoon jojoba oil
optional: 2 drops lavender essential oil

Make infusion with herbs and water, let steep overnight and strain. Gently warm infusion if desired, then add essential oils and jojoba oil. Apply infusion to scalp and hair, making sure to massage it in thoroughly. When pouring rinse onto head, hold a bowl at the end of the hair strands to catch the liquid and reapply. Repeat this several times. Rinse out if desired. Makes enough for 1–2 treatments.

Herbal-Infused Vinegar Hair Rinses

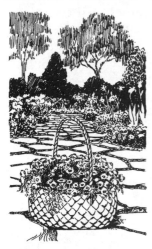

The following recipes are adaptations of the herbal-infusion hair rinses found in the preceding section. The advantage of herbal vinegars is that they can be made ahead of time and remain well preserved for a year or so. However, they do require a steeping period of 3–6 weeks. They are especially good for oily hair, and for treating fungal infections, itchy scalp and overalkaline conditions. They help remove soap residue and make the hair softer and easier to detangle. Note that vinegars may not be good for very dry hair, although they can be helpful for controlling dandruff. These herbal-infused vinegars are very concentrated, so only small amounts are needed to condition the hair and scalp, which makes them convenient for travel. When diluted with water, these herbal-infused vinegars also make excellent facial astringents. Some of these formulas, such as the Golden, Defunk and Garden Blend Vinegars, also make excellent culinary vinegars when the essential oils are omitted. They can be added to soups, stews, marinades and salad dressings. The formulas that follow are based on choice herbal blends that make excellent conditioners. However, you can also use just a single herb at a time — such as chamomile, rosemary or nettle — or look through the Botanicals section and formulate your own vinegar blends. Keep in mind that plain vinegar can also serve as a useful and simple hair rinse.

DIRECTIONS FOR HERBAL-INFUSED VINEGARS WITH DRIED HERBS. Place freshly crushed or powdered herb into a glass jar with a tightly fitting plastic lid. Pour vinegar over the herbs; stir the vinegar into the herb until thoroughly saturated, then cap tightly. Label the jar with the date and contents, and keep in a dark place. Shake daily and let steep for 3 weeks or longer. Strain vinegar when needed.

DIRECTIONS FOR HERBAL-INFUSED VINEGARS WITH FRESH HERBS. Use a glass jar with a plastic well-fitting lid and pack it tightly with fresh herbs of choice. Pour vinegar over the herbs and let it filter down through them. Keep pouring in vinegar until the herbs are completely covered by the vinegar, then cap tightly. Label the jar with the date and contents, and keep in a dark place. Let steep for 3 weeks or longer and strain when needed.

APPLYING VINEGAR HAIR RINSES. Apply 1–2 tablespoons vinegar to damp hair and scalp, thoroughly massaging it in. Leave it in for a few minutes. Rinse with plain water. You may prefer to dilute the vinegar prior to use in order to make it less caustic. Use 1 tablespoon of vinegar per cup of water, increasing the proportions as needed. Rinse with the diluted vinegar by pouring it onto your head over a bowl or basin, making sure that the ends of your hair are either in or over the container in order to catch the solution as it drains. Repeat the process several times. Make sure that the entire scalp and hair are saturated. Follow with a freshwater rinse. Be careful to keep the solution out of your eyes, since the vinegar will sting.

Basic Vinegar Rinse ALL/OILY

For short hair: 1 tablespoon organic
   apple cider vinegar
optional: 1 cup water

For long hair: 2 tablespoons organic
   apple cider vinegar
optional: 2 cups water

Massage vinegar into scalp and hair and leave in for a few minutes, or dilute vinegar with water and pour water-vinegar solution onto head. Place a bowl at the end of the hair strands to catch the liquid. Repeat several times until hair and scalp are well soaked. Rinse with freshwater.

Variations: Add essential oils to the Basic Vinegar Rinse to produce an array of delicious-smelling and more effective products. Add 1–2 drops of essential oil of choice per 1–2 tablespoons of vinegar. Some good essential oil choices are rosemary, lavender, chamomile and sage.

Golden Vinegar LIGHT HAIR

1 tablespoon chamomile flowers
1 tablespoon calendula flowers
1 teaspoon fenugreek seed
1 tablespoon marshmallow root
   (powdered or cut)

6 oz. organic apple cider vinegar
optional: water

Proceed to Directions for Herbal-Infused Vinegars with Dried Herbs. Makes about 4½ oz.

Optional: To make the vinegar smell of citrus while increasing its antimicrobial effect, add 1 drop of lemongrass essential oil, 1 drop of grapefruit essential oil and 1 drop of tea tree essential oil for every 2 oz. of strained herbal-infused vinegar.

Massage 1–2 tablespoons of vinegar into scalp and hair and leave in for a few minutes, or dilute vinegar with water, using 1 tablespoon of vinegar to 1 cup of water for short hair and 2 tablespoons of vinegar to 2 cups of water for long hair. Pour water-vinegar solution onto head and place a bowl at the end of the hair strands to catch the liquid. Repeat several times until hair and scalp are well soaked. Rinse with plain water.

Dilute the vinegar with 1–2 parts distilled water and you have a wonderful facial astringent. Use the vinegar (without the optional essential oils) for a delicious and therapeutic addition to food. *Variation follows:*

Golden Vinegar with Fresh Herbs
To make vinegar with fresh herbs fill a pint (16-oz.) jar with equal parts of each herb and follow Directions for Herbal-Infused Vinegars with Fresh Herbs. Add optional essential oils to strained vinegar. Note that fenugreek seeds will rarely be found fresh, so use 2 teaspoons of dried seeds per pint jar. Makes about 12 oz. of vinegar. The yield will vary depending on how tightly you pack the jar, how much moisture the herbs contain and how well you press the herbs during the straining process.

Midnight Beauty Vinegar
DARK HAIR

1 tablespoon black walnut hull
1 tablespoon sage
1 tablespoon comfrey root (cut or powdered)

1 tablespoon rosemary
6 oz. organic apple cider vinegar
optional: water

Proceed to Directions for Herbal-Infused Vinegars with Dried Herbs. Makes about 4½ oz.

Optional: To every strained ounce of herbal-infused vinegar add 1 drop of tangerine essential oil and 1 drop of nutmeg essential oil.

Massage 1–2 tablespoons of vinegar into scalp and hair and leave in for a few minutes, or dilute vinegar with water, using 1 tablespoon of vinegar to 1 cup of water for short hair and 2 tablespoons of vinegar to 2 cups of water for long hair. Pour water-vinegar solution onto head and place a bowl at the end of the hair strands to catch the liquid. Repeat several times until hair and scalp are well soaked. Rinse with plain water. *Variation follows:*

Midnight Beauty Vinegar with Fresh Herbs
To make vinegar with fresh herbs fill a pint (16-oz.) jar with equal parts of each herb and follow Directions for Herbal-Infused Vinegars with Fresh Herbs. Add optional essential oils to strained vinegar. Makes about 12 oz. of vinegar. The yield will vary depending on how tightly you pack the jar, how much moisture the herbs contain and how well you press the herbs during the straining process.

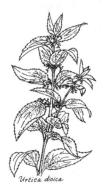

Urtica dioica

Garden Blend Vinegar
ALL HAIR COLORS

1 tablespoon nettle leaf
1 tablespoon comfrey root (cut or powdered)
1 tablespoon basil
6 oz. organic apple cider vinegar
optional: water

Proceed to Directions for Herbal-Infused Vinegars with Dried Herbs. Makes about 4½ oz.

Optional: To every strained 2 oz. of herbal vinegar add 1 drop of sweet basil essential oil and 2 drops of lavender essential oil.

Massage 1–2 tablespoons of vinegar into scalp and hair and leave in for a few minutes, or dilute vinegar with water, using 1 tablespoon of vinegar to 1 cup of water for short hair and 2 tablespoons of vinegar to 2 cups of water for long hair. Pour water-vinegar solution onto head and place a bowl at the end of the hair strands to catch the liquid. Repeat several times until hair and scalp are well soaked. Rinse with plain water.

Dilute the vinegar with 1–2 parts water and make a wonderful facial astringent. Use the vinegar without the essential oils for a delicious and therapeutic addition to food. *Variation follows:*

Garden Blend Vinegar with Fresh Herbs

To make herbal-infused vinegar with fresh herbs fill a pint (16-oz.) jar with equal parts of each herb and follow Directions for Herbal-Infused Vinegars with Fresh Herbs. Add optional essential oils to strained vinegar. Makes about 12 oz. of vinegar. The yield will vary depending on how tightly you pack the jar, how much moisture the herbs contain and how well you press the herbs during the straining process.

Defunk Vinegar   ITCHY/FUNGAL SCALP

1 tablespoon mugwort	1 tablespoon burdock root (cut or
1 tablespoon oregano	powdered)
1 tablespoon thyme	6 oz. organic apple cider vinegar
1 tablespoon calendula	*optional:* water.

Proceed to Directions for Herbal-Infused Vinegars with Dried Herbs. Makes about 4½ oz.

Optional: Add 1 drop of tea tree essential oil, 1 drop of rosemary essential oil and 2 drops of lavender essential oil to every ounce of strained herbal-infused vinegar.

Massage 1–2 tablespoons of vinegar into scalp and hair and leave in for a few minutes, or dilute vinegar with water, using 1 tablespoon of vinegar to 1 cup of water for short hair and 2 tablespoons of vinegar to 2 cups of water for long hair. Pour water-vinegar solution onto head and place a bowl at the end of the hair strands to catch the liquid. Repeat several times until hair and scalp are well soaked. Rinse with plain water.

Dilute the vinegar with 1–2 parts water and make a wonderful facial astringent. Use the vinegar without the essential oils for a delicious and therapeutic addition to food. *Variation follows:*

Defunk Vinegar with Fresh Herbs

To make herbal-infused vinegar with fresh herbs fill a pint (16-oz.) jar with equal parts of each herb and follow Directions for Herbal-Infused Vinegars with Fresh Herbs. Add optional essential oils to strained vinegar. Makes about 12 oz. of vinegar. The yield will vary depending on how tightly you pack the jar, how much moisture the herbs contain and how well you press the herbs during the straining process.

HAIR AND SCALP EMOLLIENTS

Hair and Scalp emollients include oils and pomades that soothe, nourish and soften the scalp and hair. They are also effective for treating dry flyaway hair, chemically or environmentally damaged hair and dry, itchy scalp, and can be used for detangling the hair. They can either be applied to the hair at room temperature or used for hot oil treatments. Hair and scalp emollients can tone down split and frizzy hair, providing deeply penetrating conditioning. Adding essential oils to carrier oils and butters helps to clean and deodorize the hair and scalp while adding extra conditioning effects.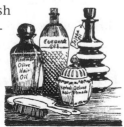

APPLYING HAIR EMOLLIENTS. To make your hair shiny, soft and more manageable, you can choose from carrier oils such as coconut, sesame, olive or jojoba, or from one of the formulas featured below. When applying oil or pomade to your hair, start by placing a very small amount on your fingertips and combing your fingers through your hair to distribute the emollient evenly. Massage the scalp as well. Apply more as needed. Beware of applying too much oil and ending up with slick, greasy hair, unless that is the effect you desire. Oil is very difficult to wash out if applied too thickly.

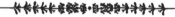

Hot Hair Oil Treatments

Hot oil treatments are used to condition dry/damaged hair as the heat helps the oil to penetrate more effectively. To use hair and scalp emollients for hot oil treatments, choose from a rich carrier oil, such as jojoba or coconut, or from one of the formulas featured below. Put the emollient in a heat-proof measuring cup and place it in a hot-water bath until the emollient reaches 100–105 degrees. Thoroughly massage the warm oil into your scalp and brush it through your hair until it is evenly dispersed. For long, thick hair use 1–2 teaspoons of oil or more as indicated. For thinner, shorter hair use ¼–½ teaspoon or more as indicated. Wrap your hair with a plastic bag or shower cap, then place a thick wool cap over that. The natural heat released from your scalp will facilitate the conditioning process. Leave your hair covered in this manner for at least an hour, then wash your hair for a shiny, luxurious result. Note that it is not absolutely necessary to wash your hair after this treatment. This procedure is also very helpful for untangling hair gnarls: Work out the knots with your fingers or a comb while the hair is saturated with oil.

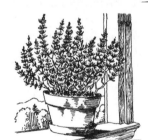

🐝 *Rosemary Olive Hair Oil*   ALL/DRY

Use as a cleansing and invigorating scalp and hair tonic for dry, brittle hair and flaky, itchy scalp.

1 oz. cold pressed olive oil
30 drops rosemary essential oil

Pour oil into jar, drop in essential oils, cap jar and shake well. The oil is ready to use. Makes 1 oz.

Variations: For drier and more damaged hair substitute jojoba oil for the olive oil. For oilier hair, replace olive oil with sesame oil.

Coconut Cedarwood Lavender Hair Oil   ALL/DRY

A rich cleansing oil for conditioning hair and scalp.

4 oz. coconut oil	25 drops lavender essential oil
10 drops cedarwood essential oil	

Scoop coconut oil into a heat-proof measuring cup and place measuring cup in a hot-water bath until the coconut oil has melted. Pour coconut oil into a wide-mouth jar and add essential oils, then quickly cap the jar to prevent essential oils from evaporating. Allow to cool and harden. Note that this oil will be looser in warmer temperatures, as coconut oil begins to melt at 76 degrees F. Makes 4 oz.

Variation: For a more masculine scent replace the lavender essential oil with 10 drops of black pepper essential oil, 10 drops of sage essential oil, and 8 drops of lemongrass essential oil.

Herbal-Infused Hair Oils

Infused herbal oils make excellent hair emollients, as they combine the nourishing and healing benefits of herbs with the lubricating and conditioning effects of oils. Plan ahead — these oils require a steeping period of 3 to 6 weeks before they are ready for use.

Sage, Rosemary and Thyme Hair Oil ALL/DRY

A cleansing and refreshing oil for dry hair with an itchy scalp. The herbs in this formula have traditionally been used for dark hair, but the amount of herb used to make this oil is not sufficient to affect one's hair color.

1 oz. freshly dried sage
1 oz. freshly dried rosemary
1 oz. freshly dried thyme
12 oz. cold pressed olive oil

Make oil following Directions for Herbal-Infused Oils with Dried Herbs. Makes about 9 oz.

Chamomile and Calendula Hair Oil ALL/DRY

A gentle, healing oil for conditioning hair and soothing flaky scalp. The herbs in this formula have traditionally been used for light hair, but the amount of herb used to make this oil is not sufficient to affect one's hair color.

2 oz. freshly dried calendula blossoms   20 oz. cold pressed olive oil
2 oz. freshly dried chamomile flowers

Make oil following Directions for Herbal-Infused Oils with Dried Herbs. Makes about 14 oz.

Comfrey, Mugwort and Nettle Hair Oil ALL/DRY/FUNGAL

A soothing, nourishing oil for itchy, funky scalp. The mugwort and nettle provide cleansing and antifungal action, while the comfrey root is reparative.

1 oz. freshly dried mugwort   1 oz. freshly dried nettle
1 oz. dried comfrey root   12 oz. cold pressed olive oil

Make oil following Directions for Herbal-Infused Oils with Dried Herbs. Makes about 9 oz.

Tropical Rosemary Hair   ALL

coconut oil
rosemary (fresh or dried)

Note: The amounts needed vary on the size jar you use for making the herbal oil.

Fill a jar with rosemary leaves (either fresh or dried), melt coconut oil and pour into the jar to cover the rosemary and to fill the jar. Then follow Directions for Herbal-Infused Oils with Heat on p. 223. Pour strained oil into wide-mouth jars and let cool and solidify. This produces a very stable oil. Yield varies.

To melt coconut oil, place oil in a heat-proof measuring cup and put cup in a pot partially filled with water over a flame. Remove from heat when oil has melted.

Note that fresh rosemary leaves, unlike most other fresh leaves, contain very little water, and that the heat used for infusion will evaporate any existing moisture. So when straining the oil no water should appear after the straining process.

Herbal Deluxe Hair Pomades

The Herbal Deluxe Hair Pomades are some of my best-selling products, and I have received many rave reviews about the results they achieve. These pomades are a thickened combination of oils that can be massaged into the scalp and hair for an excellent treatment that moisturizes, nourishes, cleans, prevents hair from splitting and increases growth and manageability. A light application can help tame wild, flyaway hair or be used to create a slick, wet look. Herbal Deluxe Hair Pomade requires advance preparation, since it contains herbal-infused oil. The herbal-infused oil recipes that follow yield about 10 oz. Only 3 oz. of this oil is needed per batch of pomade, so you will have about 7 oz. of oil left over to use directly on hair and scalp, for subsequent batches of pomade or for creating other formulas.

Herbal Deluxe Hair Pomade   ALL/DRY/DARK HAIR

1 oz. dried burdock root (cut)	3 oz. shea butter
1 oz. dried comfrey root (cut)	2 oz. beeswax
1 oz. dried nettle root (cut)	3 oz. jojoba oil
1 oz. dried salvia apiana leaf	1 oz. sesame oil
1 oz. freshly dried black walnut hull	1 teaspoon rosemary essential oil
15 oz. cold pressed olive oil	¾ teaspoon sage essential oil
3 oz. coconut oil	

Coarsely grind herbs and make herbal-infused oil with ground herbs and olive oil. See Directions for Herbal-Infused Oils with Dried Herbs. Combine 3 oz. of the strained herbal-infused oil with the rest of the ingredients (except the essential oils) in a heat-proof measuring cup and place in a hot-water bath over medium-high heat. Stir until the oils, butter and wax melt into a uniform liquid free of lumps. When it is completely melted pour liquid into a wide-mouth jar, add essential oils and cap immediately to prevent them from evaporating. When solidified it is ready for use. Makes 15 oz.

Note: You will have an extra 7 oz. of herbal-infused oil to use for another batch of pomade or to use directly on hair and scalp. It is better to make extra herbal-infused oil and have it on hand.

Herbal Deluxe Hair Pomade

ALL/DRY/LIGHT HAIR

Use 1 oz. dried burdock root (cut),
1 oz. dried comfrey root (cut),
1 oz. dried nettle root (cut), 2 oz.
freshly dried calendula blossoms,
1 oz. freshly dried chamomile
flowers
15 oz. cold pressed olive oil
3 oz. coconut oil

3 oz. shea butter
2 oz. beeswax
3 oz. jojoba oil
1 oz. sesame oil
¾ teaspoon rosemary essential oil
¾ teaspoon lavender essential oil
50 drops lime or other citrus essential
oil

Coarsely grind herbs and make herbal-infused oil with ground herbs and olive oil. See Directions for Herbal-Infused Oils with Dried Herbs. Combine 3 oz. of the strained herbal-infused oil with the rest of the ingredients (except the essential oils) in a heat-proof measuring cup and place in a hot water bath over medium-high heat. Stir until the oils, butter and wax melt into a uniform liquid free of lumps. When it is completely melted pour liquid into a wide-mouth jar, add essential oils and cap immediately to prevent them from evaporating. When solidified it is ready for use. Makes 15 oz.

Note: You will have an extra 7 oz. of herbal-infused oil to use for another batch of pomade or to use directly on hair and scalp. It is better to make extra herbal-infused oil and have it on hand.

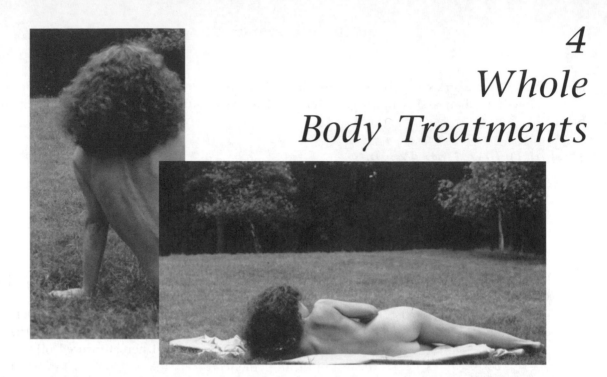

4
Whole
Body Treatments

Although the skin on the body is generally not as sensitive or exposed as that of the face and neck, it too can benefit from some special forms of care and treatment. While frequent soap-and water-showers may be the preferred method of cleansing the body in our society, this is also one of the surest routes to dry, scaly, depleted skin. Like the face, the body generally responds well to a much gentler approach to cleansing.

An effective way to improve the condition of your skin overall is to try one of the body scrubs or packs offered in the first section of this chapter on a weekly basis for exfoliation and deep cleansing, with showers or baths in between only as needed for cleansing and/or therapeutic purposes. If you do feel the need to use soap or another cleanser, try limiting its use to select areas, such as your underarms and genital region, rather than your entire body.

Whether or not you change your basic approach to cleansing the body, you can always take advantage of the emollient and therapeutic baths offered in the second section of this chapter. These baths draw on the cleansing properties of various minerals and foodstuffs and the therapeutic properties of different herbs and essential oils.

Body splashes, analogous to facial toners or astringents, though generally more diluted, are dealt with in the third section of this chapter. These can be used to gently tone the skin either after bathing or in between cleansings. They can also be used as mild deodorants and mild perfumes, and are especially refreshing when misted on with a spray bottle.

The fourth section of this chapter offers a variety of oils, creams and balms to smooth and soften your skin, replacing lost oils and moisture. Some form of body emollient is often desirable to use after bathing, exposure to sun or wind or whenever your skin is feeling dry, depleted or irritated.

The fifth section offers formulas for some gentler, more natural liquid and powdered alternatives to the harsh chemical deodorants available on the commercial market.

In the final section you will find formulas and treatments for sore muscles, achy bones and frazzled nerves.

BODY SCRUBS AND PACKS

Body scrubs, like those for the face, are used to exfoliate and cleanse the skin. Some scrubs have a more nutritive effect and are meant to be left on the skin for a period of time, allowing them to penetrate more deeply. They are often referred to as body packs, and are analogous to facial masques. They help to increase circulation while softening and smoothing the skin and imparting a healthy, radiant glow. Body scrubs are made in the same basic manner as facial scrubs, though the former can be more abrasive and stronger-acting since the skin over most of the body is not as sensitive as facial skin. Many of the gentler body scrubs and packs can even be used for the face, and many of the facial scrubs and masques can also be used for the body. I suggest using a body scrub only about once a week, since overuse can strip the skin of its protective oils. Likewise, too vigorous rubbing when applying a scrub can irritate the skin. Apply a scrub or pack just before taking a shower, bath or swim. Scrubs and packs tend to be quite messy, so you may want to perform them while standing in the tub or shower. To use a scrub or pack, moisten the formula, then gently massage it into the skin, spending more time on the areas of the body where the skin is rough or bumpy. Rinse thoroughly. If you are using a more nourishing scrub or pack, you may want to leave it on for about 20 minutes before rinsing.

Salt Scrubs

Salt's abrasive quality makes it excellent for exfoliation and cleansing. Its stimulating effects increase circulation and benefit tired, cold and dull skin. Salt scrubs are also well suited for oily, bumpy or dirty skin, but can be very drying if not used in conjunction with an emollient. Salt scrubs are not recommended for the face or for very dry, damaged or delicate skin. Moist salt may be used alone as a scrub or mixed with other ingredients. Note that salt will sting open skin. Although it is beneficial for wounds, it causes temporary discomfort.

Basic Salt Scrub

ALL/OILY/BUMPY

> **3–5 tablespoons sea salt**
> **water or herbal infusion**

Place salt in a saucer and moisten it with a little water. Gently massage damp salt into the skin for a few minutes. Rinse off. Makes enough for 1 application.

Variation: For dry skin moisten salt with oil or cream.

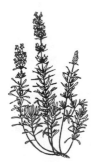

Lavender Salt Scrub

ALL/OILY

A deep-cleansing, skin-toning, invigorating scrub.

5 tablespoons sea salt **½ teaspoon olive oil**
4 drops lavender essential **water**
oil

Place salt in bowl, drop in the lavender essential oil, stir thoroughly, add the olive oil and stir thoroughly again. Sprinkle in a small amount of water, just enough to moisten the salt mixture, and then massage into the skin. Rinse off. Makes 1 treatment. *Variations follow:*

Peppermint Salt Scrub   ALL
For a stimulating and energizing treatment replace lavender essential oil with peppermint essential oil.

Hot Lava Salt Scrub   ALL
For warming the body and increasing circulation replace lavender essential oil in the above recipe with 2 drops of cinnamon essential oil, 2 drops of ginger essential oil, and 1 drop of patchouli essential oil.

Experiment with other essential oils and refer to the Essential Oils section in the Ingredients chapter to create your own custom salt scrub blends.

Salt Clay Scrubs

Combining salt and clay offers the exfoliating and cleansing properties of salt and the drawing and tightening properties of clay. The drying effects of these substances can be balanced with the addition of emollients.

Basic Salt Clay Scrub   ALL/OILY

3 tablespoons clay   4 tablespoons water
2 tablespoons sea salt

Mix salt and clay, add water and stir into a loose paste. Add more water to loosen the paste or more clay to thicken it. Massage into skin (this will not cover the surface of the body but is meant to scrub with) and leave on for 5 minutes or until the skin feels taut and tight. Rinse well. Makes enough for 1 application.

Variation: For dry skin use cream instead of water in the above formula and add 1 teaspoon of olive oil for a more soothing and lubricating treatment; allow to stay on the skin for 20 minutes.

Herbal Sea Salt Scrubs

By combining salt with dried herbs, various therapeutic effects can be produced. These scrubs tend to have a crumbly consistency. Some beneficial herbs to use for making salt scrubs are comfrey leaf and root, calendula, sage, nettle, chamomile, rose blossoms, mint, oregano, basil and lavender. You can also use a combination of herbs in a scrub formula. Refer to the Ingredients chapter for more information about the therapeutic properties of specific herbs.

Basic Herbal Salt Scrub   ALL

1 large handful of freshly dried herb   ½ teaspoon olive oil
   of choice   about 4 tablespoons water
2–3 tablespoons sea salt

Grind the herb into a powder and mix with the salt, add the water, then add the olive oil. Mix everything thoroughly. It will have a crumbly texture. Massage the scrub into the skin, (bits of the herb may fall off; just reapply) and allow to stay on for 10 minutes. Rinse off. Makes enough for 1 treatment.

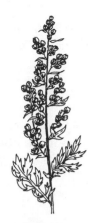

Mugwort Sea Salt ALL

A warming, cleansing skin treatment that is also good for fatigued muscles.

1 large handful of freshly
   dried mugwort leaves
   or flowering tops

2–3 tablespoons sea salt
½ teaspoon olive oil
4 tablespoons water

Grind the mugwort into a powder (mugwort grinds into a fluffy consistency) and mix with the salt, add the water, then add the olive oil. Mix everything thoroughly. It will have a crumbly texture. Massage the scrub into the skin, (bits of the mugwort will fall off, just reapply) and allow to stay on for 10 minutes. Rinse off. Makes enough for 1 treatment.

Clay Body Packs

Clay can be used alone or in combination with other ingredients to cleanse and absorb dirt and oil from the skin. It can help to facilitate the release of subdermal toxins. Clay is drying, and may be mixed with lubricating ingredients such as oil or cream to offset its drying effects.

❦ Basic Clay Body Pack ALL/OILY

1 cup clay
1 cup water

Mix clay and water till a smooth paste results. Add more water to loosen the paste or more clay to thicken it. Massage the clay into the skin and then apply it over the surface of the skin. Allow the clay to dry and then rinse off. Makes enough for 1 treatment. *Variations follow:*

Aromatic Clay Body Pack ALL

By adding essential oils to the Basic Clay Body Pack you can create a wide assortment of body packs to suit various needs.
Add 3–6 drops of essential oils to the Basic Clay Body Pack. Drop essential oils into the clay-water paste and stir in thoroughly.

Loosen Up Clay Body Pack ALL

For tense muscles add 2 drops of tangerine essential oil, 2 drops wintergreen essential oil and 1 drop of thuja essential oil to the Basic Clay Body Pack.

Rosemary Black Pepper Clay Body Pack ALL

For refreshing antimicrobial and circulatory action add 3 drops of rosemary and 2 drops of black pepper to the Basic Clay Body Pack.

Cream Clay Body Pack ALL/DRY/MATURE

A rich, nourishing body treatment for dry and mature skin.

1 cup clay
2 cups cream

1 teaspoon jojoba oil
3 drops sandalwood essential oil

Mix clay and cream until a smooth paste results, add jojoba and sandalwood oils and mix thoroughly. Add water to loosen the paste or more clay to thicken it. Massage the paste into the body and then apply a smooth coat over the surface of the skin. Leave on for as long as possible, at least 20 minutes. This paste will not dry as thoroughly as the clay packs wet with water because the addition of the cream and oil keep the clay elastic. Rinse off. Makes enough for 1 treatment.

More Nourishing Body Packs

These body treatments gently exfoliate, nourish and soothe the skin. They are appropriate for all skin types, especially dry, damaged and mature skin. They can be applied more than once a week if desired. These gentle packs are excellent for the face as well.

Golden Egg Treatment   ALL

A delicious, nourishing and drawing pack for most skin types. It can also be used on the face.

2 egg yolks
2 tablespoons sea salt
¾ cup clay
½ cup raw sunflower seeds freshly
   ground

2 tablespoons water
½ cup full-fat yogurt
4 drops nutmeg essential oil

Beat egg yolks and mix with water and yogurt. Combine salt, clay and sunflower seed meal. Mix the liquid ingredients with the dry ingredients and stir until a smooth paste results. Add more water to loosen the paste or more clay to thicken it. There will be some texture to the paste from the salt crystals and sunflower meal. Massage the paste into the body and then apply it over the surface of the skin. Leave on for as long as possible, at least 20 minutes. Rinse off. Makes enough for 1 treatment.

Ocean Lavender Treatment   ALL

A nourishing, soothing and cleansing treatment that combines the minerals and mucilage of the seaweed with the volatile oils and astringency of the lavender. An excellent treatment for the face as well as the body.

6 tablespoons finely ground seaweed
   (you can use any seaweed available
   — the slimier the better)
6 tablespoons finely ground lavender

4 tablespoons arrowroot powder or
   cornstarch
2 teaspoons olive or jojoba oil
⅔ cup water

Mix powdered seaweed, lavender and arrowroot powder, add water by the tablespoon till a loose paste is formed, let stand for about 10 minutes to let the seaweed release its mucilage (this will also make the paste thicken), then add the jojoba oil. Massage the paste into the body and then apply a thin coat of paste over the surface of the skin. Leave on for as long as possible, at least 20 minutes. Rinse off. Makes enough for 1 treatment.

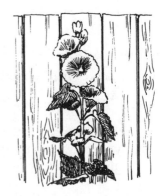

Banana Flour Treat ALL

A soothing, nutritive, moisturizing, cleansing and toning treatment for most skin types. An excellent treatment for the face as well as the body.

1 ripe banana
¾ cup whole-wheat flour,
  oat flour or buckwheat flour
⅓ cup cornmeal

½ to ¾ cup water
½ teaspoon jojoba oil
  peanut oil or other rich oil of
  choice

Mix flour and cornmeal, add water a little at a time until a smooth paste results, mash banana and add to the water-flour paste, stirring in thoroughly, then add oil, stirring in thoroughly once again. If the paste is too loose sprinkle in more flour, if too thick add water a little at a time. Massage the body with the paste and then apply a thin coat of paste over the surface of the skin. Leave on at least 20 minutes. Rinse off. Makes enough for 1 treatment. *Variation follows:*

Avocado Spread ALL/DRY

For a more skin-softening and moisturizing effect, replace the banana with ½ cup of mashed avocado pulp.

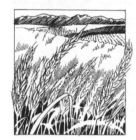

Ceres Delight ALL

A nourishing, absorbent and soothing pack for all skin types. This is an excellent scrub and mask for the face as well as the body.

¼ cup cornmeal
¼ cup whole wheat
  flour

¼ cup flaxseeds
¼ cup fennel or anise seeds
1 cup water

Mix the flours, grind the flax and fennel seeds, add ground seeds to the flour mixture and mix in thoroughly, then pour water into the dry mixture, a few tablespoons at a time, till a smooth paste the consistency of pancake batter results. Note that the paste will have grit in it due to the cornmeal and flax and fennel seeds. The finer you grind the seeds the less grit will be in the final product. Grit is desirable, as it helps exfoliate the skin, yet sensitive skin may become irritated from too much abrasion. If the paste is too loose sprinkle in more flour, if too thick add water a little at a time. Massage the body with the paste and then apply a thin coat of paste over the surface of the skin. Leave on for as long as possible, at least 20 minutes. Rinse off. Makes enough for 1 treatment. *Variations follow:*

Ceres Delight with Chamomile ALL/IRRITATED

For irritated and inflamed skin replace the fennel seeds with ⅓ cup of dry chamomile flowers ground finely, and add 1 teaspoon of jojoba and 2 tablespoons of aloe vera gel to the paste.

Ceres Delight with Cream ALL/VERY DRY/MATURE

For very dry skin replace the water with cream, replace fennel seeds with sunflower seeds and add 1 teaspoon of avocado oil; be sure to grind the seeds very finely.

Fresh Garden Body Pack ALL/DAMAGED

This is a wonderful, cooling, soothing and healing treatment for damaged, eczematous, irritated and inflamed skin. The herbs in this treatment have traditionally been used to heal wounds, burns and skin rashes. This pack makes an excellent poultice where the skin has been damaged.

2 handfuls fresh plantain leaves
2 handfuls fresh comfrey leaves
2 handfuls fresh violet leaves (the combined herbs when chopped should equal 1 well-packed quart)

1 cup water
1 teaspoon olive oil
5 drops lavender essential oil

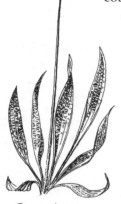

Plantago lanceolata

Chop leaves and place in food processor. (You can use a blender but I find that food processors work best for pureeing herbs.) Turn on processor and drizzle water into greens till a smooth puree results. Add more water if needed. Scoop out the puree and add the oils. Massage the body with puree and then apply a thin coat of puree over the surface of the skin. Apply thickly where skin is damaged. If the puree doesn't adhere to the skin sprinkle in some clay, cornstarch or arrowroot powder to make it stick. Leave on for as long as possible, at least 20 minutes. This pack is messy and if the herbal puree drips off just reapply.

The Fresh Garden Body Pack also makes an excellent poultice for burns and wounds. To make a poultice apply the puree thickly to the damaged skin and wear it for 20 minutes or longer. Wrap a cloth around the herbal puree to secure it against the skin. Rinse off. Makes enough for 1 application. *Variations follow:*

1. For irritated skin add 1 handful of jewelweed to the above formula.
2. For an invigorating, astringent, toning and cleansing pack replace the plantain, violet and comfrey leaves with fresh berry leaves, fresh sage leaves and fresh mint leaves. More water may be needed to form a puree with these herbs.
3. Replace the herbs with other fresh herbs of choice or availability, such as basil, lemon balm and mugwort. Refer to Ingredients chapter for further information.

BATHS

Bathing is a wonderful way to relax while cleansing and rejuvenating your entire body. There are many preparations than can be added to the water to increase both the therapeutic action and your enjoyment of the bath. Salt, minerals, herbs, essential oils, carrier oils and foodstuffs can all be added to a bath to yield various benefits.

Bath Oils

Oil added to the bath helps to soften and nourish dry, damaged or stressed skin. The warmth of the bath helps the oil to be absorbed into the skin and provides an excellent moisturizing effect. You can add any plain, herbal-infused or scented carrier oil to your bath. The carrier oils offer emolliency and nourishment for your skin, while essential oils promote various subtle energetic effects. Oil may also be added to a bath for nervous conditions, since it is said to nourish and protect the nerves.

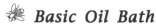

 ## Basic Oil Bath   ALL/DRY

> Use 1–2 oz. of plain carrier oil per bath

Add oil to bathwater prior to immersion. Some good choices are coconut, olive, sesame or jojoba oil.

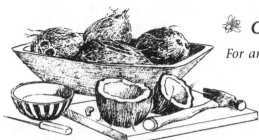

Coconut Oil Bath   ALL/DRY

For an emollient and soothing bath after sunbathing or when skin feels dry and hot.

Add 1–2 oz. coconut oil per bath

Melt the coconut oil by placing it over very low heat and then add it to the bathwater.

 ## Olive Oil Bath   ALL/DRY

All-purpose emollient for general nourishment and skin softening.

> **Add 1–2 oz. olive oil per bath**

Basic Bath Oil Blend   ALL/DRY

This is a well-balanced oil blend for most skin types. It is nourishing and soothing and is not too heavy or light. It provides an excellent base for the Aromatherapy Bath Oils that follow. This oil blend may also be used directly on the skin.

1½ oz. olive oil	1 oz. canola oil
3 oz. almond oil	½ oz. wheat germ oil
1 oz. sesame oil	

Pour oils in a jar, cap with a tight fitting lid and shake well. Add 1 oz. oil per bath. Makes 7 oz.

AROMATHERAPY BATH OILS. You can create a wide assortment of aromatherapy oils for the bath by adding essential oils to the Basic Bath Oil Blend just described, or to any other carrier oil of your choice. These oils can also be used for massage. Use 1–2 teaspoons of Aromatherapy Bath Oil per bath. Note that the concentrated essential oils make the carrier oil stronger, so less oil is needed for the bath.

 ## Basic Aromatherapy Bath Oil   ALL/DRY

> **15–30 drops essential oil of choice**
>
> **1 oz. Basic Bath Oil Blend or other carrier oil of choice**

Fill small-mouth jar with carrier oil, leaving ⅛ inch of space at the top. Add the essential oils drop by drop, cap the jar with a tight-fitting lid and shake well. Use 1–2 teaspoons of oil per bath.

Warming Bath Oil
ALL

Use this oil when you feel chilled and your muscles and bones hurt from the cold. It can also help improve poor circulation.

15 drops ginger essential oil
10 drops nutmeg
15 drops black pepper

7 drops lemongrass essential oil
4 oz. Basic Bath Oil Blend or other carrier oil of choice

Pour oil into a jar and add the essential oils, drop by drop. Cap jar with a tight-fitting lid and shake well. Add 1–2 teaspoons of oil per bath. Makes 4 oz., enough for 12–24 baths. *Variations follow:*

Sensual Bath Oil
ALL

The essential oils in this blend have been traditionally used for aphrodisiac and euphoric effects. Of course, what turns one on is a very personal thing, but this blend has a good track record.

Replace the essential oils in the above formula with 25 drops of ylang-ylang, 25 drops of sandalwood and 15 drops of sweet basil essential oils.

Energizing Bath Oil
ALL

A wake-up oil that is refreshing and stimulating.

Replace the essential oils in the above formula with 25 drops of rosemary, 25 drops of peppermint and 12 drops sweet orange or tangerine essential oils.

ESSENTIAL OILS IN THE BATH. Essential oils can also be added to a bath by simply dropping them directly into the water immediately prior to immersion. Be careful when adding essential oils directly to the bathwater, as they can burn and irritate the skin if added in too high a quantity.

🐝 Basic Essential Oil Bath
ALL

Depending on the strength of the essential oil you use, you can add anywhere from 2–8 drops per bath. Add essential oils just prior to immersion.

Variations: Add 4 drops of lavender or 2 drops of chamomile essential oil for a relaxing effect, add 3 drops of rosemary essential oil for a circulatory and decongestant effect, or add 5 drops of sandalwood essential oil for a sensual bath. Refer to the Ingredients chapter for more information on essential oils. Caution: Citrus oils can irritate the skin.

🐝 Honey and Cream Bath
ALL/DRY

This is a rich emollient bath for dry, irritated skin. The honey is a skin-soothing agent and a humectant, which means it helps draw moisture to the surface. The cream is the fat or oil of the milk and is very nourishing and softening to the skin.

½ cup heavy cream (organic if possible)
3 tablespoons honey

Combine honey and cream in a small bowl or cup, stirring until the honey is dissolved into the cream. You may need to warm them if the honey is too thick by placing the bowl into a hot-water bath as you stir. Then add the mixture to the bathwater.

Nectar Bath Oil ALL/DRY

A super rich oil with additional nutritive and emollient properties.

2 oz. wheat germ oil	2 oz. sesame oil
2 oz. peanut oil	2 oz. jojoba oil
2 oz. castor oil	

Pour oils into a glass jar, cap with a tight-fitting lid and shake well. Add 1 oz. oil per bath. Makes 10 oz.

Variation: You may add essential oils to this oil blend; add 1–2 teaspoons essential oil per 10 oz. batch and add only 1–2 teaspoons oil blend per bath.

Sea Salt Baths

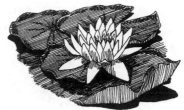

Sea Salt Baths are cleansing and detoxifying. Salt baths are drying to the skin, so be sure to apply a good moisturizer afterward. Alternatively, you can add 2 tablespoons of carrier oil to the bathwater to help counteract the drying effects of the salt.

Basic Sea Salt Bath ALL

Sea Salt Baths are made by adding 1–2 cups of salt to the bathwater.

Basic Aromatherapy Bath Salts ALL

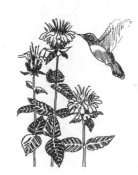

You can add essential oils to the salt to enhance its therapeutic action while also creating an array of pleasing scents.

20 drops essential oil of choice
2 oz. sea salt

Place salt in a small jar and add essential oil. Stir and shake until the essential oils are well mixed and dispersed throughout the salt. Cap tightly and store in a dark, cool place. You can use the salt right away, adding 1–2 tablespoons to the bathwater. Or allow the salt to age with the essential oils and smell how the aroma changes with time. Makes 2 oz., enough for 2–4 baths.

Note that when using essential oil-enhanced sea salt, add only 1–2 tablespoons to the bathwater, since the essential oils increase the salt's potency.

Deep Muscle Relaxation Salt Soak

ALL

For tense, sore muscles that are tight from stress or lactic acid buildup due to physical exertion.

7 drops white pine essential oil
30 drops tangerine essential oil
20 drops lavender essential oil

20 drops thuja essential oil
8 oz. epsom salt or sea salt

Place salt in a jar and add essential oils. Stir and shake until the essential oils are well mixed and dispersed throughout the salt. Cap tightly and store in a dark, cool place. You can use the salt right away, adding 1–2 tablespoons to the bathwater. Or allow the salt to age with the essential oils and smell how the aroma changes with time. Makes 8 oz., enough for 16 or more baths.

BAKING SODA BATHS. Baking soda softens the bath water and helps to soften and smooth the skin. It also has an alkalinizing and deodorizing effect. Essential oils can be added for their pleasurable aromas and to increase the soda's therapeutic action. A baking soda bath in tepid water can be especially refreshing in hot, sticky weather.

Basic Baking Soda Bath

ALL

Use ½ cup baking soda per bath.

Basic Aromatherapy Soda Bath

Add essential oils to baking soda to augment the bath's therapeutic action while producing an array of delightful fragrances.

20 drops essential oil
1 cup (8 oz.) baking soda

Place baking soda in a glass jar, and add the essential oils, drop by drop, stirring them in well. Cap the jar tightly and shake to continue mixing. Pour ¼ cup of mixture into the bathwater prior to immersion. Store in a glass jar with a tight-fitting lid. Makes 1 cup, enough for 4 baths. *Variation follows:*

Silky Smooth Soak

ALL

A refreshing, sensual-smelling soak that leaves the skin feeling smooth and soft. The reparative and hydrating properties of lavender and sandalwood may help irritated and inflamed skin.
Use 1 cup of baking soda, 9 drops of lavender essential oil and 11 drops of sandalwood essential oil.
Options: Add 3 drops chamomile essential oil for soothing inflamed or irritated skin. Replace the lavender with peppermint oil and the sandalwood with tea tree oil for a cooling, energizing and cleansing bath.

MINERAL BATHS. You can combine sea salt with other minerals such as clay, baking soda or borax to soften the water and make the bath more cleansing and softening to the skin. Essential oils and herbs can be added to these mixtures to further their therapeutic effects.

Jean Argus' Mineral Salts Mustard Bath

ALL

This therapeutic blend utilizes the warmth of mustard to open pores and release toxins, as well as providing the drawing and cleansing action of the salts and clay; combined with essential oils, these bath salts leave your skin feeling soothed and refreshed. They can be purchased ready-made from Jean's Greens (see Resources).

3 cups borax
2 cups epsom salt
½ cup sea salt
⅓ cup kaolin clay
⅓ cup mustard powder

1 dropperful (approximately 50 drops) of each of the following essential oils: wintergreen, eucalyptus, rosemary and white thyme

Mix ingredients thoroughly and crumble up any lumps in the mixture. Add the essential oils one at a time and blend them thoroughly into the mineral salt mixture. Store in a glass jar with a tight-fitting lid to prevent the essential oils from evaporating. Add 1–2 tablespoons per bath. This recipe fills a ½-gallon jar, enough to get a family through the winter.

Detoxification Soak   ALL

A drawing, deep-cleansing soak for sweating out impurities. Good to do before sleep, this soak uses significantly more ingredients than the other soaks and should be done only once a week or once a month, as it is very potent.

¼ cup sea salt
¼ cup baking soda
⅛ cup clay
¼ cup epsom salts

¼ cup borax
¼ cup sesame oil
3 drops thyme essential oil

Combine salts, baking soda, clay and borax, add and mix the sesame oil in thoroughly, then drop and mix in the thyme essential oil. Pour entire mixture into the bathwater and soak for at least a half hour. Makes enough for 1 strong treatment.

Vinegar Baths

Add vinegar to the bath to relieve aches and pains or to increase the bath's cleansing action. Vinegar baths are especially effective after heavy physical activity to remove lactic acid buildup in the muscles. Please be aware that the high acid content of vinegar may sting open skin. Also note that vinegar can be quite drying to the skin, so you might want to apply an emollient after the bath. You can also use a variety of herbal-infused vinegars, such as those made with mugwort, chamomile or lavender, to enhance the vinegar's therapeutic action.

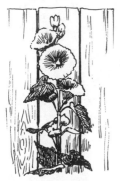

❧ Basic Vinegar Bath   ALL

Add 1–2 cups of vinegar per bath

Pour into the bathwater prior to immersion. Soak for 20 minutes or longer.

Lavender Vinegar Bath   ALL

Make lavender-infused vinegar and add to the bathwater.

3 oz. dried lavender flowers
15 oz. raw apple cider vinegar

Follow Directions for Herbal-Infused Vinegars with Dried Herbs using the lavender and the vinegar. Add ½ cup to the bathwater. Makes 10–12 oz., enough for 2–3 baths.

Variations: Replace the lavender with chamomile, mint or thyme.

Herbal Infusions for the Bath

Herbal infusions, made from one or more herbs, can turn a bath into a wonderfully aromatic and therapeutic experience. I suggest making a strong infusion of the herbs, then straining and adding it to the bathwater in order to avoid a clogged drain. Add ½ to 1 gallon of infusion per bath; either fresh or dried herbs can be used for making it. The recipes that follow call for dried herbs, with the exception of the ginger bath. If you wish to use fresh herbs instead, use 4 times as much fresh herb as dried.

Lavender Chamomile Hops Relaxation Bath ALL

A sweetly fragrant bath for releasing tension and soothing the skin.

2 handfuls lavender
2 handfuls chamomile flowers

1 handful hop strobiles
about 1 gallon boiling water

Place herbs in a jar, pour boiling water over them, cap tightly and steep for a minimum of 1 hour. Strain and add to bathwater. Set aside a cup of the infusion and sip some as you bathe for a relaxing tea blend. Makes enough for 1 bath.

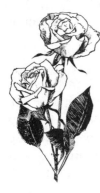

Rose, Mugwort and Sage Bath Blend ALL

An astringent, cleansing, skin-toning bath. Mugwort has been used in Native American rituals for cleansing and centering one's energy. In addition, it has muscle-relaxant properties. As you relax you can also open to the healing of the herbs.

1 handful roses
2 handfuls mugwort

1 handful sage
about 1 gallon boiling water

Place herbs in a jar, pour boiling water over them and cap tightly. Steep for a minimum of 1 hour. Strain and add to bathwater. Makes enough for 1 bath.

Mint Rosemary Bath ALL

A refreshing, stimulating bath for when you feel hot and fatigued. A good blend anytime of year but especially summer.

3 handfuls mint leaves
1 handful rosemary sprigs

1 handful basil leaves
about 1 gallon boiling water

Place herbs in a jar, pour boiling water over them and cap well. Steep for a minimum of 1 hour. Strain and add to bathwater. Set aside a cup of the infusion and sip some as you bathe. Makes enough for 1 bath.

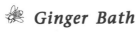

Ginger Bath   ALL

A warming bath for increasing circulation and counteracting chilled bones and muscles.

6 oz. fresh ginger root
1 gallon boiling water

Grate the ginger root, place in a gallon jar, pour water into the jar and let steep for a minimum of 1 hour. Strain and add the liquid to the bathwater. Set aside a cup of the infusion and sip some as you bathe. Ginger tea warms your insides and stimulates circulation and metabolic activity. Makes enough for 1 bath.

Variation: Substitute 2 oz. of dried powder ginger root for the fresh root, although the resulting bath may not be as potent.

BODY SPLASHES

Body Splashes are made like facial astringents. When applied to the skin they are refreshing, toning and deodorizing. I find that splashes work best if misted onto the skin with a spray bottle. You can also pour a little into the palm of your hand and splash it on. Use splashes after a shower or bath, or anytime you feel the need for a refreshing pick-me-up. Body splashes can also be applied to the face and head.

Scented Water Body Splashes

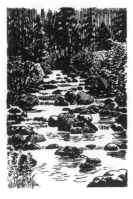

These refreshing splashes combine essential oils with distilled water. They have antimicrobial and antiseptic properties, and act as mild deodorants and perfumes. Since essential oils are not water-soluble, they will separate from the water and will need to be shaken vigorously before each use. These splashes are susceptible to bacterial contamination when they are made without alcohol; adding a small amount of alcohol will extend their shelf life. If they contain no alcohol, these splashes should be made in small batches, stored in the refrigerator and used quickly. Storage in a spray mist bottle helps to reduce the possibility of bacterial contamination. Misting also provides a pleasurable and effective way to apply the splash.

Basic Scented Water Body Splashes   ALL

20 drops essential oil of choice
2 oz. distilled water

Pour water into a jar, add essential oil, drop by drop, cap and shake. It is ready to use. Makes 2 oz.

Optional: Add 2 teaspoon of vodka to preserve the splash and also to produce a more astringent and cleansing effect. Replace the distilled water with sparkling spring water for a tingling sensation and a more stimulating effect.

Peppermint Water   ALL
A cooling, refreshing splash, especially for hot summer days.
Use 20 drops of peppermint essential oil and 2 oz. of distilled water.

Sensual Splash   ALL
Use 10 drops of ylang-ylang essential oil, 10 drops of sandalwood essential oil and 2 oz. of distilled water.

Variations: Make body splashes with chamomile essential oil for irritated skin, fennel essential oil for dry skin, lemongrass essential oil for oily skin and rosemary and lavender essential oils combined for invigoration and cleansing. Refer to the Ingredients chapter for further information on essential oils.

Herbal Infusion Body Splashes

These splashes combine the therapeutic action of herbs with the toning, tightening and cleansing properties of alcohol. They can be more drying than the Scented Water Body Splashes due to the alcohol content, and are less aromatic since they are made without essential oils. You can enhance the therapeutic and aromatic properties of these formulas with the addition of essential oils if desired. The following formulas are well preserved and require no refrigeration.

Chamomile Burdock Body Splash   ALL

A soothing, refreshing splash that is excellent for helping heal rashes and other irritated skin.

Combine the following freshly dried herbs to equal 1 large handful or a total of 1 ounce: chamomile flowers, burdock root (crushed or powdered prior to use), comfrey root (crushed or powdered prior to use), violet leaf

16 oz. water
about 12 oz. 80 proof vodka

Make an infusion with herbs and water, let steep for 4 hours and strain. Pour strained herbal infusion into a measuring cup and add an equal amount of vodka. Pour liquid mixture into a jar, cap and shake well. It is ready to use. Makes about 24 oz.

Variation: To strengthen the formula and intensify its aroma, add ¼ teaspoon of chamomile essential oil.

Spearmint Blend Body Splash   ALL

An invigorating, cleansing and hydrating body splash for all skin types.

Combine the following freshly dried herbs to equal 1 large handful or a total of 1 ounce: spearmint, nettle leaf and fennel seeds crushed with a mortar and pestle prior to use

16 oz. water
about 12 oz. 80 proof vodka

Make an infusion with herbs and water, let steep for 4 hours and strain. Note that the more spearmint used for the infusion the stronger the spearmint aroma will be. Pour strained herbal infusion into a measuring cup and add an equal amount of liquor. Pour liquid mixture into a jar, cap and shake well. It is ready to use. Makes about 24 oz.

Variation: To strengthen the formula and intensify its aroma, add ½ teaspoon of spearmint essential oil and ¼ teaspoon of fennel essential oil.

BODY EMOLLIENTS

Body emollients—oils, creams and balms—are formulas that moisturize, nourish and lubricate the skin. Apply emollients after bathing, before and after exposure to sun or wind or whenever the skin feels dry or irritated. Dry or scaly areas benefit from spot applications of an emollient throughout the day, and especially before night slumber.

Body Oils

Body oils can be used for baths, as just described; for massage; or as an emollient moisture barrier that helps to keep your skin hydrated, lubricated and nourished. Choose from among the various bath oils listed in the Baths section or from the following formulas. For the best results, allow the skin to air-dry after a bath or shower and apply the oil when the skin is still slightly moist.

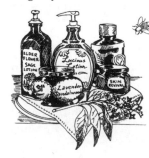

🐝 *Tropical Body* ALL/DRY

Use coconut oil for a cooling, soothing skin softener.

2–3 tablespoons coconut oil

Scoop out 1 tablespoon of coconut oil at a time, let it melt into the palm of your hand and then massage it into the skin. Repeat until skin is well lubricated. Makes enough for 1 treatment.

🐝 *Mediterranean Body* ALL/DRY

Olive oil makes an excellent topical treatment for keeping the skin soft and lubricated.

2–3 tablespoons of olive oil (more or less as needed)

Massage olive oil into slightly damp, warm skin. Makes enough for 1 treatment. *Variations follow:*
1. The olive oil scent may not appeal to some folks, and by adding 2 drops of essential oil of choice per tablespoon of olive oil you can produce a more agreeable aroma.
2. Try sesame oil, almond oil, jojoba oil or other carrier oil of choice.

Nourishing Oil

ALL/DRY

A rich, nourishing oil that leaves the skin feeling silky smooth. The lecithin makes the oil slide and spread more evenly and also provides the skin with nutrients.

1 oz. jojoba oil	½ oz. lecithin
1 oz. peanut oil	½ oz. wheat germ oil
1 oz. almond oil	

Pour oils and lecithin into a spouted cup and stir all the ingredients until a uniform liquid results, making sure the lecithin is well dissolved in the oils. Pour the mixture into a jar, cap tightly and store in a cool, dark place. Massage small amounts of Nourishing Oil into the skin. Makes 4 oz.

Comfrey Comfort

ALL/DRY/DAMAGED

A healing, nourishing oil for damaged and weathered skin. This oil is thick and heavy and will take a few minutes to soak into the skin. The odor — wheat germ oil, olive oil and herbs — can be quite strong. You may want to add essential oils to produce a more appealing aroma.

4 oz. comfrey leaf-infused olive oil	3 oz. avocado oil
4 oz. comfrey root-infused olive oil	1 oz. wheat germ oil
4 oz. calendula-infused olive oil (see Luscious Lotion p. 29)	

To make comfrey leaf-infused olive oil, use 2 oz. of comfrey leaf, freshly dried and coarsely ground, and 8 oz. of cold pressed olive oil and follow Directions for Herbal-Infused Oils with Dried Herbs. Yields about 5 oz. of oil.

To make comfrey root-infused olive oil, use 2 oz. of comfrey root, freshly dried and coarsely ground, and 8 oz. of cold pressed olive oil and follow Directions for Herbal-Infused Oils with Dried Herbs. Yields about 5 oz. of oil.

Once you have obtained your herbal-infused oils, pour all the oils into a pint-size jar, cap and shake well. Massage the skin with the oil as needed. Makes 16 oz.

Variation: Add 1 teaspoon of lavender or other essential oil of choice.

Creamy Rose Chamomile Oil

ALL/DRY/DAMAGED

An excellent oil for dry, rashy, cracked and irritated skin. The shea butter in this recipe makes this oil thick, creamy and opaque. It is a heavy oil that requires a little bit of time to soak into the skin.

3 oz. rose-infused olive oil	2 oz. violet leaf-infused olive oil
3 oz. chamomile-infused olive oil	3 oz. shea butter

Pour oils into a heat-proof measuring cup and add the shea butter. Place cup into a hot-water bath. Stir the oils and shea butter and wait till the shea butter has melted. Then remove from water and pour into a squeeze bottle or wide-mouth jar. Massage the skin with oil as needed. Don't pour the oil into a small-mouth glass jar, as the thickness of this oil will keep it from pouring, especially in colder temperatures. Makes 11 oz.

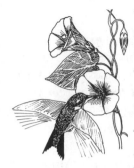

To make rose-infused olive oil, use 2 oz. of roses, freshly dried and coarsely ground, and 10 oz. of cold pressed olive oil. Then follow Directions for Herbal-Infused Oils with Dried Herbs. Yields about 7 oz.

To make chamomile-infused olive oil, use 2 oz. of chamomile flowers, freshly dried and coarsely ground, and 10 oz. of cold pressed olive oil. Then follow Directions for Herbal-Infused Oils with Dried Herbs. Yields about 7 oz.

To make violet leaf-infused olive oil, use 2 oz. of violet leaf, freshly dried and coarsely ground, and 8 oz. of cold pressed olive oil. Then follow Directions for Herbal-Infused Oils with Dried Herbs. Yields about 5 oz.

Basic Body Oil Blend
ALL

This basic oil blend provides a well-balanced, nourishing base that is not too heavy or light and easily absorbed by the skin. It can be used alone or combined with essential oils to create different effects.

12 oz. almond oil
12 oz. canola oil

1 oz. wheat germ oil
4 oz. St. Johnswort-infused olive oil

Combine oils in quart jar, cap and shake well. The oil is ready for use and can be massaged into the skin, added to the bath or used as a base for the recipes that follow.

To make St. Johnswort-infused olive oil, use fresh St. Johnswort flowers and buds and cold pressed olive oil and follow Directions for Herbal-Infused Oils with Fresh Herbs.

Springtime Blend
ALL

An uplifting, healing, floral-scented oil that can be used anytime of year.

4 oz. Basic Body Oil Blend (preferred)
   or other carrier oil of choice
24 drops basil essential oil

8 drops ylang–ylang essential oil
15 drops lavender essential oil

Pour Basic Body Oil Blend or carrier oil of choice into a jar and add the essential oils, drop by drop. Cap jar with a tight-fitting lid and shake well. The oil is ready to use. Makes 4 oz.

Heaven & Earth
ALL

A festive, spicy, fruity blend for pleasing the senses. I made this blend up as a gift for a friend who did not like floral smells.

4 oz. Basic Body Oil Blend
15 drops lemongrass essential oil
20 drops tangerine essential oil
5 drops bay essential oil

20 drops anise essential oil
5 drops patchouli essential oil
15 drops sweet basil essential oil

Pour Basic Body Oil Blend or carrier oil of choice into a jar and add the essential oils, drop by drop. Cap jar with a tight-fitting lid and shake well. The oil is ready to use. Makes 4 oz.

Rosemary Basil and Peppermint Wake-Up Oil   ALL

A stimulating, refreshing blend for invigorating circulation and waking up. This essential oil blend can be used as a smelling blend to wake up the brain during long nights of work or study. To use simply inhale the odor of the blend straight out of the bottle or place some oil on a tissue and keep near nose or you can apply some oil directly under your nose but be sure it is not too strong for you.

4 oz. Basic Body Oil Blend (preferred) **or other carrier oil of choice** **35 drops rosemary essential oil**	**25 drops basil essential oil** **15 drops peppermint essential oil**

Pour Basic Body Oil Blend or carrier oil of choice into a jar and add the essential oils, drop by drop. Cap jar with a tight-fitting lid and shake well. The oil is ready to use. Makes 4 oz. *Variation follows:*

Rosemary & Lavender Blend
For a more relaxing yet still rejuvenating body oil omit the peppermint and basil essential oils and add 30 drops of lavender essential oil.

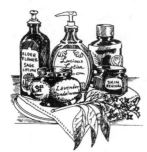

Moisturizing Creams and Lotions

Moisturizing creams — emulsions that combine the emollient effects of oil with the hydrating action of water — provide the same benefits for the body as for the face, as described in the first chapter. You can use any of the face cream formulas as a body cream, or try some of those that follow. Please refer to the Techniques and Definitions chapter for detailed instructions on making creams.

Lavender Sandalwood Moisturizing Cream   ALL/DRY

An excellent face and body cream for most skin types, with a truly delicious aroma. When making this formula for the body more essential oils are used than when making it for the face as illustrated in the first chapter. The addition of essential oils in the quantity given here helps preserves the cream for 6 months to a year outside refrigeration.

Use 2 teaspoons of lavender essential oil, ¾ teaspoon of sandalwood essential oil and see formula p. 29.

Luscious Lotion   ALL/OILY

An excellent face and body moisturizer for normal to oily skin with the added healing properties of calendula and St. Johnswort. When making this formula for the body more essential oils are used than when making it for the face, as illustrated in the first chapter. This cream is preserved for 6 months outside refrigeration when made with the quantities of essential oils mentioned in the following recipe.

Use 1 teaspoon ylang-ylang essential oil, 1 teaspoon lavender essential oil, ½ teaspoon lemongrass essential oil and see formula p. 29.

Skin Revival

ALL/DRY/MATURE

A nourishing, protective, healing moisturizer for dry, aged and damaged skin, eczema and dermatitis. Has some ultraviolet protection: SPF-4. When making this formula for the body more essential oils are used than when making it for the face, as illustrated in the first chapter. on pp. 29–30.

1 teaspoon of lavender essential oil **20 drops of cedarwood essential oil**
30 drops of geranium egypt essential oil

BODY LOTIONS. The following lotions are thinner and lighter than the cream formulas offered in this book due to the higher water content and the omission of solid oils. They are made with the same basic ingredients as creams, but the addition of borax as an emulsifying agent allows for the greater proportion of water to oil and beeswax. These lotions glide on easily, and may be the best choice for people with oily skin.

Basic Lotion Formula

ALL

8 oz. carrier oil of choice **½ oz. beeswax**
11 oz. water **1 teaspoon borax**

Place beeswax and carrier oil in a heat-proof measuring cup in a hot-water bath. Stir occasionally until the wax is completely melted into the oil. Let cool to body temperature. Meanwhile dissolve borax into water and warm to body temperature. Pour oil-wax mixture into a bowl and blend with a handheld mixer with one beater, add the water-borax mixture a little at a time, then beat until creamy and thick, about 5 minutes. Add essential oils and stir in thoroughly by hand. Pour into pump jars, squeeze bottles or wide-mouth jars. Makes about 19 oz.

Variations: You can produce an assortment of lotions based on the Basic Lotion Formula by using different herbal infusions for the water part and different carrier oils for the oil part, as well as by varying the essential oils.

Elder Flower Sage Lotion

ALL/OILY

Use the following freshly dried herbs: 2 tablespoons of elder flower, 2 tablespoons sage, 2 tablespoons yarrow; 16 oz. of water, 4 oz. of grapeseed oil, 4 oz. of canola oil, 1 teaspoon of borax, and ½ oz. of beeswax; *optional:* 30 drops of sage essential oil, 60 drops of lime essential oil.
Make herbal infusion with herbs and water, let steep for 4 hours and strain. Use 11 oz. of strained infusion as your water part and follow directions for Basic Lotion Formula. Makes 19 oz.

Rose Calendula Lotion

ALL

Use the following freshly dried herbs: 3 tablespoons of roses, 3 tablespoons of calendula; 16 oz. of water, 4 oz. of almond oil, 4 oz. of peanut oil, 1 teaspoon of borax, ½ oz. of beeswax; *optional:* 40 drops of essential oil of rose geranium or other essential oil of choice.
Make herbal infusion with herbs and water, let steep for 4 hours and strain. Use 11 oz. of strained infusion as your water part and follow directions for Basic Lotion Formula. Makes 19 oz.

Fennel Marshmallow Lotion

ALL/DRY/DAMAGED

Use the following freshly dried herbs: 3 tablespoons of marshmallow root (cut), 3 tablespoons of fennel seeds; 16 oz. of water, 2 oz. of jojoba oil, 4 oz. of peanut oil, 1 oz. of avocado oil, 1 oz. of wheat germ oil, 1 teaspoon of borax, ½ oz. of beeswax; *optional:* 40 drops of essential oil of fennel or other essential oil of choice.

Make herbal infusion with herbs and water, let steep for 8 hours, and strain. Use 11 oz. of strained infusion as your water part and follow directions for Basic Lotion Formula above. Makes 19 oz.

For Elbows, Knees and Other Dry Spots

The following formulas are concentrated, thick balms that are made with reparative ingredients. They are meant to be used on parts of the body that require extra attention.

Plantain Coconut Balm   ALL/DRY/DAMAGED

A soothing reparative balm for cracked, itchy, hot and dry skin.

3 oz. plantain-infused olive oil
2 oz. coconut oil
1 oz. beeswax

optional: 20 drops chamomile
essential oil

In a heat-proof measuring cup, combine plantain-infused olive oil with the coconut oil and beeswax. Place the measuring cup in a hot-water bath and allow the oils and beeswax to melt together and become a uniform liquid free of lumps. When it is completely melted, pour oil-wax mixture into a wide-mouth jar and immediately drop in essential oil. Quickly cap jar to prevent essential oil from evaporating. Leave balm undisturbed to harden. When completely hard, it is ready for use. Apply to skin as often as needed and especially before night slumber. Makes 6 oz.

Note: Make plantain-infused olive oil using 2 oz. of fresh plantain leaves and 4 oz. of cold pressed olive oil and follow Directions for Herbal-Infused Oils with Fresh Herbs. Yields about 4 oz.

Skin Soothe Balm   ALL/DRY/DAMAGED

A healing balm for dry, cracked skin. Apply throughout the day and especially before night slumber.

2 oz. comfrey-infused olive oil (see
   Comfrey Salve/Loose Version p. 36)
2 oz. calendula-infused olive oil (see
   Luscious Lotion p. 29)
2 oz. of chamomile-infused olive oil
   (see Creamy Rose Chamomile Oil
   pp. 82–83)
3 oz. jojoba oil

2 oz. shea butter
1 oz. cocoa butter
½ oz. lecithin
3 oz. beeswax
100 drops lavender essential oil
100 drops fennel essential oil
50 drops sandalwood essential oil

In a heat-proof measuring cup, combine strained herbal-infused oils, jojoba oil, shea butter, cocoa butter, lecithin and beeswax. Place the measuring cup in a hot-water bath and while stirring allow the ingredients to melt together and become a uniform liquid free of lumps. When it is completely melted, pour mixture into a wide-mouth jar and immediately drop in essential oils. Quickly cap jar to prevent essential oils from evaporating. Leave balm undisturbed for several hours or overnight to cool and solidify. The consistency of this balm is loose, somewhat like petroleum jelly, which allows it to spread over the skin without much friction. If you want to make it harder add more beeswax. Be aware that this balm may become grainy in colder temperatures, but this does not reduce its effectiveness.

DEODORANT LIQUIDS AND POWDERS

Commercial deodorants are filled with nasty chemicals and other ingredients like aluminum that can have deleterious health effects. These preparations can be some of the most allergenic products both to the wearer and to those in the wearer's proximity. Heavily perfumed deodorants can aggravate chemical sensitivities and provoke sinus irritation, headaches or nausea. Fortunately, it is surprisingly simple to make gentle but effective products to prevent or clear body odor. It is my opinion that body odor is a natural phenomenon that is not offensive in and of itself. A healthy body produces a healthy odor. Body odors convey a great deal about an individual's emotional state and carry hormonal and pheromonal information. However, people in our society are often intolerant of other people's, or even their own, body odor. Many people thus find it desirable to mask or minimize their natural scent. Following is an array of deodorant formulas that combine natural antimicrobial, absorbent and cleansing ingredients such as alcohol, botanicals, essential oils, clay and other substances. The guiding principle behind these formulas is to gently minimize or neutralize body odor. Some formulas incorporate natural fragrances that subtly blend with one's own personal scent.

Liquid Deodorants

Deodorants can be made with a combination of teas, tinctures, water, juices, essential oils and alcohol, such as vodka or brandy. One important rule is to add enough alcohol to act as a preservative when using perishable liquids such as tea, water or juice. To offset the alcohol's drying effects you may want to add small amounts of glycerin. For the strongest cleansing action, apply liquid deodorant with a cotton ball or cloth or for convenience, place the deodorants in a fine-mist spray bottle.

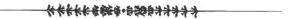

Using Alcohol as Preservative Basic Formula

As a general rule, ¼ cup of water-based liquid such as juice or an infusion will be preserved by ¼ cup of 80 proof liquor. A product needs to contain 15–20 percent alcohol to stay preserved.

WITCH HAZEL DEODORANTS. Distilled witch hazel, available at pharmacies, makes an adequate deodorant on its own or used as a base to which essential oils can be added.

🐝 *Basic Witch Hazel Deodorant*   ALL

Witch Hazel, distilled and store-bought, applied to a cotton swab or cloth and rubbed into the underarms cleanses and neutralizes body odor. Variation follows:

Witch Hazel Tea Tree Double Whammy   ALL
Add 10 drops of tea tree essential oil to every ounce of witch hazel to increase the antimicrobial and deodorizing action of the witch hazel.

Ken's Deodorant   All

My friend Ken was dissatisfied with commercial soaps and deodorants. He found these products to be ineffective at clearing body odor, while also containing offensive synthetic scents and other irritating chemical ingredients. He did a little experimenting and was thrilled to discover this simple formula that far surpasses deodorants and soaps for cleansing action. Ken also feels that applying the deodorant to a cotton ball or cloth and wiping the underarms does a better job than spraying it on.

4 oz. witch hazel	5 drops rosemary essential oil
8 drops lavender essential oil	2 drops patchouli essential oil

Pour ingredients into a 4-oz. jar and shake well. It is ready to use. Apply to cotton ball and wipe underarms after bathing and as needed throughout the day. Shake before use. Makes 4 oz.

VODKA DEODORANTS. Food-grade alcohol, such as vodka, is cleansing and mildly deodorizing. You can use straight vodka, but you may find it to be too drying to the skin. Dilute the vodka with water and a less drying effect results. The diluted vodka provides a simple deodorant that can be used on its own or as a base for the various formulas that follow.

Basic Vodka Deodorant   All

¼ cup 80 proof vodka	*optional:* ¼–½ teaspoon vegetable
¼ cup distilled water	glycerin

Pour vodka, water and glycerin (optional) into a jar or spray mist bottle, cap and shake. It is now ready for use. Makes 4 oz.

Variations: The addition of essential oils augments the deodorizing effects while also producing appealing aromas. The following are some choice examples.

Woodland Deodorant   All

An excellent choice for both men and women. Combines the disinfectant and deodorizing effects of the alcohol and the essential oils. It also offers a gentle, pleasant aroma.

¼ cup 80 proof vodka	16 drops cedarwood essential oil
¼ cup distilled water	20 drops sandalwood essential oil
10 drops tea tree essential oil	

Pour vodka and water into a jar, drop in essential oils, cap and shake. Apply deodorant onto a cotton swab or cloth and wipe underarms for cleaning and neutralizing body odor. You can also put the deodorant into a spray bottle and mist underarms. Makes 4 oz.

Variation: If the deodorant feels too drying add ¼–½ teaspoon of vegetable glycerin.

Exotic Deodorant   All

A strongly scented effective deodorant. This can also be used as an exotic air freshener when misted around the room or onto upholstered furniture and curtains.

¼ cup 80 proof vodka
¼ cup distilled water
10 drops geranium egypt essential oil

10 drops patchouli essential oil
15 drops lavender essential oil

Pour vodka and water into a jar, drop in the essential oils, cap and shake. Apply deodorant onto a cotton swab or cloth and wipe underarms for cleaning and neutralizing body odor. You can also put the deodorant into a spray bottle and mist underarms. Makes 4 oz.

Variation: If the deodorant feels too drying add ¼–½ teaspoon of vegetable glycerin.

TINCTURE DEODORANTS. You can make effective, pleasantly aromatic deodorants by tincturing antimicrobial and deodorizing herbs, then diluting them and adding essential oils. You must plan ahead when making these formulas, since making a tincture requires a minimum of 3 weeks.

Mugwort Deodorant   ALL

4 oz. mugwort tincture
3 oz. distilled water
½ teaspoon glycerin

optional: 20 drops fennel or
    other essential oil of choice

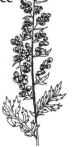

Pour mugwort tincture, water and glycerin into a jar, add essential oils, cap and shake. Apply deodorant onto a cotton swab or cloth and wipe underarms. You can also put the deodorant into a spray bottle and mist underarms. Makes 7 oz.

Note: Make mugwort tincture with fresh mugwort flowering tops or leaves and 80–100 proof vodka. Follow Directions for Alcohol Tinctures Using Fresh Herbs.

Variations: Lavender, sage and thyme are good choices for deodorants. Substitute one of these herbs for the mugwort in the preceding recipe.

Artemesia vulgari

Vanilla Deodorant   ALL

This is my favorite deodorant that smells delicious.

2 oz. vanilla tincture
2 oz. sage tincture
½ teaspoon glycerin
4 oz. water

20 drops tea tree essential oil
40 drops lavender essential oil
16 drops cedarwood essential oil

Pour vanilla and sage tincture, water and glycerin into a jar, add essential oils, cap and shake. Apply deodorant mixture onto a cotton swab or cloth and rub into underarms for cleaning and neutralizing body odor. You can also put the deodorant into a spray bottle and spray mist underarms. Makes 8 oz.

Note: Make vanilla tincture with 10 vanilla bean pods and 10 oz. of pure grain alcohol or as high-proof an alcohol as you can find. If you are using 190 proof alcohol add 2 oz. of water to the alcohol. The vanilla resins need a menstrum with a high alcohol and low water content to be efficiently extracted. Follow Directions for Alcohol Tinctures Using Dried Herbs. This will give you enough vanilla tincture for several batches of deodorant, and some to use in food preparations. This vanilla extract is much more potent and delicious than the store-bought extracts and is worth making if only for the sole purpose of food flavoring.

Make sage tincture using fresh sage leaves and 100 proof vodka and follow Directions for Alcohol Tinctures Using Fresh Herbs.

Herbal-Infusion and Spirit Deodorants. These deodorants, which combine water extracts of herbs with alcohol, are quick and satisfying to make, and offer a ready means of accessing the cleansing and deodorizing properties of various herbs. The possibilities for creating effective customized deodorants by this method are vast. You will need to plan ahead for the time the herbal infusion needs to steep, usually from 1 to 8 hours. Refer to the Directions for Infusions for detailed instructions on pp. 218–219. Note that these deodorants are mild, and the addition of essential oils enhances their deodorizing effects. The following formulas can also be used as mouth rinses.

Sage and Brandy   All

The water extract of the sage provides astringent and cleansing action and the alcohol disinfects and deodorizes.

¼ cup 80 proof brandy
¼ cup sage infusion (use 1 tablespoon
   sage leaf and 4 oz. water)

½ teaspoon glycerin
20 drops sage essential oil for further
   deodorizing action

Make herbal infusion with sage leaf and water, steep for 8 hours and strain. Pour 2 oz. of sage infusion, brandy, glycerin and essential oil into a jar, cap and shake. Apply deodorant mixture onto a cotton swab or cloth and rub into underarms for cleaning and neutralizing body odor. You can also put the deodorant into a spray bottle and mist underarms. Makes 4 oz. *Variations follow:*

Clove and Brandy Deodorant   All
The cloves have strong cleansing and deodorizing action, and their its scent is also appealing.
Substitute cloves for sage and 2 drops of clove oil for sage oil and proceed as above.
Other good choices of herbs for making herbal infusion deodorants are basil, lavender, mint, thyme and yarrow. Choose from one of these and substitute them in the above formula.

Deodorant Body Powders

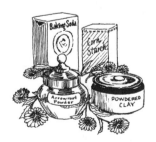

🐝 Basic Body Powders   All
Body powders act as antiperspirants and deodorants.

Clay, cornstarch, arrowroot powder or baking soda can either be used alone as absorbent body powders or as a base for deodorizing powder formulas. Use spice shakers for sprinkling on body powders, or apply by hand. The following formulas may include essential oils and other botanical ingredients.

Orange Baking Soda Body Powder   ALL

A refreshing, deodorizing body powder with a spicy, sweet orange scent. This recipe yields a small amount that can easily be increased by multiplying the ingredients.

5 drops orange essential oil	1 drop cassia essential oil
3 drops tea tree essential oil	1 tablespoon baking soda

Put baking soda in a small jar, add essential oils and stir them in thoroughly. Cap and shake jar to continue combining the ingredients. Apply powder to underarms and wherever needed. To store powder, cap jar with a tight-fitting lid. Makes ½ oz., enough for 2 applications.

Variations: You can substitute the baking powder with cornstarch or arrowroot powder.

Peppermint Arrowroot Body Powder   ALL

A refreshing, strongly antimicrobial body powder with a peppermint aroma for sweaty, strongly scented body odor. If you find this powder pleasing and effective you may want to multiply the ingredients and make a larger batch.

4 drops peppermint essential oil	2 drops sage essential oil
4 drops tea tree essential oil	1 tablespoon of arrowroot powder

Put arrowroot powder in a small jar, add essential oils and stir them in thoroughly. Cap and shake the jar to continue mixing the ingredients. It is ready to use. To store powder, cap jar with a tight-fitting lid. Makes ½ oz., enough for 2 or more underarm applications.

Variation: Cornstarch can be used in place of the arrowroot powder in the above recipe.

Cinnamon Rosemary Body Powder   ALL

A spicy, refreshing-smelling absorbent body powder that also has antiseptic properties.

16 drops cinnamon essential oil	10 drops thuja essential oil
25 drops rosemary essential oil	4 tablespoons clay

Put clay in a small jar, add essential oils and stir them in thoroughly. Cap and shake the jar to continue mixing the ingredients. To store powder, cap jar with a tight-fitting lid. Makes 2 oz.

Sandalwood Body Powder   ALL

A mildly scented absorbent body powder that both men and women really like.

1 cup clay	¼ cup slippery elm powder
½ cup baking soda	100 drops sandalwood essential oil
½ cup arrowroot powder	20 drops tea tree essential oil

Place clay, baking soda, arrowroot powder and slippery elm powder into a jar, mix the powders thoroughly and add the essential oils while stirring them in. Cap and shake jar. To use, sprinkle into underarms and wherever needed. Makes about 2¼ cups.

Lavender Rose Thyme Body Powder ALL

A sweet-smelling body powder to keep dry and deodorized.

1 cup clay
½ cup baking soda
½ cup arrowroot powder
½ cup freshly dried herbs (lavender, rose blossoms and thyme leaf combined)

¼ cup slippery elm powder
60 drops lavender essential oil
30 drops rose geranium essential oil

Powder herbs, except the slippery elm, in a coffee grinder used exclusively for herbs and seeds. Sift herbs through a fine-mesh strainer over a bowl and regrind the coarser particles as needed. It is important to get the herbs as fine as possible so the powder feels soft and silky against the skin. Place all ingredients except the essential oils into a jar, mix the powders thoroughly and add the essential oils while stirring them in. Cap and shake jar. Makes about 2½ cups.

PREPARATIONS FOR SORE MUSCLES, BONES AND NERVES

Many of the recipes for bath and body oils are helpful for treating sore muscles, aching bones and frazzled nerves. For example, the salt and vinegar baths are excellent for soreness, while the warming ginger bath is very helpful for alleviating bone-penetrating chills. Following are some recipes formulated specifically for their therapeutic effects.

St. Johnswort Oil ALL/DAMAGED

This herbal-infused oil is excellent for strained and pained muscles and nerves. Massage into skin and repeat throughout the day or as needed. This oil is used in a variety of other formulas, and it would be wise to make a pint or quart of it to last for the year.

Make St. Johnswort-infused olive oil with fresh St. Johnswort flowers and buds and cold pressed olive oil and follow Directions for Herbal-Infused Oils with Fresh Herbs.

St. Johnswort Tincture ALL

This is an excellent remedy that is ingested for the relief of muscular and nerve pain. St. Johnswort is a cellular oxygenator that helps remove lactic acid buildup in the muscles and can help release nerve tension. After a strenuous workout, to prevent my muscles from getting sore I take about ¼ teaspoon of St. Johnswort tincture, and I repeat the dose at 2-4 hour intervals for the following 24 hours.

To make see St. Johnswort Tincture for Pain p. 49.

Relaxation Salve ALL/DAMAGED

This is another product based on the healing properties of St. Johnswort, with the added emolliency of the coconut oil. A topical nervine for helping restore nerve health, it can also be used for stiff, sore muscles and back, abrasions, burns and sunburns. The salve is also more convenient to travel with and less messy to work with than St. Johnswort oil.

1 oz. beeswax	3 oz. St. Johnswort-infused olive oil
2 oz. coconut oil	(see formula p. 92)

Pour St. Johnswort oil into a heat-proof measuring cup, then add first the coconut oil and next the beeswax, noting the level of the measure after each addition. Place the cup in a hot-water bath and while stirring allow the beeswax and coconut oil to melt and become a uniform liquid free of lumps and solids. Pour into a wide-mouth jar, let solidify undisturbed and then cap. It is now ready to use. Store in a cool, dark place for longer storage. Salves keep for a period of 1–2 years if stored properly. Makes 6 oz.

Arnica Oil   ALL/DAMAGED

Arnica is the oil of choice for bruised soreness. Massage it gently into pained and injured area.

Make arnica-infused olive oil with arnica flowers and cold pressed olive oil. You can use fresh or dried flowers depending on what is available. If the flowers are dried, use 1 oz. of flower to 5 oz. of oil and proceed to Directions for Herbal-Infused Oils with Dried Herbs. If the flowers are fresh, proceed to Directions for Herbal-Infused Oils with Fresh Herbs.

Loosen-Up Body Oil   ALL

A therapeutic blend for tight sore muscles. Place 1–2 tablespoons in bathwater just prior to immersion or massage into skin.

1 oz. St. Johnswort-infused olive oil	40 drops tangerine essential oil
(see formula p. 92)	8 drops thuja essential oil
1 oz. peanut oil	4 drops white pine essential oil
2 oz. canola oil	

Pour St. Johnswort-infused olive oil, peanut oil and canola oil into a jar and add the essential oils, drop by drop. Cap jar with a tight-fitting lid and shake well. The oil is ready to use. Makes 4 oz. *Variation follows:*

Analgesic Oil   ALL/PAINED
Another oil used for the relief of aches and pains.
Replace the essential oils in the Loosen-Up Body Oil with 40 drops of wintergreen essential oil, 40 drops of lavender essential oil and 28 drops of black pepper essential oil.

Fire and Ice Liniment Balm   ALL/PAINED

This is a very concentrated balm that makes the body feel hot and cold. It can help alleviate muscular pain and soreness. Try it on rheumatic or stiff muscles and joints. Apply it to the skin before engaging in strenuous activity to stimulate the muscles and joints. It can also be used as a decongestant and placed in a vaporizer for steam inhalation.

4 oz. olive oil (peanut or sesame oil may also be used)

1 tablespoon wintergreen essential oil

1 tablespoon lavender essential oil

1 tablespoon rosemary essential oil

1 tablespoon ginger essential oil

1 tablespoon thuja essential oil

1 tablespoon camphor essential oil

2 teaspoons cassia cinnamon essential oil

2 teaspoons black pepper essential oil

1–2 tablespoons menthol crystals

2½ oz. beeswax

Place menthol crystals in 2 oz. of olive oil overnight. This will dissolve the crystals into the oil. Put remaining 2 oz. of olive oil and beeswax in a heat-proof measuring cup and place in a hot-water bath. Combine essential oils. When beeswax has melted, slowly pour essential oils and the menthol crystal-oil mixture into the oil-beeswax mixture. Stir until completely dissolved and free of any lumps. Pour into jar and cap to prevent essential oils from evaporating. Apply to the skin in very small amounts. Makes about 11 oz.

Note: This balm may be too stimulating and strong-scented for some people, so check and see how you respond to it.

Herbal Body Care Baskets

These make wonderful and useful gifts that delight most recipients. Your friends or family members will feel truly cared for when you give them a personalized basket of body care products that you have made yourself. A gift basket also encourages the recipient to take the time to indulge in simple yet luxurious bodily pleasures. To make an herbal basket, place your choice of herbal body care products in a basket, then decorate it with dried flowers and leaves. You may also wish to include other items such as a loofah sponge, a handmade washcloth or a natural sea silk sponge. Be sure to include a list of ingredients and directions for using each of the products. Below I offer ideas for three different gift baskets composed of products from this chapter grouped according to skin type. You can also choose from the various other formulas in this chapter to create your own customized Gift Basket.

Herbal Body Care Basket for Oily Skin

Lavender Salt Scrub, Rosemary Black Pepper Clay Body Pack, Energizing Bath Oil, Deep Muscle Relaxation Soak, Peppermint Water, Elder Flower Sage Lotion, Exotic Deodorant.

Herbal Body Care Basket for Normal Skin

Hot Lava Salt Scrub, Ceres Delight Body Pack, Silky Smooth Soak, Spearmint Blend Body Splash, Rose Calendula Lotion, Woodland Deodorant.

Herbal Body Care Basket for Dry Skin

Ocean Lavender Treatment, Sensual Splash, Comfrey Comfort, Fennel Marshmallow Lotion, Skin Soothe Balm, Sandalwood Body Powder.

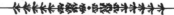

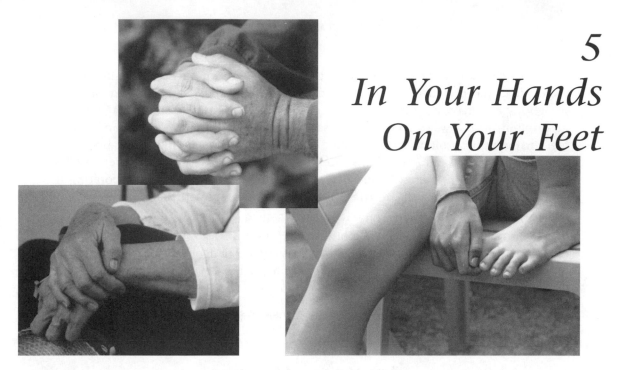

5
In Your Hands On Your Feet

Our hands are often the most abused, and our feet the most neglected, parts of our body. This is ironic as much of our identity is bound up in how we use our hands, and since everything from the simplest daily routine to the most specialized professional activity can involve their use. An individual's uniqueness is even embossed on the hands, in the form of their fingerprints and the lines on their palms. Yet many of us take our hands for granted as we go about our daily business, whether it involves slicing onions, digging trenches, typing at a word processor, painting on a canvas or changing diapers. The activities that involve the hands can lead to anything from dryness and chapping to cramping and swelling. My own hands often feel tired, achy and dried out from garden work, harvesting wild plants and making formulas, on top of the daily round of cooking and washing dishes. The first part of this chapter covers preparations and techniques that can help prevent and alleviate some of the common problems that affect our busy hands. These include soaks, oils, salves and moisturizers, preparations for cuticle care and special formulas to help heal minor cuts and wounds.

The feet, like the hands, are complex structures consisting internally of a series of small bones swathed in a highly complex network of muscles and nerves. To think that such relatively small structures bear the full weight of a body, often for many hours each day! Most people's feet literally take a pounding during the course of a typical day, and the effects are often exacerbated by the shoes they wear. The second part of this chapter offers an array of soaks, oils, creams, balms and powders to help rejuvenate tired feet and treat such conditions as cracked heels and athlete's foot.

A Word About Massage

One of the most therapeutic and rejuvenating methods for treating tired, cramped or swollen hands or feet is a simple massage. You might want to begin with a therapeutic soak (see the next section), then follow up with a massage using one of the oil formulas provided later in this chapter. It is especially satisfying to have somebody else massage your hands or feet for you, but it is also something you can do on your own. A warm soak and massage improves the circulation to hands and feet, bringing fresh blood to the tissues and helping to remove metabolic by-products that can lead to cramping, swelling and pain. Because massage benefits the hands and feet both internally and externally, I highly recommend incorporating it into your natural body care routine — your hands and feet will thank you for it.

I like to massage my feet with Energizing Foot Oil (see p. 111) as part of my wake-up exercise ritual. During the winter months the Hot Lava Foot Oil (see p. 113) is especially pleasing. And before bed, a foot massage exchange with a friend or partner can prove to be the best nightcap. Try using the Lavender Chamomile Foot Oil (see p. 113) for additional tranquilizing effects.

IN YOUR HANDS

Hand Soaks

Hand soaks offer a pleasant and relaxing way to rejuvenate tired, swollen or painful hands. They are also good for loosening and cleansing away dirt from under the fingernails and for treating split cuticles and cuts, abrasions or bruises. To prevent the skin from drying out, especially when doing the vinegar or salt soaks that follow, you can apply an emollient prior to soaking, or add a teaspoon of rich oil like jojoba or olive to the water.

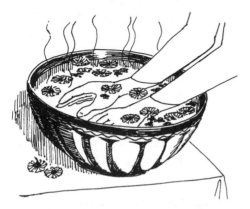

BASIC HAND SOAK TECHNIQUE. Choose a bowl that both of your hands fit into comfortably and fill it with water or herbal infusion, as hot as you can comfortably tolerate. Keep your hands in the water for at least 10 minutes. For a more therapeutic soak, try one of the following formulas.

VINEGAR SOAKS. Vinegar acts as an antifungal and disinfectant while helping to relieve aches and pains. Herbal-infused vinegar combines the positive attributes of vinegar with the healing properties of herbs. For example, mugwort-infused vinegar is great for soreness or aches and pains, calendula increases the vinegar's antimicrobial action and evergreens add an uplifting and invigorating quality.

Basic Vinegar Soak ALL

For a simple soak, add 2 tablespoons of vinegar to the hand-soak water. Note that vinegar can be quite drying to the skin, so you might want to apply a moisturizing formula to your hands afterward. Caution: Vinegar may sting raw and open skin.

Chamomile-Infused Vinegar ALL/PAINED/INFLAMED

Chamomile vinegar is an excellent, relaxing, anti-inflammatory preparation when added to the soaking water. This is also the recipe for an excellent hair rinse for light-haired folks.

Use 2 handfuls of freshly dried chamomile flowers to 10 oz. of organic raw apple cider vinegar and follow Directions for Herbal-Infused Vinegars with Dried Herbs. Or use fresh chamomile flowers and follow Directions for Herbal-Infused Vinegars with Fresh Herbs. Add 1–2 tablespoons of chamomile vinegar per soak. Using dried chamomile, the yield is approximately 7–8 oz. of vinegar, enough for 8–16 soaks; using fresh, the yield will vary according to the size of the jar used for the vinegar infusion.

Mugwort-Infused Vinegar ALL/PAINED

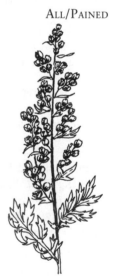

Add mugwort vinegar to soak water for pain relief and cleansing. This is also a culinary vinegar, as the mugwort is related to tarragon and adds a pleasing aromatic flavor to salad dressings and other dishes, as well as increasing digestive power.

To make the mugwort vinegar, use 2 handfuls of freshly dried mugwort leaves to 10 oz. of organic raw apple cider vinegar and follow Directions for Herbal-Infused Vinegars with Dried Herbs. Or use fresh mugwort and follow Directions for Herbal-Infused Vinegars with Fresh Herbs. Add 1–2 tablespoons of mugwort vinegar per soak. Using dried mugwort, the yield is approximately 7–8 oz. of vinegar, enough for 8–16 soaks; using fresh, the yield will vary according to the size of the jar.

Variations: For other possible herbal vinegars, use lavender, rosemary or mint, or refer to the Botanicals section in the Ingredients chapter for more ideas.

SEA SALT SOAKS. Use sea salt and herbal salt soaks for swollen, achy and painful hands. These soaks can also help heal wounds, but note that the salt will sting open skin. Salt soaks are drying to the skin, so a good moisturizer should be applied afterward. You can also apply an oil to the hands before a salt soak to prevent them from drying out.

Basic Salt Soak for Hands ALL

Add 1–2 tablespoons of sea salt to hand-soak water

HERBAL SEA SALT SOAKS. Combine sea salt with essential oils to produce an array of therapeutic and aromatically pleasing herbal salts. When using herbal salts you will only need to add 1–2 teaspoons of salt to the hand-soak water, since the potency of the salt is increased by the addition of the essential oils.

 ## *Basic Herbal Sea Salt*   ALL

**15–30 drops essential oil
6 tablespoons sea salt**

Place salt in a glass jar with a tight-fitting, nonmetallic lid, then drop essential oils into the salt a few drops at a time, stirring in thoroughly after each dropping; when done adding the oils, cap tightly and shake the jar to continue mixing the ingredients. It is important to cap the jar tightly so the volatile oils do not evaporate and the salt continues to absorb them. You may use them right away or store them in a cool, dark place. Add 1–2 teaspoons of salt to the hand-soak water. Makes about 3 oz. of herbal salt, enough for 9–18 soaks.

Variations: Use your nose and the information in the Essential Oils section to guide your personal formulations. Variations follow:

Stimulating Salt Soak   ALL
A refreshing, cooling and invigorating blend for tired and achy hands. It is also cleansing and disinfecting and smells uplifting and delicious.
Use 10 drops of peppermint essential oil, 10 drops of rosemary essential oil, 5 drops of lemongrass essential oil and 6 tablespoons of sea salt.
Follow directions for Basic Herbal Sea Salt above. Add 1–2 teaspoons of the salts per hand soak. Apply a moisturizer afterward. Makes enough for 9–18 soaks.

Tea Tree Lavender Salt Soak   ALL/INFECTED
A strong disinfectant, antifungal hand soak with muscle- relaxing properties. Good to use on wounded, broken skin, although it may sting.
Replace essential oils in above formula with 10 drops of tea tree essential oil, 10 drops of lavender essential oil, and 5 drops of melissa essential oil.

Calming Salt Soak   ALL
This exotic, spicy, woody blend relaxes and soothes overworked, tense hands that are irritated and inflamed. A good soak to use before going to bed.
Replace essential oils in above formula with 10 drops of sandalwood essential oil, 5 drops of patchouli essential oil, 5 drops of nutmeg essential oil and 5 drops of chamomile essential oil.

HERBAL-INFUSED HAND SOAKS. You can use strong herbal infusions, made by simply steeping herbs in water, for therapeutic hand soaks. The unstrained infusion is poured into a pot, gently reheated and placed in the soaking bowl. Additional warm water may be added so that hands are completely immersed.

Basic Herbal-Infused Hand Soak   ALL

Use 1 oz. (approximately 3-6 tablespoons) of freshly dried herb to 16 oz. water, and make a strong infusion. Pour the unstrained infusion into a pot, then gently reheat and pour it into the bowl. Top off with additional warm water. Below are some good choices for hand soaking.

Marshmallow-Violet-Elder Soak ALL/DRY

A soothing, skin-softening hand soak for dry, chapped and damaged skin.

1 tablespoon or ⅓ oz. freshly dried
marshmallow root (cut)

1 tablespoon or ⅓ oz. freshly dried
crushed violet leaf

1 tablespoon or ⅓ oz. freshly dried
crushed elder flowers

16 oz. water

Combine the herbs and make herbal infusion with herbs and water. Steep for at least 4 hours to allow the marshmallow to release its mucilage. Pour unstrained infusion into pot, gently reheat, then pour it into the bowl. Top off with additional warm water. Makes enough for 1 treatment.

Mint Soak ALL

A refreshing, stimulating soak for fatigued, overheated and worn-out hands.

1 large handful dried mint leaves (or
3–4 large handfuls fresh mint leaves)

16 oz. water

Make herbal infusion with mint and water and let steep for at least 1 hour. Pour unstrained infusion into pot, gently reheat and pour it into the bowl. Make a little extra infusion and set aside a cup for drinking as you relax into the hand soak. Makes enough for 1 treatment.

Flaxseed Hand Soak ALL/DRY/DAMAGED

This soak is extremely gummy and is very helpful for dry, inflamed, irritated and itchy hands.

¼ cup flaxseeds
16 oz. water

optional: ¼ teaspoon rich carrier oil,
like olive, peanut or avocado

Make herbal infusion with flaxseeds and water and let steep for 8 hours. Pour unstrained infusion into a pot and gently reheat, then add to the bowl and top off with additional warm water. Add optional rich carrier oil such as olive or peanut. If your hands are very damaged you will want to do this soak several times a week and follow it up with a rich cream application.

ANTIMICROBIAL SOAKS FOR CUT AND WOUNDED HANDS. Minor cuts and wounds to the hands can be encouraged to heal more quickly with an antimicrobial soak made from various herbal tinc-tures. Be aware that the alcohol content in the tinctures may sting open wounds if used undiluted. Remember that tinctures must be prepared several weeks in advance of using them to allow for optimal extraction of the active ingredients in the herbs. Once made, they are easily pre-served for future use if stored out of direct heat and sun-light, and can be used for many purposes. If you don't have the time or inclination to make your own tinctures, use this section as a reference guide for purchasing and using ready-made tinctures available at health food stores and via mail order (see Resources).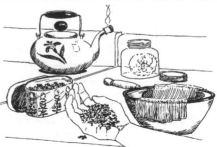

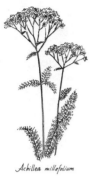

Yarrow Tincture

DAMAGED/INFECTED

Yarrow is a strong antiseptic, styptic analgesic with astringent properties, making it an excellent herb to use on wounds.

Fresh yarrow leaves and flowers
100 proof vodka

Follow Directions for Alcohol Tinctures Using Fresh Herbs. Add 3–4 dropperfuls of yarrow tincture to soak water or apply directly to the wound area. Yield varies depending on the size of the jar in which you make the tincture.

Achillea millefolium

Calendula Tincture with Fresh Blossoms

DAMAGED/INFECTED

Calendula helps heal cuts, bruises and scrapes, as well as split cuticles.

> **Fresh calendula blossoms**
> **190 proof grain alcohol (preferred) or 100 proof vodka**

Follow Directions for Alcohol Tinctures Using Fresh Herbs. Add 3–4 dropperfuls of calendula tincture to soak water or apply directly to the injured area. Yield varies depending on the size of the jar in which you make the tincture.

Calendula Tincture with Dried Blossoms

DAMAGED/INFECTED

> **2 oz. dried calendula blossoms**
> **10 oz. 140 proof grain alcohol (preferred) or 100 proof vodka**

Follow Directions for Alcohol Tinctures Using Dried Herbs.

Add 3–4 dropperfuls of calendula tincture to soak water or apply directly to the injured area. This will make about 7–8 oz. of calendula tincture.

Defense Formula

DAMAGED/INFECTED

This formulation is based on a combination of herbs traditionally used for their antimicrobial action. It can be used to help clear infections inside and outside the body. (This is a recipe offered premade through Earthly Extracts, a medicinal tincture line I formulate (see Resources).

> **Use freshly dried herbs:**
> 1 oz. echinacea angustifolia root (cut), 1 oz. goldenseal root (cut), ½ oz. echinacea purpurea seed,
>
> ½ oz. spilanthes, ¼ oz. calendula blossoms, ¼ prickly ash bark (cut)
> 14 oz. 100 proof vodka

Grind the herbs into a coarse powder with a coffee/seed grinder and follow Directions for Alcohol Tinctures Using Dried Herbs. Add 3–4 dropperfuls of Defense Formula tincture to the hand-soak water or apply directly to the injured area. Makes 10–11 oz. of tincture.

Note: If you don't have a scale and the herbs are chopped into fine pieces, substitute 6 tablespoons for 1 oz., 3 tablespoons for ½ oz. and 1½ tablespoons for ¼ oz.

When I make compound tinctures like the Defense Formula, I tincture the herbs separately and then combine them after they are pressed. I use different water and alcohol ratios for the different herbs to maximize the extraction of soluble constituents. And I also use fresh spilanthes and echinacea angustifolia roots. I feel this provides the best tincture. However, the results from the technique described above will be more than adequate.

Hand Softeners or Emollients

Emollients for lubricating and moisturizing the hands include carrier oils, salves and creams. These are good formulas to use for massages as well as for healing dry, chapped or damaged skin. Emollients also help to soften and heal split or dried cuticles.

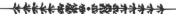

Hand Rejuvenating Night Treatment

If your hands are very dry and cracked, try applying a generous amount of rich oil, cream or salve at bedtime and wearing gloves to bed. This will help to seal in the moisture along with the restorative and nourishing properties of the formula. The gloves also hold in the heat generated by your hands, which aids in the penetration of the treatment. Your hands will feel like new in the morning. Some excellent choices for this overnight treatment are plain shea butter, Manna Hand Cream, Superhealing Hand Balm and Skin Revival.

 Mediterranean Hands   ALL

A simple but effective way to nourish and soften the hands. To help hands hydrate and seal in moisture apply oil after washing hands when they are still moist.

    1–2 teaspoons cold pressed olive oil
    optional: **1 drop lavender essential oil**

Massage oil into hands. Add 1 drop of essential oil of lavender for fragrance and therapeutic value. Makes enough for 1 treatment.

 South Sea Island Hands   ALL

A skin-softening and cooling treatment. The coconut oil will melt as it is applied to the skin.

    1–2 teaspoons coconut oil
    optional: **1 drop essential oil of rosemary**

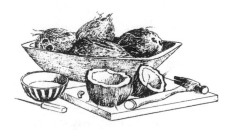

Massage oil into hands. You can add 1 drop of rosemary essential oil for added therapeutic value. Makes enough for 1 treatment.

Shea Butter Hands
ALL/DRY/DAMAGED

My favorite for dry, cracked, bruised and hurting hands. Shea butter was introduced to me by West African drummers, who use it religiously on their hands to heal splits and bruises and general damage that occurs from constant banging on the djembes (drums). I recommend shea butter particularly for gardeners and carpenters.

1–2 teaspoons of shea butter

For best results, massage into hands before and after engaging them in work. Shea butter is available via mail order (see Resources) and in health food and African specialty stores.

AROMATHERAPY OILS FOR HANDS. Combining essential oils with nourishing carrier oils and butters provides healing for various conditions while soothing the soul with delightful aromas. These oils are easy to make and immediately ready for use. You can massage these formulas directly into the hands, or add them to water for a hand soak, using ½ teaspoon per 16 oz. of warm water. Many of these oils can also be used on other parts of the body.

🐝 Basic Aromatherapy Oil for Hands
ALL

15–30 drops essential oil
1 oz. carrier oil

Pour carrier oil into a 1-oz. small-mouth glass jar (preferably blue or amber) with a well-fitting lid. Leave an ⅛-inch of space at the top for the essential oils. Add these oils drop by drop, cap jar and shake well. Label with ingredients and its ready for use. Makes 1 oz.

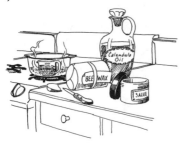

SALVES FOR HANDS. You can turn any oil into a salve by thickening it with beeswax. Salves are especially good for chapped, dried skin, and healing salves can be made for eczema and other conditions by adding the appropriate herbs. Salves can be more convenient to work with than oils, because they don't spill and are ideal for tucking into a handbag or travel kit. To use a salve, massage a small amount into the affected area at least twice daily. If necessary, wipe away excess with an absorbent cloth, but do not wash it off. To make the following formulas, please refer to Directions for Salves and Balms on p 224.

Comfrey Salve
ALL/DAMAGED

Comfrey, also known as "knit bone," contains allantoin, a cell proliferant that helps close or knit things back together. Use on sprains, wounds, scar tissue and cracked skin.

3 oz. comfrey-infused olive oil
1 oz. beeswax

In order to make this salve you first need to make comfrey-infused oil, as follows: Use 1 oz. of comfrey leaf, freshly dried and coarsely ground; 1 oz. of comfrey root, freshly dried and coarsely ground; 8 oz. cold pressed olive oil, and follow Directions for Herbal-Infused Oils with Dried

Herbs. Makes about 6 oz. of comfrey-infused olive oil, more than called for in this salve recipe. Note: Comfrey oil is useful for other preparations, so it's a good idea to have extra on hand. Once you have made the oil, follow Directions for Salves and Balms.

All-Purpose Salve   ALL/DAMAGED

This broad-spectrum healing salve is useful on minor skin irritations, inflammations, burns, diaper rash and chapped, cracked skin.

> 1 oz. plantain-infused olive oil
> 1 oz. St. Johnswort-infused olive oil
> 1 oz. calendula-infused olive oil
> 1 oz. beeswax

It is necessary to make or purchase the herbal-infused oils before preparing the salve.

To make plantain-infused olive oil, use fresh plantain leaves and cold pressed olive oil and follow Directions for Herbal-Infused Oils with Fresh Herbs. To make St. Johnswort-infused olive oil, use fresh St. Johnswort flowers and buds, or flowering tops, and cold pressed olive oil and follow Directions for Herbal-Infused Oils with Fresh Herbs. To make calendula-infused olive oil, use 2 oz. of freshly dried calendula flowers and 10 oz. of cold pressed olive oil and follow Directions for Herbal-Infused Oils with Dried Herbs. You will end up with about 7 oz. of calendula-infused olive oil. After you have obtained the infused oils, proceed to Directions for Salves and Balms. Makes 4 oz. of salve.

Note: It is wise to make a large quantity of these herbal-infused oils, as they are used in numerous other formulas.

Superhealing Hand Balm   ALL/DAMAGED/DRY

Use this balm to keep hands from drying and cracking by applying before and after engaging them in work or to repair cracked and chapped skin.

> 1 oz. plus 1 tablespoon jojoba oil
> 2 oz. plus 1 tablespoon shea butter
> 2 oz. comfrey-infused olive oil (see
>   Comfrey Salve pp. 102-103)
> 1 oz. beeswax
> ¾ teaspoon lavender essential oil

Place all ingredients except the lavender essential oil in a heat-proof measuring cup and place cup in a hot-water bath. Stir until ingredients are thoroughly melted. Remove from heat and stir for a couple of minutes to cool but not thicken; this also helps to evenly distribute the ingredients. Pour into a wide-mouth jar, add essential oil and quickly cap the jar with a tight-fitting lid to prevent the essential oil from evaporating. Allow butter to sit undisturbed for several hours or overnight to completely cool. Massage Superhealing Hand Balm into hands as often as you can; try to do it at least twice a day. Apply balm before night slumber for greatest reparative action, and if hands are really chapped sleep with gloves. Makes about 7 oz. of balm.

Variations: Replace the lavender oil with ¾ teaspoon of tea tree essential oil for antiseptic properties when hands are infected or cut. Or, replace the lavender oil with ¾ teaspoon of wintergreen essential oil for analgesic properties when hands are painful and sore.

MOISTURIZING CREAMS FOR HANDS. Creams, which are emulsifications of water and oil, are luxurious preparations to soften and soothe the skin. The formulas presented here are for hydrating, lubricating and nourishing dry, chapped hands. Even people who have oily skin on their face or other areas of their body frequently have dry hands that can benefit from one of these rich creams. Tuck a jar of cream into your bag and carry it with you to use throughout the day as needed.

Manna Hand Cream   ALL/DRY/DAMAGED

A rich, delicious-smelling hand cream for dry, chapped, cracked and irritated skin. The cocoa butter helps hold moisture in the skin and gives the cream a chocolate aroma. The sandalwood contributes to the hydrating, anti-inflammatory and antiseptic effects of the cream.

- 2 oz. jojoba oil
- 1 oz. comfrey root-infused olive oil (preferred) or plain olive oil
- 2 oz. peanut oil
- 1 oz. avocado oil
- 1 oz. shea butter
- 1½ oz. cocoa butter

- ½ oz. coconut oil
- 1 oz. beeswax
- 2 teaspoons sandalwood essential oil
- 7 drops cinnamon essential oil
- 10 drops orange essential oil
- 9 oz. distilled water

Follow Directions for Creams. Makes 19 oz. Note that this cream may become slightly granular in cold temperatures.

To make comfrey root-infused olive oil, use 2 oz. of comfrey root, freshly dried and coarsely ground, and 8 oz. of cold pressed olive oil. Then follow Directions for Herbal-Infused Oils with Dried Herbs.

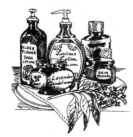

Skin Revival   ALL/DRY/DAMAGED

A nourishing, protective, healing moisturizer for dry, aged and damaged skin, eczema and dermatitis. Excellent on any part of the body and very beneficial on dry, chapped and cracked hands. Has some ultraviolet protection; SPF-4. See formula pp. 29–30.

Silk Hands   ALL/DRY/DAMAGED

This preparation is an incredibly rich and soothing formula for dry, chapped, inflamed and irritated hands. The seeds and cream provide important skin nourishment, the slippery elm powder and flaxseeds contain significant amounts of mucilage to help soothe and soften the skin and the glycerin acts as a humectant to help draw moisture to the skin.

- 1 teaspoon glycerin
- 1 teaspoon slippery elm powder
- 1 tablespoon flaxseeds
- 1 teaspoon sunflower seeds

- 6 walnut halves crushed
- 1–2 tablespoons dairy cream (organic preferred)

Grind and sift flaxseeds, sunflower seeds and walnuts, add slippery elm powder, mix thoroughly, add cream and stir until a smooth paste is reached, then add the glycerin and stir again. Massage this paste into the hands and evenly apply another coat of paste, put on gloves and leave on for at least 1 hour or, if possible, overnight. This also makes an excellent face masque for dry, damaged skin. Makes enough for 1 treatment.

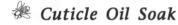

Cuticle Care

Cuticles have a tendency to dry out, harden and split. Under very dry or harsh conditions they may feel sore or split deeply enough to bleed. Cuticle care is as easy as rubbing a healing, reparative oil, cream or salve into the cuticle tissue. If the cuticles are very dry or damaged, soak them in warm oil and massage them with an emollient several times a day, and especially before bedtime. Here are a few good suggestions.

Cuticle Oil Soak   DRY/DAMAGED

To help heal and soothe dry and split cuticles, soak them in oil. Choose from any rich carrier oil such as jojoba, peanut, or olive, or from an herbal-infused oil such as comfrey, St. Johnswort or plantain. Gently warm the oil and pour it into a small bowl; add enough to submerse your cuticles. Soak for 20 minutes or longer, and repeat once or twice a day. After soaking, cover oil and reuse for following soaks. Discard oil after a few soaks or when it no longer appears fresh.

Calendula Salve   ALL/DAMAGED

This salve helps heal damaged, split and cracked cuticles and protect the skin from further damage.

> **2 oz. freshly dried whole calendula blossoms**
>
> **10 oz. cold pressed olive oil**
> **2 oz. beeswax**

Grind calendula blossoms and using olive oil, follow Directions for Herbal-Infused Oils with Dried Herbs. This makes approximately 7 oz. of calendula-infused oil. To make salve use 6 oz. of calendula oil and 2 oz. of beeswax and follow Directions for Salves and Balms. Makes 8 oz. of salve.

Lavender Sandalwood Jojoba Oil   ALL/DRY/DAMAGED

A wonderful-smelling reparative oil for healing and hydrating the skin and cuticles.

> **2 oz. jojoba oil**
> **20 drops lavender essential oil**
>
> **10 drops sandalwood oil**

Pour jojoba oil into a 2-oz. small-mouth bottle with a lid, leaving an ⅛-inch space at the top, add essential oils a few drops at a time, cap and shake well before use. Store out of direct heat or light source. Makes 2 oz.

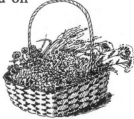

Variation: Substitute another rich oil like olive or peanut for the jojoba.

Manna Hand Cream

This rich emollient cream is excellent for massaging into damaged cuticles. See formula p. 104.

Skin Revival

Another rich nutritive cream for protecting and healing cuticles. See formula pp. 29–30.

Nails

Nails are good indicators of our general health. Nail strength is directly linked to how well nourished we are, especially with regard to protein and mineral intake. If we are not consuming enough of these nutrients we tend to have soft and easily broken nails. Including seaweeds in the diet, about ½ oz. per day, can bring about a positive and noticeable change. Seaweed nourishes the thyroid gland and supplies the body with high concentrations of minerals that can invigorate the metabolism and speed up the rate of nail and hair growth.

ON YOUR FEET

Foot Soaks

Soaks are a pleasant and relaxing way to thoroughly cleanse the feet. They are also excellent for alleviating the discomforts of tired, achy feet. Soaking your feet at the end of a long day seems to miraculously refresh and rejuvenate your entire being. The quantities given are for one strong footbath, but many of the recipes can easily be doubled or quadrupled and stored for future soaks. I like to soak my feet for at least 20 minutes and up to about 1 hour. If you choose to soak for longer than 20 minutes, keep a kettle of simmering water on hand to add to your footbath in order to maintain the desired level of heat.

BASIC FOOT SOAK TECHNIQUE. To prepare a foot soak, choose a vessel that accommodates both your feet comfortably and that is deep enough to reach the level of your mid-calf. For a plain soak, fill the vessel with water that is as hot as you can comfortably tolerate, or use one of the following formulas for increased therapeutic effects.

HERBAL-INFUSED FOOT SOAKS. If you are using dry herbs in your foot soak, first infuse them by placing about 2 oz. of herb (approximately 2–3 handfuls) into a ½-gallon jar with a lid. Note that less herb is used in making these infusions than is called for in the Directions for Herbal Infusions in the Techniques and Definitions chapter. Pour boiling water over the herbs, cap the jar tightly and let the solution steep for a minimum of 1 hour. The longer you allow the herbs to steep, the stronger and more effective the infusion will be. You can skip the step of straining the infusion and simply pour the entire contents of the jar into the soaking vessel, adding hot water up to the mid-calf level. I prefer to leave the infusion unstrained, and enjoy the sensation of squishing the herbs beneath my feet and between my toes during the soak. Here are some of my favorite soak formulas:

 ## Ginger Feet ALL

A warming, stimulating footbath that also seems to make you feel healthier all over. It's great during cold weather and flu season.

> **2 oz. fresh ginger root grated per footbath**
> **64 oz. water**

Make herbal infusion with ginger root and water. Pour unstrained infusion into the soaking vessel, adding hot water up to the mid-calf level. Add grated ginger directly to the footbath for a quicker (although somewhat less potent) bath. *Variation follows:*
Dried Ginger Feet
Use 2–3 teaspoons of dried ginger root powder or add dried root directly to the bathwater.

 ## Evergreen Feet ALL

A fabulous year-round foot soak made with fresh plant matter. This is especially nice in the winter months, and also useful as a decongestant.

Clip off the tips of some white pine, spruce and/or hemlock trees. Think green: You can even recycle your Christmas tree or wreaths for soaking.

> **4 large handfuls plant material per foot soak**
> **64 oz. water**

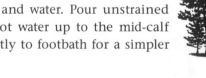

Make herbal infusion with evergreen tips and water. Pour unstrained infusion into the soaking vessel, adding hot water up to the mid-calf level. You can also add evergreen tips directly to footbath for a simpler if less potent preparation.

 ## Kitchen Cupboard Soak ALL

This soak utilizes what is already in the house to provide effective results. Look in the Botanicals section in the Ingredients chapter for specific information on the herbs that are in your cupboard.

Go to your cupboard and see what culinary herbs and spices you have. Rosemary, thyme, basil, oregano, bay, tarragon and savory make enjoyable soaks and also have cleansing and immune- and circulatory-enhancing properties. Use 2 oz. or 2 handfuls of herb per soak. The measure of the herb in handfuls varies in relation to the cut of the herb. If the herb has been cut small or powdered you will measure a smaller amount than if using whole pieces of herbs. You may need to add more, depending on the strength of the herbs and how long they've been sitting in the cupboard. Mustard, clove, cinnamon and ginger are all very concentrated, so use these with caution, adding only 2–3 teaspoons per footbath. Peppers like cayenne and black are extremely potent, and I would use only ½–1 teaspoon per foot-

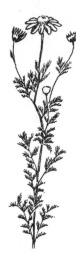

bath. Be careful not to touch your eyes after handling the pepper; better yet, use a spoon to scoop out the pepper to keep it off your fingers.

Make herbal infusion with herb and water. Pour unstrained infusion into the soaking vessel, adding hot water up to the mid-calf level. Or add the powdered herbs directly to the footbath for a simpler if less potent preparation.

"Rock-a-Bye Baby" ALL/DRY

A calming, soothing and healthful blend for overworked, dry, chapped and pained feet.

1 oz. chamomile   1 oz. comfrey root or marshmallow
½ oz. lavender   root

Make infusion with herbs and water. Pour unstrained infusion into the soaking vessel, adding hot water up to the mid-calf level.

Athlete's Foot Soak ALL/DAMAGED

An antifungal soak for athlete's foot and other microbial problems.

½ oz. black walnut hull   ¼ oz. myrrh powder
½ oz. thuja   64 oz. water
1 oz. calendula (whole blossoms)

Make infusion with herbs and water. Pour unstrained infusion into the soaking vessel and add hot water up to the mid-calf level.

ESSENTIAL OIL FOOT SOAKS. Adding essential oils directly to the water can increase a foot soak's therapeutic action while providing a refreshing or mood-enchancing aroma. Refer to the Essential Oils section in the Ingredients chapter for more suggestions.

🐝 *Basic Essential Oil Foot Soak* ALL

Use a vessel that accommodates both your feet comfortably and that is deep enough to reach the level of your mid-calf. Fill it with water that is as hot as you can comfortably tolerate. Add 2–5 drops of essential oil to the water just prior to immersion. The essential oils evaporate quickly, so you may need to add more during the soak. *Variations follow:*

🐝 *Tea Tree Feet* ALL

Tea tree essential oil is a strong antifungal agent and general disinfectant. Use on smelly, moldy or infected feet.
Add 4 drops of tea tree essential oil directly to the footbath immediately prior to immersing feet.

Pepped-Up Feet

ALL

A refreshing, stimulating foot soak.
Use 2 drops of peppermint essential oil, 1 drop of wintergreen essential oil and 1 drop of rosemary essential oil.
Add essential oils directly to the bathwater immediately before immersing feet.

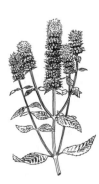

Far East Feet   ALL
A warming, spicy blend for improving circulation.
Use 1 drop of cassia cinnamon essential oil, 2 drops of ginger essential oil and 1 drop lemongrass
essential oil.
Add essential oils directly to the bathwater immediately before immersing feet.

VINEGAR SOAKS. Ordinary vinegar acts as an antifungal agent and disinfectant. Herbal-infused
vinegar combines the positive attributes of vinegar with the healing properties of herbs. For
example, mugwort-infused vinegar is great for soreness, aches and pains, spilanthes increases
the vinegar's antimicrobial action and mint adds an uplifting and invigorating quality. Note
that vinegar can be quite drying to the skin, so you might want to apply a moisturizing formula to your feet afterward. Caution: Vinegar may sting open skin.

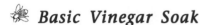 ## Basic Vinegar Soak   ALL

*Use a vessel that accommodates both your feet comfortably and that is deep enough to reach the
level of your mid-calf. Fill it with water that is as hot as you can comfortably tolerate.*

   ¼ cup of vinegar

Add vinegar to the water just prior to immersion.

HERBAL VINEGAR SOAKS. Plan ahead when making these formulas, as they require a steeping
period of 3 weeks or longer. Once they are made, however, herbal vinegars will keep for many
months without refrigeration. I have even made herbal-infused vinegars that were still good
after 3 years.

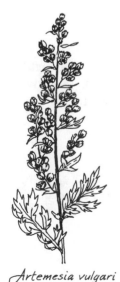

Artemesia vulgari

Autumn Soak   ALL

*A good antifungal and relaxing foot soak that needs to be made in the autumn
as the black walnuts fall from the tree and the mugwort is in flower. This vinegar also makes an excellent hair rinse for dark hair.*

**Equal amounts fresh black walnut hulls and fresh flowering mugwort
   tops and vinegar**

Using herbs and vinegar, follow Directions for Herbal-Infused Vinegars with
Fresh Herbs. Use the outer green hull of the black walnut; make sure to use
gloves when handling them, as they can stain your hands. Add ¼ cup of
vinegar per foot soak.

Variation: If you don't have black walnuts in your neighborhood or it's not
autumn you can make the recipe with dried herbs; it just won't be as potent. If the herbs are dried: Use 2 oz. of dried black walnut hulls, 2 oz. of
dried mugwort and 18 oz. of vinegar and follow Directions for Herbal-Infused Vinegars with Dried Herbs. Add ¼ cup of vinegar per foot soak. Makes
about 14 oz. of herbal-infused vinegar.

Black Mint Vinegar

ALL

A delightful-smelling and refreshing vinegar for tired and achy feet. May also be used for salad dressing and other culinary needs.

2 oz. dried black mint or other mint of choice
8 oz. vinegar

Use herb and vinegar and follow Directions for Herbal-Infused Vinegars with Dried Herbs. Add ¼ cup per foot soak. Makes about 6 oz. of vinegar.

SEA SALT SOAKS. Use sea salt and herbal salt soaks for swollen, achy and painful feet. Salt soaks can also help heal wounds, but note that the salt will sting open skin. Salt is drying to the skin, so a good moisturizer should be applied before soaking and after if needed.

 ## Basic Salt Soak for Feet

ALL

Add 2 oz. or 4 tablespoons of sea salt per foot soak

HERBAL SEA SALTS SOAKS. Combine sea salt with essential oils and produce an array of therapeutic and aromatically pleasing herbal salts. When using herbal salts you will only need to add ½ oz. or 1 tablespoon of salt to the foot-soak water, since the potency of the salt is increased by the addition of essential oil.

 ## Basic Herbal Sea Salt

ALL

15–30 drops essential oil
6 tablespoons sea salt

Place salt in a glass jar with a tight-fitting nonmetallic lid and drop essential oils into the salt a few drops at a time, stirring in thoroughly after each dropping. When done adding the essential oil, cap tightly and shake to continue mixing the ingredients. It is important to cap tightly so the essential oils don't evaporate and the salt continues to absorb them. You may use them right away or store them in a cool, dark place. Add ½ oz. or 1 tablespoon of salt to the water. Makes about 3 oz., enough for 6 soaks.

Note: Use your nose and the information in the Essential Oils section to guide your formulations. *Variations follow:*

Energizing Salts

ALL

A refreshing, cooling and invigorating blend for tired and achy feet that is also cleansing and deodorizing.
Use 8 drops of peppermint essential oil, 8 drops of rosemary essential oil, 5 drops of eucalyptus essential oil, 10 drops of tangerine essential oil and 6 tablespoons sea salt.
Follow directions for Basic Herbal Sea Salt above.

Antimicrobial Salts

ALL

A strong disinfectant, deodorizing, antifungal foot soak with muscle-relaxing properties.
Use 10 drops of tea tree essential oil, 10 drops of lavender essential oil, 5 drops of white pine essential oil and 6 tablespoons sea salt.
Follow directions for Basic Herbal Sea Salt above.

A Hard Day's Salt Soak
ALL

This spicy, woody blend relaxes and soothes overworked, tense feet. A good soak to do before going to bed.
Use 5 drops of sandalwood essential oil, 5 drops of fir essential oil, 5 drops of patchouli essential oil, 5 drops of black pepper essential oil, 5 drops of chamomile essential oil and 6 tablespoons sea salt. Follow directions for Basic Herbal Sea Salt above.

FOOT OIL SOAKS. Oil soaks are made by adding a carrier oil to the foot-soak water. The carrier oil provides nourishment and lubrication. Oil soaks are good if you have dry, scaly or cracked skin. You can also add oil to any other foot-soak formula to counteract the drying action of ingredients like salt and vinegar.

 ## Basic Foot Oil Soak
ALL/DRY

Use a vessel that accommodates both your feet comfortably and that is deep enough to reach the level of your mid-calf. Fill it with water that is as hot as you can comfortably tolerate.

2–3 tablespoons of carrier or herbal-infused oil

Add oil to the water just prior to immersion.

 ## Basic Aromatherapy Foot Oil
ALL

A carrier oil may be enriched with essential oils to offer various aromas and therapeutic effects. Higher concentrations of essential oils can be used when making foot oils than when making oils for other parts of the body, since the feet are rather callous and thick-skinned. Aromatherapy oils are also nice for foot massages. Keep in mind that less oil is added to the footbath water when using aromatherapy oils than when adding plain carrier oils.

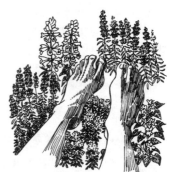

20–30 drops essential oil of choice
1 oz. carrier oil

Pour carrier oil into a jar, add essential oils, cap and shake well. Add 1–2 teaspoons per footbath. Makes 1 oz., enough for about 3–6 soaks.

Note: The essential oil combinations listed in the herbal salt soaks are also applicable to foot oil formulas. Here are some examples:

Energizing Foot Oil
ALL

A refreshing, cooling and invigorating blend for tired and achy feet that is also cleansing and deodorizing. The olive oil provides nourishment and emolliency for the skin.
Use 12 drops of peppermint essential oil, 13 drops of rosemary essential oil, 5 drops of lemongrass, essential oil and 1 oz. cold pressed olive oil.

Antimicrobial Foot Oil
ALL

A strong disinfectant, deodorizing, antifungal foot soak with muscle-relaxing properties. The olive oil provides nourishment and emolliency for the skin.
Use 12 drops of tea tree essential oil, 13 drops of lavender essential oil, 5 drops of white pine essential oil and 1 oz. cold pressed olive oil.

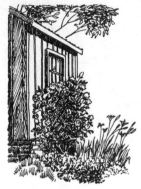

Grapefruit Feet

ALL

Grapefruit seed extract is an excellent antimicrobial, antifungal agent. By the way, it does not smell like grapefruit, and actually has very little odor.

Add 10–20 drops of grapefruit seed extract directly to footbath

 ### Borax Soak

ALL

A foot soak for antifungal, disinfectant and deodorant purposes.

Add ¼ cup of borax per foot soak

Variations: You can add different essential oils to the borax before adding it to the soak water to produce various aromas and therapeutic effects. For additional cleansing add 2 drops of tea tree essential oil and 2 drops of lavender essential oil to the borax before adding to water. Or add 4 drops of peppermint for a stimulating, cooling soak.

Foot Emollients

Emollients — oils, salves and creams — offer the same benefits to the feet as to the hands, operating to nourish, soothe and heal dry, damaged skin. A foot emollient can also be specially formulated to have analgesic, antifungal, warming or stimulating properties. When applying the emollient, massage it well into your feet to promote absorption and to stimulate circulation and metabolic activity. The amount of emollient required per treatment depends on the condition of the skin — skin that is very dry or cracked will absorb more oil. Start with a small amount and massage in more as needed. The following oil recipes can also be used for foot soaks (see Foot Oil Soaks).

 ### Mediterranean Feet

ALL/DRY

A simple and nourishing moisturizer to massage into the feet for general skin conditions.

2–3 teaspoons of olive oil

Oil Feet Treat

ALL/DRY/DAMAGED

A rich, nourishing foot oil for dry, cracked and damaged skin.

2 oz. jojoba oil
2 oz. peanut oil
1 oz. avocado oil

2 oz. comfrey root-infused olive oil
(see Comfrey Comfort p. 82)

Combine oils in a narrow-mouth glass bottle with a lid, cap and shake well before using. Apply 1–2 teaspoons to feet per treatment. Makes 7 oz., enough for 20 or more applications.

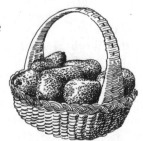

Hot Lava Foot Oil

ALL

This warming oil is great for feet that are cold due to poor circulation or cold weather.

2 oz. peanut oil or other carrier oil of
  your choice
12 drops ginger essential oil

8 drops cinnamon essential oil
4 drops patchouli essential oil

Pour carrier oil into a small-mouth glass bottle with a lid, leaving an ⅛-space at the top, add your essential oils, cap and shake before use. Apply 1–2 teaspoons per foot treatment. Makes 2 oz., enough for 6 or more treatments.

Lavender Chamomile Foot Oil

ALL

A great oil for unwinding and relaxing strained and tired feet, as well as for feet that are dry, irritated and sensitive. The oil possesses antiinflammatory and antiseptic properties as well.

2 oz. lavender-infused peanut oil
  (although less effective, plain
  peanut oil may also be used),

25 drops lavender essential oil
5 drops chamomile essential oil

Pour carrier oil into a small-mouth glass bottle with a lid, leaving an ⅛-inch space at the top, add your essential oils, cap and shake before use. Apply 1–2 teaspoons per foot treatment. Makes 2 oz., enough for 6 or more treatments.

Antifungal Healing Oil

ALL/DAMAGED

A strong disinfectant oil for fungal and other microbial problems. It may also may be used on cold sores to keep them from spreading and to diminish their duration and intensity. Apply directly to the cold sore with a Q-Tip and repeat applications throughout the day. You will find many other uses for this healing formula as well.

2 oz. black walnut-infused olive oil
  (although less effective, plain olive
  oil may be used)
10 drops tea tree essential oil

10 drops thuja essential oil
10 drops rosemary essential oil
10 drops cajeput essential oil

Pour carrier oil into a small-mouth glass bottle with a lid, leaving an ⅛-inch space at the top, add your essential oils, cap and shake before use. Apply 1–2 teaspoons per foot treatment. Makes 2 oz., enough for 6 or more treatments.

Note: To make black walnut-infused olive oil, use fresh black walnut hulls and cold pressed olive oil and follow Directions for Herbal-Infused Oils with Fresh Herbs. In addition, I suggest using the Herbal-Infused Oil with Heat method found in the Techniques and Definitions chapter to minimize the chances of spoilage. You can also use dried hulls; add 3 oz. of black walnut hulls, freshly dried and coarsely ground, and 12 oz. of cold pressed olive oil. Then follow Directions for Herbal-Infused Oils with with Dried Herbs. Yields about 8 oz. of oil.

SALVES FOR FEET. Salves are especially effective for very dry skin conditions, such as cracked heels. Herbal salves can also be formulated to help combat such conditions as foot fungus and inflammations. To use a salve start by massaging a small amount — about the size of a small pea will do — into the problem area, applying more as needed. Apply the salve a minimum of twice a day, without washing it off.

Black Walnut and Tea Tree Salve   ALL/DAMAGED

This is a strong-acting salve for fungal, viral and septic skin conditions as well as cold sores and bug bites.

3 oz. black walnut-infused olive oil
  (see Antifungal Healing Oil p. 113)

1 oz. beeswax
½ teaspoon tea tree essential oil

Follow Directions for Salves and Balms. Makes 4 oz.

All-Purpose Salve   ALL/DAMAGED

This is a broad-spectrum healing salve useful on minor skin irritations, inflammations, burns, diaper rash and chapped, cracked skin.

See formula p. 103.

Superhealing Foot Butter   ALL/DRY/DAMAGED

This rich, thick butter is excellent for dry, cracked and damaged skin. It's great for dancers and barefoot walkers.

2 tablespoons shea butter
2 tablespoons coconut oil
1 tablespoon grated cocoa butter
1 tablespoon plus 1 teaspoon grated beeswax

4 tablespoons jojoba oil
optional: 30 drops lavender essential oil

Place ingredients, except lavender essential oil, in a heat-proof measuring cup and place cup in a hot-water bath. Stir until ingredients are thoroughly melted. Remove from heat and continue to stir for a couple of minutes until the mixture is slightly cooled but not thickened; this also helps to evenly distribute the ingredients. Pour into a wide-mouth jar; if adding essential oil, do so now, and quickly cap the jar with a tight-fitting lid to prevent it from evaporating. Allow butter to sit undisturbed for several hours or overnight to completely cool. Massage the butter into problem area as often as you can; try to do it at least twice a day. It is also beneficial to apply it generously onto feet before night slumber. Makes about 4 oz.

Note: You may want to add an additional teaspoon of beeswax in warm weather to thicken the consistency

Shea Butter Feet
ALL/DRY/DAMAGED

Shea butter alone is excellent for healing dry, chapped, cracked, hot and bruised feet. I like to massage my feet with it during the dance camp I attend every summer, when dancing on wooden floors for days at a time rips up my feet. It also helps to cool down and heal the blisters that result from constant dancing.

Shea butter is available from health food stores and natural body care shops and via mail order (see Resources).

FOOT CREAMS. Foot creams combine the emollient properties of oil with the hydrating effects of a water-based liquid. The liquid component can be water, herbal tea and/or floral water. You can also add small amounts of an herbal tincture or vinegar, according to the therapeutic effects you desire. Foot creams are easy to make once you get the hang of it, but as with any cream you must follow the instructions closely. Don't be discouraged if your first few attempts don't work out perfectly. Even a poorly emulsified cream can be used, since it will still contain all the beneficial ingredients — it just may not look very professional. When you do get it right, creams are heavenly both to the touch and to the eye. For detailed instructions on making creams, refer to the Techniques and Definitions chapter page 224.

Peppermint Foot Cream
ALL

An invigorating, delicious-smelling cream for tired and dry feet.

3 oz. peanut oil	1½ oz. shea butter
1 oz. jojoba oil	½ oz. beeswax
2 oz. almond oil	1½ teaspoons peppermint essential oil
1½ oz. cocoa butter	9 oz. distilled water

Follow Directions for Creams. This recipe uses less beeswax than the Basic Cream Formula due to the presence of the cocoa butter. Makes 19 oz.

Healing Foot Cream
ALL

This rejuvenating antifungal foot cream is simple to make as it doesn't contain herbal-infused oils but relies on the essential oils for its medicinal properties. The sweet birch essential oil adds a nice aroma as well as its analgesic qualities. It is a very stable cream, lasting 6 months to a year outside refrigeration.

6 oz. expeller pressed canola oil	40 drops tea tree essential oil
3 oz. coconut oil	1 teaspoon sweet birch essential oil
1 oz. beeswax	1 teaspoon tangerine essential oil
¼ teaspoon thuja essential oil	¼ teaspoon of nutmeg essential oil
	9 oz. distilled water

Betula lenta

Follow Directions for Creams. Makes 19 oz.

Black Walnut Chaparral Foot Cream   ALL/DRY/DAMAGED

This is a potent cream with antifungal and nutritive properties. Good for smelly, damaged feet. You will need to make or purchase the herbal-infused oils before preparing the cream.

2 oz. black walnut-infused olive oil
2 oz. chaparral-infused olive oil or 4
   oz. combined infused oil
2 oz. jojoba oil
1 ½ oz. shea butter
1 ½ oz. coconut oil
1 oz. beeswax

½ teaspoon peppermint essential oil
40 drops rosemary essential oil
40 drops tea tree essential oil
¼ teaspoon thuja essential oil
40 drops cajeput essential oil
9 oz. distilled water

Make a combined infused oil of black walnut and chaparral. Use 1 oz. of freshly dried black walnut hulls and 1 oz. of chaparral. Crush and coarsely powder the herbs in a mortar and pestle or coffee grinder used exclusively for herbs and seeds. To the 2 oz. of powdered herbs, use 8 oz. of olive oil and follow Directions for Herbal-Infused Oils with Dried Herbs. When oil is strained you will have 4–6 oz. of infused olive oil of chaparral and black walnut. Note that when making herbal-infused oils with dried plant material, some of the oil gets lost from the final product due to its being absorbed into the dried herb.

Now follow Directions for Creams. Makes 19 oz.

Skin Revival   ALL/DRY/DAMAGED

A nourishing, protective, healing moisturizer for dry, aged and damaged skin, eczema and dermatitis. Excellent on any part of the body and especially on dry cracked feet. Has some ultraviolet protection: SPF-4. (See formula pp. 29–30).

Foot Powders

Feet that are encased in shoes and socks for long periods of time are often exposed to excess moisture, which can promote fungal infections or foul odor from bacterial growth. Foot powders can help to prevent fungal and bacterial growth by absorbing this excess moisture. Various ingredients can also be added to the formula to make it deodorizing and disinfecting. Foot powders are generally made with one or a combination of ingredients such as baking soda, clay, cornstarch, arrowroot powder and powdered herbs; essential oils can be added to any of them. You may choose to use a foot powder with varying therapeutic properties depending on the type and intensity of the problem. Apply the foot powder as the final step in any foot treatment program. You can also apply foot powder throughout the day. Sprinkle the powder directly into your shoes at night to help reduce odor. Use spice shakers or powder canisters for sprinkling on foot powder, or simply apply by hand.

❧ Basic Foot Powder

ALL

Use clay, cornstarch, arrowroot powder, baking soda or other absorbent powder, sprinkling it onto the feet, especially between the toes. This basic procedure will help keep the feet dry. If you use baking soda, it will also offer a mild deodorizing effect. *Variation follows:*

❧ Basic Foot Powder with Essential Oils

ALL

You can augment the deodorizing and disinfecting action by adding essential oil to the powder prior to application.

Place 1–2 teaspoons of powder, such as cornstarch or baking soda, in palm of hand, add 1–2 drops of essential oil and apply to feet. Makes enough for 1 application.

Citrus Soda Foot Powder

ALL

A refreshing, deodorizing, antifungal foot powder with a grapefruit scent. This recipe makes enough for a couple of applications. If you like the formula multiply the ingredients to create more.

4 drops grapefruit essential oil	2 teaspoons baking soda
2 drops tea tree essential oil	

Put baking soda in a small jar, add essential oils and stir them in thoroughly. Apply to feet, particularly between toes and on soles. Sprinkle into shoes as well. Store powder in shaker with a top or jar with a tight-fitting lid. Makes enough for 2 applications.

Peppermint Foot Powder

ALL

A refreshing, strongly antimicrobial foot powder with a peppermint aroma for sweaty, smelly feet. This recipe makes enough for a few applications. If you like the formula multiply the ingredients to create more.

4 drops peppermint essential oil	3 teaspoons
4 drops tea tree essential oil	arrowroot powder
2 drops sage essential oil	(or cornstarch)

Put arrowroot powder in a small jar, add essential oils and stir them in thoroughly. Cap jar and shake to continue mixing the ingredients. Apply powder to feet, particularly between toes and on soles. Sprinkle into shoes as well. Store powder in a shaker with a top or jar with a tight-fitting lid. Makes enough for 3 applications.

Lavender Cinnamon Foot Powder

ALL

A spicy, refreshing-smelling absorbent foot powder for damp, smelly feet. It also has antiseptic properties.

40 drops cinnamon essential oil	20 drops thuja essential oil
½ teaspoon lavender essential oil	½ cup clay

Put clay in a small jar, drip in essential oils while stirring them in thoroughly. Cap the jar and shake to continue mixing the ingredients. Apply powder to feet, especially between toes and on soles. Sprinkle into shoes as well. Store powder in shaker with a top or jar with a tight-fitting lid. Makes ½ cup.

Happy Feet from Jean's Greens

A foot powder specially formulated by Jean Argus to keep feet dry and free of bacteria that cause odor and fungal infection. The herbal ingredients are excellent antifungal, antimicrobial disinfectants.

½ cup cornstarch
1 cup clay (bentonite or French green)
1 tablespoon goldenseal powder
1 tablespoon myrrh gum powder
2 tablespoons black walnut hull
   powder

3 tablespoons chaparral
2 tablespoons thyme
20 drops peppermint essential oil

Grind the chaparral and thyme into a powder and thoroughly mix all the ingredients together. Stir in the peppermint essential oil and store in an airtight container or shaker. Sprinkle onto feet, especially between the toes. May also be sprinkled directly into shoes. Makes about 2 cups, enough for a few months.

Lavender Chamomile Rose Foot Powder

A sweet-smelling powder to keep feet dry. It will gently deodorize most feet.

1 cup clay
½ cup baking soda
½ cup arrowroot powder
½ cup freshly dried herbs (lavender, chamomile and rose blossoms combined)

¼ cup slippery elm powder
100 drops lavender essential oil
65 drops rose geranium essential oil
90 drops rosemary essential oil
optional: 100 drops tea tree oil for stronger antimicrobial effect

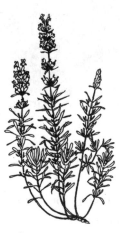

Lavandula angustifolia

Powder herbs, except the slippery elm, in a coffee grinder used exclusively for herbs and seeds, then sift herbs through a fine-mesh strainer, over a bowl, regrinding the coarser particles as needed. It is important to get the herbs as finely powdered as possible so the foot powder feels soft and silky against the skin. Place powdered herbs, clay, baking soda, arrowroot and slippery elm powder in a jar, mix thoroughly and add the essential oils a few drops at a time while stirring them in. Cap and shake jar. (Note that if baking soda is clumpy press through sifter.) To use powder, sprinkle onto feet, especially between the toes. May also be sprinkled into shoes. Store powder, in shaker with a top or jar with a tight-fitting lid. Makes about 2¾ cups. *Variation follows:*

Thyme Mint Foot Powder

You can replace the ½ cup of freshly dried herbs of lavender, chamomile and rose blossoms with ¼ cup of thyme and 1 /4 cup of mint. And replace the essential oils with 30 drops of peppermint essential oil, 50 drops of rosemary essential oil and 10 drops of thyme essential oil. Try experimenting with other herb and essential oil combinations to create personalized formulas.

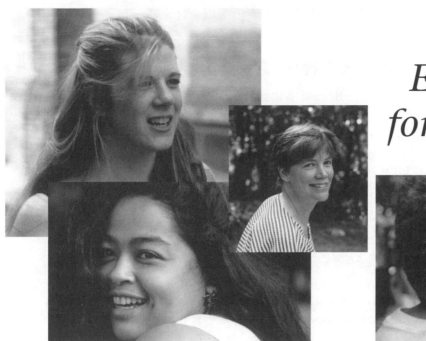

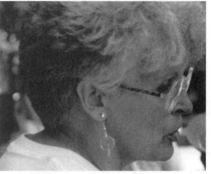

6
Especially for Women

While most of the body care preparations and principles in this book can be used by men and women alike, women have certain special needs based on the demands of the menstrual cycle, pregnancy, birth, lactation and menopause. This chapter deals with some natural preparations and treatments that can help to ease women through the different phases of their reproductive cycle, and offers some suggestions about natural breast care.

BREAST HEALTH

Gently massaging the breasts is an important ritual for women, because it aids in the circulation of blood and lymph fluid, which is responsible for maintaining healthy breast tissue. Regular breast massage can help prevent the buildup of lymph fluid, which may cause discomfort and lead to other more serious problems. It can also be incorporated into your regular breast self-exam. Breast massage is also a way to love and admire our own bodies. Our society gives women the message not to touch ourselves or experience our own beauty, so we often end up feeling alienated from our bodies. On the other hand, our breasts are sexualized, objectified and given a central place in the standard, media-driven image of feminine beauty. Many women end up feeling unattractive or inadequate because their breasts diverge from this artificial standard. By treating our breasts to a gentle massage we not only reap the physical benefits, but can also urge ourselves toward greater appreciation of the bodies we are born with. Massaging the breasts can also be very helpful for alleviating premenstrual problems. Breast massage is simultaneously relaxing and invigorating. As an extra incentive to incorporate breast massage into your body care routine, remember that it will make your breasts more healthy and vibrant. When massaging your breasts, be very gentle, since the breast tissue is fragile and easily damaged.

Breast Massage

Sage Blue from Wolf Howl Herbals, in Vermont, who has been a massage therapist for over two decades, has agreed to share with us her excellent technique for breast massage. You will find her favorite breast balm recipe to use while doing these strokes, as well as her ideas on breast health.

"Breast Cancer is increasing at an alarming rate. We can do something about it! We can take responsibility for our own breast health, learning about our breasts, recognizing normal breast changes that occur during our cycle and getting comfortable with the natural lumpiness of breasts. We can do this in a natural, most loving way with breast massage.

"Bras, particularly tight sports bras, constrict movement of fluids in the breasts and may cause the surrounding lymph-drainage system to fill with toxins, which then feel lumpy. Regular (once a week or once a month) breast massage helps the lymph system surrounding the breast tissue to drain toxins from the tissues into the bloodstream, where they are cleansed from the body."

Sage Blue's Breast Massage Techniques

Find a comfortable, private place where you can sit, recline or lie down; for instance, you can do the massage while soaking in the bathtub. Apply just enough oil or balm to help your hands glide over your breasts without sticking, but still maintaining enough resistance to allow deep strokes. Try all or any combination of the following massage strokes:

Sternum Stroke. With fingers together and hands slightly cupped, place your hands over your breasts at the heart level, letting your fingers touch at the center of the breastbone (sternum). Using moderate pressure, draw your fingers toward your palms. When your fingers touch your palms, move your hands up about a ½ inch and repeat the stroke, and so on all the way up to the collarbone. Repeat.

Nipple Stroke. Place the fingers of both hands on either side of one nipple and stroke from the nipple to the underarm with one hand and to the breastbone with the other. Move your hands around the nipple, stroking outward in all directions, like the spokes of a wheel.

Underarm Stroke. Reach across to one underarm with fingers together and hand cupped and stroke with moderate pressure toward your breast. Move your fingers down (away from the underarm) about an inch and repeat the stroke. Continue until your hand is underneath the breast. Now, go back up to the underarm and make circles all around this lymph-rich area with the flat of your hand. Massage the other side in the same manner. Repeat several times.

Merry-Go-Round Stroke. Cup your breast in your hands and slowly and gently move it in circles in all directions.

Heart Stroke. With fingers together and hands cupped, place your hands over your breasts at heart level, letting your fingers touch at the breastbone. Slide your hands up over your breasts and around the sides until they meet together underneath (make a heart). Repeat.

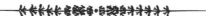

Breast Massage Oils, Balms and Creams

The following formulas are ideal for breast massage. They contain herbal-infused and essential oils that increase lymphatic circulation, as well as nourishing substances that soften and lubricate the skin. You can also use a simple carrier oil, such as coconut or olive oil, or another cream or balm offered elsewhere in the book, as long as it glides well and is not sticky. Some good choices are Calendula Cream, Comfrey Salve (Loose Version), Plantain Coconut Balm or Skin Soothe Balm. The following choice formulas have been created especially for the breasts:

Sage Blue's Breast Balm ALL

This balm contains herbal-infused oils that are gentle, soothing and effective lymphatic movers. It must be made in the spring or summer, when the required flowers are in bloom. Breast Balm is available ready-made from Wolf Howl Herbals (see Resources).

¼ cup violet blossom-infused olive oil (helps decongest lymph system)

1 cup dandelion blossom-infused olive oil (penetrates deeply with its golden magic)

½ cup red clover blossom-infused olive oil (inhibits the spread of cancer)

½ cup calendula blossom-infused olive oil (lymphatic cleanser; reduces swollen glands)

4 oz. beeswax

1 tablespoon vitamin E

½ teaspoon tangerine essential oil (decongests the lymphatic system)

½ teaspoon sandalwood essential oil (supports the lymphatic system)

To make herbal-infused oils according to Sage Blue's method: Fill jars with the freshly picked blossoms (use a different jar for each type) and cover with cold pressed olive oil. The violet blossoms should be placed in the jar whole. Pick dandelion blossoms at mid-morning and remove all the green parts before placing in the jar. Pick vibrant, red clover blossoms just as soon as they are dry from dew, and use them whole. Pick calendula flowers at their peak and break them apart before placing in the jar. Set the jars in the sun for 2–3 days (and nights too, provide for moon energy). Several times during the day, open the jar and wipe off any moisture condensation from the inside of the lid with a paper towel. Strain the oil and squeeze the flowers to get the last bit of oil. Store in the refrigerator until you are ready to prepare the balm.

Follow Directions for Salves and Balms. When the beeswax has thoroughly melted remove the heat-proof cup from the hot-water bath. Add the vitamin E along with the essential oils, stirring them in. Quickly pour the mixture into a wide-mouth jar and cap with a tight-fitting lid. When completely cooled, it is ready for use. This balm should be just firm enough to hold a shape and soft enough to dip your finger in easily. Makes 22 oz.

Wendy's Beauty and the Breast Oil   All

This formula uses herbs that support the immune system and lymphatic functioning. It is excellent for lymphatic circulation and helps alleviate pain and swelling of breast tissues. It can also be used for swollen lymph glands elsewhere in the body (Available from "Sweet Melissa Botanicals," see Resources).

Use the following herbs dried and freshly ground: ½ oz. yarrow, ½ oz. calendula, ½ oz. red clover blossoms	1 oz. fresh poke root 5 oz. castor oil 5 oz. olive oil

1. Combine the castor and olive oils.

2. Make herbal-infused oils with each dried herb, using 2½ oz. combination of castor and olive oil, as your menstrum per ½ oz. of herb. Follow Directions for Herbal-Infused oils with Dried Herbs.

3. Make infused poke oil by grinding the fresh poke root with 2½ oz. combination of castor and olive oil and then follow Directions for Herbal-Infused oils with Fresh Herbs.

4. Allow these oils to steep or infuse on a source of heat no greater than 125 degrees, such as a warming tray or radiator. You can strain the oils after 2 weeks. Note that the addition of heat speeds up the oil-infusion process.

5. Combine the strained oils and massage into breasts a few times a week or as needed. Makes about 7 oz. of oil.

Healthful Breast Oil   All

2 oz. almond oil	10 drops ylang-ylang essential oil
1 ½ oz. peanut oil	5 drops fennel essential oil
½ oz. wheat germ oil	5 drops ginger essential oil

Pour almond, peanut and wheat germ oils into a jar, add essential oils drop by drop, cap and shake well. It is ready for use. Makes 4 oz.

Beautiful Breast Cream   All

A rich, soothing cream for nourishing and massaging breasts.

2 oz. jojoba oil	9 oz. distilled water
2 oz. avocado oil	¼ teaspoon geranium egypt essential
2 oz. canola oil	oil or other geranium available
2 oz. coconut oil	¼ teaspoon fennel essential oil
1 oz. shea butter	40 drops ylang-ylang essential oil
1 oz. beeswax	

Follow Directions for Creams. Makes 19 oz.

PREGNANCY AND BIRTH

Pregnancy and childbirth place incredible demands on women's bodies, and the rigors of these processes stand as a testament to our strength and resiliency. There are a number of ways that we can gently and naturally support our bodies through the pregnancy and childbirth experiences, in order to ease some of its stresses and strains.

As the skin stretches and expands to accommodate your growing baby, you may need extra help in keeping it supple and elastic to prevent tearing, scarring and stretch marks. Eating generous amounts of skin-nourishing nutrients — appropriate oils and fats in particular — will help to keep the skin elastic from the inside out, preventing or minimizing stretch marks. You can also apply nourishing and emollient substances to the skin to reduce or prevent scarring. I always believed that stretch marks were badges of motherhood, and therefore desirable. So when I was pregnant with my son I applied nothing to my skin. This, combined with my rather spartan vegan diet, which included very little fat and virtually no animal products, resulted in my developing the marks of a mother. Stretch marks, which result from the skin's tearing as it is stretched, tend to happen in the last month of pregnancy — all of mine occurred in my last three overdue weeks. I do not wish to promote the idea here that stretch marks are undesirable, but only that women should have the choice of being scarred or not. Although I might make a different choice if I were pregnant for the first time today, at this point I'm happy to bear the marks of motherhood.

Emollients for preventing or minimizing stretch marks, such as oils, balms and creams, should be applied daily to the abdominal skin, breasts, buttocks and thighs. Although the majority of stretching occurs in the latter part of a pregnancy, it can help to nourish and lubricate these areas with topical emollients in the earlier stages as well, particularly if you are prone to dry skin. Note that pregnant women should avoid using scented products, even those scented with natural essential oils. This is because essential oils are absorbed into the skin and can cross the placental barrier. Some essential oils, such as pennyroyal, can actually bring on a miscarriage. Although most essential oils do not have such dramatic effects, all are highly concentrated and powerful. If essential oils are used they should be added in very diluted amounts, 2–5 drops per 1 oz. of oil, balm or cream. If you do choose to use essential oils during pregnancy, please proceed with extreme caution.

Belly Oils, Balms and Creams

Choose from rich carrier oils, such as jojoba, peanut, olive or avocado, using them alone or in combination to massage the abdominal skin surface, breast, thighs and buttocks. See the Ingredients chapter for further information about the different carrier oils. You may also want to try any of the following formulas:

Smooth Belly Combo
All/Dry

A rich, nourishing oil to prevent stretch marks, apply daily to the abdominal skin surface, breasts, buttocks and thighs.

4 oz. jojoba oil   4 oz. almond oil
4 oz. avocado oil

Pour oils into a jar, cap and shake. It is ready to use. Makes 12 oz.

Creamy Belly Balm
All/Dry

A solid oil for rich nourishment and emolliency, excellent for preventing stretch marks.

2 oz. jojoba oil   3 tablespoons (1½ oz.) olive oil
2 oz. coconut oil   1 oz. beeswax
2 oz. shea butter

Pour liquid oils into a heat-proof measuring cup and add the shea butter and coconut oil, measuring after each addition. Melt, break or grate beeswax into small pieces and add to the oil mixture, enough to bring the level of the measuring cup up 1 oz. Place the measuring cup in a hot-water bath and while stirring allow everything to melt and become a uniform liquid free of lumps and clumps. When all the ingredients have melted and thoroughly combined, pour the liquid into a wide-mouth jar, let cool undisturbed and cap when solidified. It is now ready to use. Makes 8½ oz.

Variation: You can use an herbal-infused olive oil made with calendula, comfrey or other herb of choice in place of the plain olive oil.

Skin Revival Cream
All

This cream, mentioned throughout the book for its skin-nourishing and reparative properties, is also excellent for preventing stretch marks. Many women have used this cream successfully to prevent stretch marks by applying it every day during their pregnancy. When you make the cream for this purpose, omit the essential oils in the original recipe (see formula pp. 29–30)

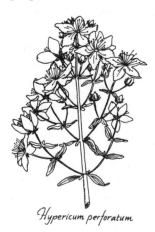

Hypericum perforatum

Birthing Recipes

Perineal Emollients. Massaging and lubricating the perineum with nourishing emollients before and during labor helps to prevent perineal tears and encourages healthy tissue so that this sensitive area can deal with the extreme stretching required of it during birth. When massaging the perineum during labor, you may find warming the oil to be comforting and helpful in stretching the skin. To warm the oil, place it in a jar or heat-proof cup in a hot-water bath until it reaches the desired temperature. You can choose a rich carrier oil, such as olive, jojoba or avocado, or some of the suggestions that follow.

Wheat Germ Oil   ALL

This oil is what my midwife suggested to use for perineal massage, and so every time I smell it I am brought back to the intense, exhilarating and deep feeling of birthing. It is a good choice for perineal massage, as it contains a significant amount of vitamin E and nourishes the skin, helping to make it elastic and strong for the stretching required when the baby's head emerges.

St. Johnswort Oil   ALL

This is another frequently used oil for perineal massage. Its anti-inflammatory and pain-relieving properties are very helpful during and after labor.

> **St. Johnswort fresh flowers and buds**
> **cold pressed olive oil**

Follow Directions for Herbal-Infused Oils with Fresh Herbs. Yield varies.

Perineum Oil Combo

A mixture of rich and reparative oils to soften and stretch the perineum.

> **4 oz. comfrey-infused olive oil (see**   **(see Luscious Lotion p. 29.)**
>   **Comfrey Salve/Loose Version p. 36)**   **1 oz. wheat germ oil**
> **2 oz. St. Johnswort-infused olive oil**

Pour oils in a jar, cap and shake. It is ready to use. Massage into the perineum throughout pregnancy and during labor. Makes 7 oz.

PERINEAL TEARS. If you do experience perineal tearing during labor, here are some formulas and procedures that can soothe the soreness and facilitate the healing process.

BASIC SITZ BATH. Sitz baths are excellent for soothing and healing perineal tears. To make a sitz bath find a tub sized to fit your whole pelvic area, big enough to comfortably sit in and deep enough to submerge your pelvic area up to the belly button. I found a plastic bucket 20 inches in diameter and 10 inches high in my local hardware store that was intended to be used for hand-washing clothes, and it was a perfect fit for my size. I suggest this as the minimum-size tub for sitz baths. Partially fill tub with water and add herbal infusion and other reparative substances. Sit in the bath for a minimum of 20 minutes. Sitz baths are also helpful for hemorrhoids, which often occur during pregnancy.

Herbal Blend Sitz Bath for Perineal Tears   ALL/DAMAGED

This blend contains antimicrobial and cell-proliferative herbs that help heal and soothe tears and irritations.

> **1 handful freshly dried yarrow**   **1 handful dried comfrey root**
> **1 handful dried calendula blossoms**   **64 oz. water**
> **1 handful dried comfrey leaves**

Make herbal infusion with herbs and water. Warm infusion and add to the sitz bath, sit in the bath for 20 minutes and repeat 1 or 2 times daily. You don't have to strain the herbs out of the infusion if you can discard the sitz bath liquid into the earth or compost pile so your drains will not be clogged. Makes enough for 1 sitz bath.

Perineal Healing Oil   ALL/DAMAGED

    1 oz. comfrey-infused olive oil (see   5 drops lavender essential oil
      Comfrey Salve/Loose Version p. 36)   4 drops tea tree essential oil
    1 oz. jojoba oil
    1 oz. calendula-infused olive oil (see
      Luscious Lotion p. 29)

Pour oils into a jar and add the essential oils drop by drop, cap and shake. Gently apply oil to the pained and torn area and reapply as needed. Makes 3 oz.

Hemorrhoid Helpers

WITCH HAZEL. Hemorrhoids are one of the most common discomforts that can occur during pregnancy and after childbirth. Witch hazel tincture (see following formula) or distilled witch hazel extract, which can be purchased at a pharmacy, can be used to wipe the anal opening throughout the day and especially after every bowel movement to help shrink hemorrhoids and reduce the associated pain, itchiness and inflammation. Moisten a piece of cotton flannel, a cotton ball or a paper towel with diluted witch hazel tincture or distilled witch hazel extract. Gently place this directly on the anus and allow it to remain there for 20 minutes.

Witch Hazel Tincture   ALL

    Witch hazel green twig and leaf   190 proof grain alcohol (preferred) or
      harvested in early spring   100 proof vodka

Harvest the new green growth of twigs and leaves in early spring and follow procedure for tincturing with fresh herbs. When using this tincture for hemorrhoid application, you may want to dilute it by half with water; otherwise it may sting too much from all the alcohol. Witch hazel tincture contains tannins and other chemical components which make it more astringent and effective than distilled pharmacy-bought witch hazel.

Chamomile Relief   ALL/DAMAGED

The soothing, anti-inflammatory action of chamomile is helpful in easing the pain and reducing the size of hemorrhoids.

    Chamomile tea bag   cup and saucer or small jar with lid
    1–2 oz. very hot water

Place tea bag in cup and cover with very hot water, just enough to saturate it. Place a saucer on top of the cup to prevent the evaporation of the herb's volatile oils. Let tea bag cool to body temperature and apply to anal opening, leaving on for 20 minutes. Makes enough for 1 application.

Variations: You can use yarrow, arnica, sage or white oak bark in place of chamomile. If using loose herbs you may want to grind them (especially the oak bark) and pour very hot water over them, just enough to saturate them, so they begin to release their properties. If using loose herbs, or to reinforce a tea bag, place wet herbs or tea bag in small muslin sack or wrap in thin porous cloth before applying.

Fresh Poultices ALL/DAMAGED

Fresh herbs can be mashed up and applied to the anal opening for relief and healing of hemorrhoids.

> **A small handful of yarrow, plantain or violet leaves**

Keep fresh herb poultice in place for 20 minutes. This procedure can be messy, so you may want to sit on an old towel or cloth. See Botanicals section for other herbs that are soothing and astringent for making fresh poultices.

Hemorrhoid Balm ALL/DAMAGED

A soothing and astringent balm. Apply after wiping a bowel movement and as needed.

> 1 oz. yarrow-infused olive oil
> 1 oz. yellow dock root-infused olive oil
> 1 oz. plantain-infused olive oil (see Plantain Coconut Balm p. 86)
>
> ½ oz. shea butter
> 1 oz. beeswax
> 20 drops thuja essential oil

Make herbal-infused oils and then follow Directions for Salves and Balms. Makes 4 ½ oz.

Note: To make yarrow-infused olive oil, use 2 oz. of yarrow flowering tops, freshly dried and coarsely ground, and 10 oz. of cold pressed olive oil. Then follow Directions for Herbal-Infused Oils with Dried Herbs. Yields about 7 oz. of oil. Or you can use fresh yarrow flowering tops and follow Directions for Herbal-Infused Oils with Fresh Herbs.

To make yellow dock root-infused olive oil, use 3 oz. of yellow dock root, freshly dried and coarsely ground, and 12 oz. of olive oil. Then proceed to Directions for Herbal-Infused Oil with Dried Herbs. Yields about 8 oz. of oil.

LACTATION

BASIC NIPPLE EMOLLIENT. The experience of breast-feeding a new baby, though one of the most wonderful and fulfilling experiences of motherhood, can also lead to painful, dry, cracked nipples. Between nursings it can be very soothing and healing to apply an emollient oil or formula to the nipples. Use rich carrier oils like jojoba, olive, coconut or shea butter, or choose one of the following formulas. Gently massage the oil or formula into your nipples, ending with a thick application after each nursing. Note that you should not apply these oils when it is near your baby's nursing time.

Throughout the book you will find various oils, creams and balms that are appropriate for massaging into your nipples. Some excellent ones are the All-Purpose Salve (see formula p. 103), Plantain Coconut Balm (see formula p. 86) and Creamy Belly Balm (see formula p. 124). If you are experiencing a lot of pain and inflammation, you may want to try the Relaxation Salve (see formula pp. 92–93). When using a product that contains essential oils, please be sure to gently wash off your nipples prior to nursing to prevent the baby from ingesting these oils. The essential oils are excellent for healing cracked, sore nipples, but not good for babies to ingest.

Comfrey Salve (Loose Version)   ALL/DAMAGED

This salve is the one most widely used for sore, cracked nipples. Note that this formula uses a 1-to-4 beeswax-to-oil ratio to produce a very loose salve, which minimizes friction during application. You may want to make this salve in large quantities, as it is useful for so many other situations.

See formula p. 36.

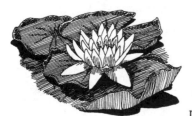

MENOPAUSE

In traditional Earth-based societies, menopause was considered an auspicious time in a woman's life. The changeover from the monthly cycle to the retention of the "wise blood" indicated that a woman was ready to assume her full feminine power. Unfortunately, menopause is essentially treated as an illness in western society, and there is a great deal of secrecy and shame surrounding the process. Instead of being encouraged to step into our power at this time in our lives, we are urged to run to the doctor for estrogen replacement therapy with the first signs of menopause. Is it any wonder? Just think what would happen if we were encouraged to step into our power as we grow older and wiser, instead of being subdued by artificial hormones! There are, of course, certain discomforts associated with menopause, just as there are with menstruation, pregnancy, childbirth and lactation. There are also some natural steps we can take to ease these discomforts without masking or denying the experience — or the power — of menopause.

In physical terms, menopause marks the end of a woman's reproductive cycle. Whether we are conscious of it or not, our adult bodies have been focusing on the exigencies of procreation up until this point. The physical changes that occur during this phase of a woman's life can be quite marked. One of the main changes is that the reduction of hormones during menopause can affect the moisture-retaining capacity of the skin and vaginal tissue. This can lead to dryness and thinning of the skin and vaginal walls, conditions that can be treated with emollient oils or creams. Menopausal discomforts can also be greatly reduced or avoided if appropriate lifestyle choices are made with regard to diet, exercise and sleep. See Resources for further information.

Oils and Creams for Dry, Mature Skin

🐝 *Basic Body Oil* ALL/DRY/MATURE

Choose rich carrier oils, such as olive, jojoba, or avocado for massaging into the skin daily. Many of the creams, oils and balms found throughout this book can be used to help keep mature skin supple. You may want to apply these formulas both morning and night to help the skin retain its moisture. Avoid using soap, except on the hands, feet, underarms and genital area when necessary. When you do use soap, choose a very mild one. A gentle liquid soap diluted to half its strength is also a good choice for mature skin.

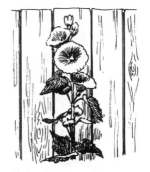

As a rule, when bathing always add a lubricating substance such as jojoba oil, olive oil or cream to the water.

Rich Body Oil ALL/DRY/MATURE

A nourishing, rich and protective oil for dry, mature skin that can also be used on the face.

3 oz. jojoba oil	10 drops sandalwood essential oil
2 oz. avocado oil	10 drops lavender essential oil
1 oz. almond oil	

Pour oils into a jar, add essential oils, cap and shake. Apply to skin after bathing, before night slumber and as needed. Makes 6 oz.

Blue Chamomile Face Cream from Jean's Greens ALL/DRY/MATURE

This cream, created by and for Jean Argus (who is a crone herself), is excellent for keeping mature, dry skin lubricated and nourished. It contains a variety of healing herbs, oils and essential oils designed to protect and revitalize aged skin (see formula pp. 30–31).

Skin Revival ALL/DRY/MATURE/DAMAGED

This cream is an excellent formula for dry, aged skin and can be used as a night cream to keep skin lubricated and protected. Since this cream is very concentrated, begin by applying small amounts and then apply more as needed. Can be used on face and body (see formula pp. 29–30).

Facial Toner for Mature Skin

In general, mature skin tends toward dryness, so any toner applied to it should contain only small amounts of alcohol or vinegar, if any at all. It is best to use water-based toners with other hydrating ingredients like glycerin and aloe. In the first chapter you will find some Hydrating Herbal Toners appropriate for mature skin. The following formula is also well suited for this purpose:

Rejuvenate-Hydrate Face Toner

All/Dry/Mature

A gentle hydrating facial mist for mature skin.

2 tablespoons plus 2 teaspoons comfrey root herbal infusion (preferred)
or distilled water
3 teaspoons aloe vera gel

1 teaspoon glycerin
4 drops lavender essential oil
3 drops fennel essential oil
4 drops sandalwood essential oil

Pour all ingredients into a spray mist bottle, cap and shake well. It is ready to use. Use up within a couple of months, checking for bacterial contamination periodically. Keep in the refrigerator for prolonged storage. Yields 2 oz.

Vaginal Emollients

Vaginal emollients are useful for preventing and soothing inflammation and irritation of the sensitive genital region. They can be applied to the vaginal walls inside the vagina and on the vaginal opening at any time. If your vagina feels dry, protect it with an emollient prior to and during sexual activity. Any of the rich carrier oils, such as coconut, olive or jojoba, are well suited for this purpose. See the Ingredients chapter for information about the specific carrier oils.
You may also wish to try any of the following formulas:

Yoni Oil

Dry

A gentle, nourishing, lubricating and soothing oil for vaginal dryness. The shea butter in this recipe makes this oil thick, creamy and opaque, and semi-solid in cold temperatures.

2 oz. chamomile-infused olive oil (see
Creamy Rose Chamomile Oil pp. 82)
2 oz. violet leaf-infused olive oil (see
Creamy Rose Chamomile Oil p. 82)

3 oz. shea butter
20 drops fennel essential oil

Place chamomile- and violet-infused olive oils in a heat-proof measuring cup and add the shea butter. Place cup in a hot-water bath (a pot filled partly with water and set on a flame). Stir the oil and shea butter until the shea butter has melted. Remove from water bath and pour into a squeeze bottle or wide-mouth jar, add the essential oil and cap the jar. When cool, it is ready to use. Apply the oil inside the vaginal walls and around the vaginal opening as needed. Note: Don't pour the oil into a small-mouth jar, because during the cooler weather the thickness of this oil will keep it from pouring. Makes 7 oz.

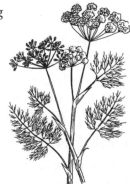

Foeniculum vulgare

Calendula Coconut Balm

DRY/IRRITATED

A soothing balm that combines the lubricating effects of the coconut oil with the healing properties of the calendula.

3 oz. calendula-infused olive oil (see
Luscious Lotion p. 29)

2 oz. coconut oil
1 oz. beeswax

In a heat-proof measuring cup, combine the calendula-infused olive oil with the coconut oil and the beeswax. Place measuring cup in a hot-water bath, stir mixture and allow to melt together and become a uniform liquid free of lumps or clumps. When completely melted, pour oil-wax mixture into a wide-mouth jar. Leave undisturbed to harden and then cap the jar. When completely hard, it is ready for use. Makes 6 oz.
Variations follow:
1. Add 15 drops of lavender essential oil and 15 drops of sandalwood essential oil to increase the soothing effects and give the balm a refreshing and appealing aroma. Add essential oils right after pouring the melted oil-wax mixture into the jar, and cap the jar quickly to prevent evaporation.
2. Replace the calendula-infused oil with another herbal-infused oil such as comfrey, chamomile, violet, etc.

OTHER LUBRICANTS. Other good lubricating choices for vaginal dryness are Comfrey Salve (Loose Version) (see formula p. 36), All-Purpose Salve (see formula p. 103) and Plantain Coconut Balm (see formula p. 86). These balms also help heal vaginal irritations and inflammations or try the following formula.

Itch Relief Oil

DRY/IRRITATED

A lubricating, soothing oil for vaginal dryness accompanied by irritation and itching.

2 oz. mugwort-infused olive oil
2 oz. plantain-infused olive oil (see
Plantain Coconut Balm p. 86)
2 oz. calendula-infused olive oil (see
Luscious Lotion p. 29)

1 oz. jojoba oil
4 drops lavender essential oil
4 drops tea tree essential oil
3 drops chamomile essential
oil

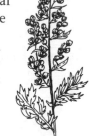

Pour oils into a jar, add essential oils, cap and shake. Gently apply oil on vaginal walls and on vaginal opening. Apply as often as needed and especially before night slumber. Makes 7 oz.

Note: To make mugwort-infused olive oil, use 2 oz. of mugwort flowering tops, freshly dried and coarsely ground, and 10 oz. of cold pressed olive oil. Then follow Directions for Herbal-Infused Oils with Dried Herbs.

Artemesia vulgari

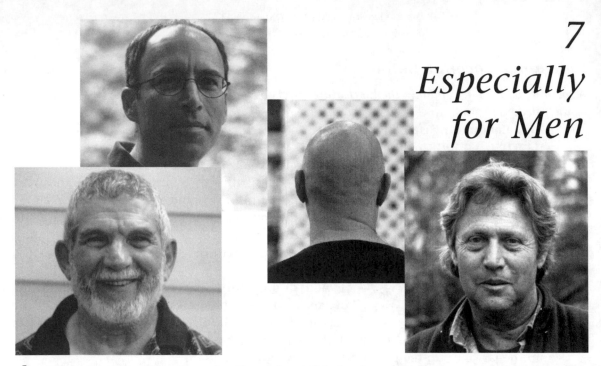

7
Especially for Men

Although most of the formulas throughout this book are for both men and women, this section will focus more specifically on men's needs and preferences. There are specific products designed for men, such as shaving products. However, what tends to make a product suitable for a man is often its scent. In some cases, men and women enjoy wearing the same aroma. Many men are more typically drawn to certain essential oils, as listed in the box below, but they should not feel limited to these. More typically feminine scents, such as floral and fruit scents, can also be added to formulas in varying quantities to produce a wide assortment of aromas to please many men, and women too.

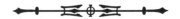

Scents for Men

The aromas most associated with the masculine are woody, spicy and fresh green scents. The essential oils that men are typically drawn to are bay, black pepper, cedarwood, fir, mint, rosemary, sage and sandalwood. Keep in mind that fruit and floral scents can be added in small quantities to produce a multitude of pleasing aromas.

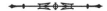

The following shaving formulas provide excellent alternatives to commercial products available on the market. They are made without synthetic chemicals, and are much more gentle on the skin.

Shaving Lotion

Herbal Shaving Lotion

ALL

This mild soap is excellent for shaving. It provides glide for smooth shaving and protects the skin from drying out, keeping it supple and soft.

Use the following dried and crushed
herbs: 2 teaspoons comfrey root,
2 teaspoons marshmallow root
1 cup water

½ teaspoon coconut oil
¼ teaspoon jojoba oil
3 oz. castile soap
60 drops rosemary essential oil

Make an infusion with herbs and water, let steep for 8 hours or overnight and strain. Gently reheat infusion to a warm temperature and add coconut oil. Stir until the coconut oil has melted. Take off heat and add liquid castile soap and jojoba oil. Pour into jar or squeeze bottle, add essential oil, cap and shake. It is ready for use. Shake prior to each application. Store in the refrigerator if not used up within a few weeks. Makes about 9 oz.

Variation: You can use plain water in place of the herbal infusion, although the resulting lotion will be less nourishing and protective to the skin. For a more moisturizing lotion, increase the coconut and jojoba oils.

Aftershave

Aftershaves are refreshing and antiseptic facial astringents that help refine and tighten the pores. They are made primarily with alcohol and water, and often contain significant amounts of essential oils which make them more like perfumes and colognes. Aftershaves are often used to perfume oneself as the final step in the shaving ritual. Although they generally have a drying effect, they can be helpful in soothing skin irritated by the shaving process. I've added glycerin and aloe to the formulas to offset the drying effect of the alcohol. You can also use less alcohol or replace the alcohol with distilled witch hazel for a less drying effect. Another way to offset the drying effect is to add a teaspoon of aftershave to a pint-size bowl of cold water and splash this mixture onto the face. The following formulas can be placed in spray bottles and misted onto the face, or stored in a blue or amber glass jar (to prevent light from degrading the essential oils) with a well-fitting lid, then applied to the face by hand. Always shake these products before use to redistribute the essential oils. When made with the amount of alcohol indicated in the formulas, these aftershaves are well preserved and require no refrigeration. These formulas also make excellent strong-scented deodorants. For a fragrance-free aftershave, omit the essential oils. However, to maintain a 4-oz. yield, replace the essential oils with 1½ teaspoons of distilled witch hazel, distilled water or herbal infusion. Following are a choice assortment of aftershaves.

Woodland Aftershave

ALL

A refreshing woodland-scented aftershave.

4 tablespoons vodka or brandy
    (80–100 proof)
2 tablespoons herbal infusion of
    choice (preferred) or distilled water
1 tablespoon aloe vera gel
½ teaspoon glycerin

1 teaspoon distilled witch hazel
½ teaspoon fir essential oil
½ teaspoon sandalwood essential oil
24 drops bay essential oil
24 drops black pepper essential oil

Pour ingredients into a 4-oz. spray mist bottle or other glass jar, cap and shake. It is ready to use. Shake prior to use. Yields 4 oz.

Note: For a less drying effect substitute the 4 tablespoons of vodka and the 2 tablespoons of herbal infusion with 6 tablespoons of distilled witch hazel. Variations follow:

Sage Lavender Aftershave

ALL

A clean smelling aftershave with the fragrant smell of sage and lavender.
Replace essentials oils with ½ teaspoon of sage essential oil, ½ teaspoon of lavender essential oil and 30 drops of cedarwood essential oil.

Lime Mint Aftershave

ALL/OILY

A stimulating and refreshing aftershave with a citrus-mint aroma. It is particularly astringent due to the citrus essential oils and is recommended for oily skin.
Replace essential oils with ½ teaspoon of spearmint or ¼ teaspoon peppermint essential oil, ¼ teaspoon of distilled water, ½ teaspoon of lime essential oil, 20 drops of grapefruit essential oil and 20 drops of orange essential oil.

Calendula Comfrey Aftershave

ALL

This aftershave is more skin-reparative than the others, as it contains the healing properties of calendula and comfrey.

2 tablespoons calendula tincture (see
    formula p. 100)
2 tablespoons comfrey leaf tincture
1 tablespoon distilled water
2 tablespoons aloe vera gel
1 teaspoon distilled witch hazel

½ teaspoon glycerin
1½ teaspoons essential oils of choice
    or if omitting essential oils add an
    additional 1 ½ teaspoons calendula
    tincture

Pour ingredients in a 4-oz. spray mist bottle or other glass jar, cap and shake. It is ready to use. Shake prior to each use. Yields 4 oz.

Note: To make comfrey leaf tincture use either fresh leaves and 100 proof vodka and follow Directions for Alcohol Tinctures Using Fresh Herbs, or use 1 oz. of comfrey leaf, dried, and 4 oz. of 100 proof vodka and follow Directions for Alcohol Tinctures Using Dried Herbs.

Skin Soother

ALL/DRY

Apply to the skin after shaving or when needed to help hydrate, heal and soothe the skin. It does not contain alcohol and is less astringent and more moisturizing than the just-described aftershaves.

Use the following dried herbs: 1
   teaspoon fennel seeds (freshly
   crushed), 1 tablespoon comfrey root
   (freshly crushed), 2 tablespoons
   chamomile, 2 tablespoons
   calendula flowers

8 oz. water
2 oz. plus 1 tablespoon glycerin
1 tablespoon aloe vera gel

Make herbal infusion with herbs, 2 oz. of glycerin and water and let steep for 4–8 hours. Pour 3 oz. of strained infusion, 1 tablespoon of glycerin, and 1 tablespoon of aloe into a jar (preferably a spray mist bottle). Shake gently. Apply after shaving and cleaning the face or as needed, and especially before night slumber. Use up within a couple of months; keep refrigerated and check for bacterial contamination periodically. You will end up with extra infusion, which you can drink or use for a hair rinse or soak. When consuming, don't add sweetener to the infusion, as the presence of the glycerin makes it sweet. Makes 4 oz.

Variation: Add 10 drops of fennel essential oil, 3 drops of chamomile essential oil and 18 drops of sandalwood essential oil to toner. The essential oils, although not necessary, add an appealing scent to the toner, help preserve it and amplify the hydrating and skin-reparative effects.

Body Powders

Body powders act as antiperspirants and deodorants. They can also soothe minor skin irritations. Clay, cornstarch, arrowroot powder or baking soda can either be used alone as absorbent body powders or as a base for deodorizing powder formulas. Use spice shakers or powder canisters for sprinkling on body powders, or apply by hand.

Sage Baking Soda Body Powder   ALL

A refreshing body powder with strong deodorizing action. This recipe makes a small amount. If you like the formula, simply multiply the ingredients for a larger yield.

4 drops sage essential oil
2 drops tea tree essential oil

1 drop black pepper essential oil
2 teaspoons baking soda

Put baking soda in a small jar, add essential oils and stir them in thoroughly. Cap jar and shake to continue mixing. Apply powder to underarms and wherever needed. To store powder, cap jar with a tight fitting lid. Makes enough for 2 applications.

Variations: You can replace the baking powder with cornstarch or arrowroot powder.

Woodland Body Powder   ALL

An absorbent and deodorizing body powder that has an appealing woodsy aroma.

1 cup clay
½ cup baking soda
½ cup arrowroot powder
¼ cup slippery elm powder
¾ teaspoon sandalwood essential oil

½ teaspoon fir essential oil
¼ teaspoon tea tree essential oil
22 drops black pepper essential oil
20 drops bay essential oil

Place clay, baking soda, arrowroot powder and slippery elm powder into a jar, mix the powders thoroughly and add the essential oils a little at a time while stirring them in. Be sure to evenly distribute the essential oils in the powder, breaking up any clumps that the essential oil makes with the powder. Cap and shake the jar vigorously to continue mixing. Sprinkle under arms and wherever needed. Makes about 2¼ cups.

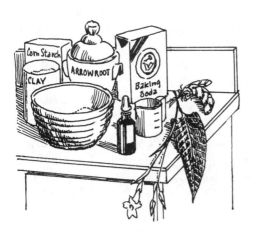

Jock Itch Remedies

Jock itch is the common name for an irritation caused by a fungus named *tinea cruris*. This fungal skin condition is characterized by an itchy, irritated rash that typically appears around the groin. Several of the antifungal powders, creams and balms mentioned throughout this book can be used for it, such as the Antifungal Healing Foot Oil, Black Walnut and Tea Tree Salve, Healing Foot Cream, Black Walnut Chaparral Foot Cream and Happy Feet Powder. You can also try the following formulas made from herbs and essential oils with healing and strong antifungal properties.

Jock Relief Powder
FUNGAL/IRRITATED

A refreshing and soothing powder formulated to keep skin dry and free of bacteria that cause odor and fungal infection. The herbal ingredients are excellent antifungal, antimicrobial disinfectants.

Use the following dried herbs:
1 table spoon slippery elm powder,
2 tablespoons calendula blossoms,
1 tablespoon goldenseal powder,
1 tablespoon myrrh powder,
2 tablespoons black walnut hull powder, 3 tablespoons chaparral,
2 tablespoons yarrow
1 cup clay (bentonite or French green)

¼ cup baking soda
¼ cup cornstarch or arrowroot powder
30 drops tea tree essential oil
30 drops rosemary essential oil
20 drops sage essential oil
20 drops wintergreen essential oil
20 drops lavender essential oil
20 drops chamomile essential oil

Grind the chaparral, calendula and yarrow into a powder and thoroughly mix all the ingredients together. Add the essential oils a little at a time and stir them in thoroughly. Place in an airtight container or shaker, cap tightly and shake to continue mixing ingredients. Sprinkle onto skin as often as needed. Makes about 2¼ cups.

Fungal Free Cream
FUNGAL

This is a strong-scented antifungal cream that relies on the essential oils for its medicinal properties. It is both soothing and cleansing. This is a very stable cream, lasting 6 months to a year outside refrigeration.

6 oz. expeller pressed canola oil
3 oz. coconut oil
1 oz. beeswax
¼ teaspoon lavender essential oil
¼ teaspoon thuja essential oil

40 drops tea tree essential oil
½ teaspoon wintergreen essential oil
¼ teaspoon chamomile essential oil
9 oz. distilled water

Follow Directions for Creams. Apply as often as needed. Makes 19 oz.

Variation: For a stronger antifungal effect replace the canola oil with black walnut hull-infused olive oil (see Antifungal Healing Oil p. 113) or chaparral-infused olive oil.

Note: To make chaparral-infused olive oil, use 3 oz. of chaparral, dried and coarsely ground, and 12 oz. of cold pressed olive oil. Then follow Directions for Herbal-Infused Oils with Dried Herbs. Yield about 9 oz. of oil.

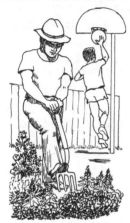

Liquid Deodorants

By combining alcohol, witch hazel, distilled water and essential oils, you can create effective and appealing deodorants, which are among the easiest and most practical formulas to make. For the strongest cleansing effect, apply deodorant onto a cotton swab or cloth and rub well over the entire underarm region. Although less cleansing, you can also put the deodorant into a spray bottle and mist the underarms. These formulas do not require refrigeration and have a shelf life of about a year. Remember to shake deodorant before each application. The following formulas are potent and refreshing.

Sage Fir Deodorant   ALL

This deodorant is an excellent choice both for men and women. It combines the disinfecting and deodorizing effects of the alcohol with the essential oils. It also offers a refreshingly pleasant aroma.

¼ cup 80 proof vodka
¼ cup distilled water
10 drops fir essential oil
10 drops sage essential oil

5 drops tea tree essential oil
6 drops black pepper essential oil
6 drops bay essential oil

Pour the vodka and the water into a jar, drop in the essential oils, cap and shake. Apply deodorant mixture onto a cotton swab or cloth and rub into underarms for cleaning and neutralizing body odor. You can also put the deodorant into a spray bottle and mist underarms. Shake well before each use. Makes 4 oz.

Variations: If the deodorant feels too drying add ¼–½ teaspoon of vegetable glycerin.

Distinctive Deodorant   ALL

This is an effective antimicrobial deodorant for strong body odor.

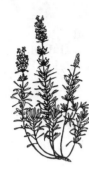

2 oz. distilled witch hazel
2 oz. vodka
½ teaspoon glycerin
24 drops tea tree oil

10 drops rosemary essential oil
6 drops cedarwood essential oil
4 drops lime essential oil
4 drops lavender essential oil

Pour the witch hazel, vodka and glycerin into a jar and drop in the essential oils. Cap and shake the jar. Apply deodorant mixture onto a cotton swab or cloth and rub and wipe underarms. You can also put the deodorant into a spray mist bottle and spray underarms. Shake well before each use. Yields 4 oz.

Body Emollients

In this section you will find oils, creams and balms that soften and soothe the skin with aromas specifically geared to men. Any of the emollients mentioned elsewhere in the book can also be used by men and feel free to adapt the essential oils in a formula found elsewhere in the book to give it more masculine appeal.

BODY OILS. The following formulas are made with essential oils diluted in a carrier oil base. The subtle fragrance and emollient effects of the oils make them suitable for applying directly to the skin after a shower or whenever the skin needs some lubrication. These oils are also great for massage. They can even be added to a bath for an aromatic treat while softening and moisturizing the skin.

Spring Green Oil for Men   ALL

A fresh-smelling oil for bath and massage that moisturizes the skin.

40 drops basil essential oil
40 drops black pepper essential oil
12 drops sage essential oil

12 drops nutmeg essential oil
4 oz. almond oil or other carrier oil of choice

Pour carrier oils into a jar and add the essential oils drop by drop. Cap jar with a tight-fitting lid and shake well. The oil is ready to use. Use 1–2 teaspoons of oil per bath. Makes 4 oz.

Oriental Express Body Oil for Men   ALL/DRY

A nourishing, refreshing and masculine-smelling blend that can be used for massage, as a bath oil or as a lubricating skin treat.

2 oz. canola oil
1 oz. peanut oil
1 tablespoon jojoba oil
1 tablespoon olive oil
30 drops fir essential oil

30 drops sandalwood essential oil
30 drops black pepper essential oil
9 drops sage essential oil
12 drops cedarwood essential oil
5 drops patchouli essential oil

Pour carrier oils into a jar and add the essential oils drop by drop. Cap jar with a tight-fitting lid and shake well. The oil is ready to use. Use 1–2 teaspoons of oil per bath. Makes 4 oz.

MUSCLE SHINE BODY EMOLLIENT. Men, and some women too, are particularly fond of their muscles and often enjoy coating them with a rich emollient that makes their skin look slick and shiny and accentuates their muscular contours. Most oils and butters can be used for this purpose. The following formula produces a thick creamy oil, that does the job exceptionally well and is also an effective emollient for the skin. During the colder months the oil will thicken into a semsolid oil. This formula also makes a nice hair conditioner.

Muscle Shine ALL/DRY

2 oz. castor oil	1 oz. lecithin
3 oz. coconut oil	1 oz. jojoba oil

Pour oils and lecithin into a heat-proof measuring cup and place in a hot-water bath. Heat until the coconut oil has completely melted. Stir the oils well during the cooling process but pour into a squeeze bottle or a wide-mouth jar before it completely cools. Yields 7 oz. of oil.

Variations: Add essential oils to create a more pleasing aroma. For a refreshing pick-me-up scent, add 50 drops of peppermint essential oil. For an inviting aroma add 50 drops of sandalwood essential oil, 20 drops of fir essential oil and 5 drops of sage essential oil. Add essential oils after the mixture has been poured into a jar. Quickly cap the jar to prevent the essential oil from evaporating.

MOISTURIZING CREAMS FOR MEN. These creams offer hydration and lubrication that help restore skin to a soft and supple condition. Apply them after shaving to keep skin from becoming dry and chapped. When making a cream, you are emulsifying water and oil to yield a product that is lighter and more quickly absorbed than pure oils or balms. Keep in mind that creams are a little tricky to make, so it is important to follow the directions closely, making certain to measure the ingredients carefully. When making the following formulas, refer to Directions for Creams on pp. 225–226.

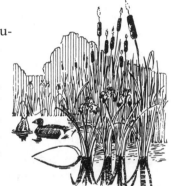

Sandalwood Black Pepper Skin Delight ALL/DRY

This nourishing and hydrating moisturizing formula may be used for the face and body for most skin types. It is excellent to apply after shaving or as needed. It has an appealing, refreshing aroma associated with the masculine but often enjoyed by women too.

3 oz. coconut oil	1½ teaspoons sandalwood essential oil
3 oz. almond oil	15 drops black pepper essential oil
3 oz. canola oil	10 drops tangerine essential oil
1 oz. beeswax	8 drops sage essential oil
9 oz. distilled water	15 drops rosemary essential oil

Proceed to Directions for Creams. Yields 19 oz.

Skin Rejuvenation Cream for Men   ALL/DRY/IRRITATED

A rich cream for dry and irritated skin. Good to use on eczematic, inflamed and aged skin, this cream contains lavender and chamomile essential oils for their anti-inflammatory properties.

2 oz. coconut oil
1 oz. shea butter   **2 teaspoons lecithin**
1 oz. plus 1 tablespoon jojoba oil   **9 oz. distilled water**
1 oz. peanut oil   **2 teaspoons glycerin**
1 oz. comfrey root-infused olive oil   **7 drops lavender essential oil**
  (see Comfrey Comfort p. 82)   **5 drops blue chamomile essential oil**
2 oz. calendula-infused olive oil (see   **20 drops cedarwood essential oil**
  Luscious Lotion p. 29)   **15 drops fir essential oil**
1 tablespoon wheat germ oil   **5 drops fennel essential oil**
½ oz. beeswax

Note: Less beeswax is used in this recipe than in the Basic Cream Formula. The addition of lecithin helps emulsify creams and therefore can be used to replace a portion of the beeswax within a cream formula. Also, when making Skin Rejuvenation Cream, add the lecithin to the liquid oil component and the glycerin to the water component. This cream is very thick and rich and is harder to pour than other creams, so you will need to scoop it out.

Proceed to Directions for Creams. Yields 19 oz.

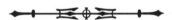

About Balding

Men tend to go bald more than women. The most common form of balding in men is an inherited trait, and many consider it to be an undesirable event when their hair begins to thin out. I am uncertain whether anything can be done about genetic balding. However, eating well, drinking plenty of water and getting sufficient exercise and rest all contribute to a healthy body, and to healthy head of hair. Reducing stress is also important for optimal health, and may play a role in preventing hair loss. Massaging the scalp feels great and increases circulation, which may help reduce the loss of hair and even stimulate its growth. If you experience irreversible hair loss, then try loving your baldness — many people find a bald head attractive and distinguished. Some men even highlight their bald scalps with oils or pomades.

Try using Rosemary Olive Hair Oil, Sage Rosemary and Thyme Hair Oil or Herbal Deluxe Hair Pomade, all found in chapter 3, to massage the scalp. For the general health of your hair and scalp, and especially when balding is a concern, it is wise to use natural hair products to eliminate synthetic and harsh chemicals from your hair care routine, since these may contribute to hair loss. See chapter 3 for alternatives to commercial hair products.

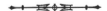

Bald Head Balm

ALL/DRY/BALD

Apply this rich and refreshing balm to the scalp as often as desired to keep skin well lubricated and nourished.

1 oz. coconut oil
1 oz. shea butter
1 oz. beeswax
2 oz. jojoba oil
1½ oz. herbal-infused oil of choice
  (such as nettle, comfrey or burdock)
  or plain olive oil

½ teaspoon rosemary essential oil
¼ teaspoon sage essential oil
½ teaspoon sandalwood essential oil

Combine ingredients, except essential oils, in a heat-proof measuring cup and place in a hot-water bath over medium-high heat. Stir until the oils, butter and wax melt into a uniform liquid, free of lumps. When it is completely melted, pour mixture into a wide-mouth jar, add essential oils and cap immediately to prevent them from evaporating. When solidified it is read for use. Makes about 7 oz.

Spirited Perfumes and Colognes

These perfumes and colognes are made by combining alcohol, water and essential oils. The fragrance derives from the essential oils. Perfumes are more concentrated and applied in smaller quantities than colognes. Colognes are diluted perfumes, containing more water and less essential oil than perfumes. Perfumes and colognes are often worn to create persona. They can make the wearer feel special, and people frequently use them to lift their spirits or alter their mood. The act of perfuming oneself is a self-healing ritual currently referred to as aromatherapy. It is fun to make customized scents that truly suit a person's taste. Men often shy away from using perfumes, but when created according to individual preferences they can be greatly enjoyed. Perfumes and colognes are easy to make, and take just a few minutes to prepare. You may want to let the perfume or cologne sit for a few weeks to allow the scent to fully blend and mature, as many perfumists suggest. Perfumes and colognes are naturally well preserved by the high alcohol and essential oil content. However, they should be kept out of direct light and heat, and stored in colored glass if possible. Shaking well before each use is important in 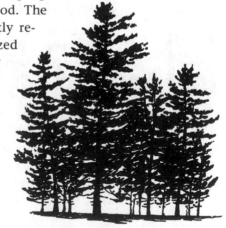 order to redistribute the essential oils. In the following section you will find perfume and cologne formulas, in addition to a basic formula that allows you to create your own custom blends. Refer to the Essential Oils section in the Ingredients chapter as you begin to blend your own scents.

Basic Perfume Formula

Use this basic formula to create various perfumes. Play around with the essential oil component to produce different aromatic results.

In parts: 7 parts 190 proof grain
　alcohol
1 part distilled water
2 parts essential oil
In spoon measurements: 1 tablespoon
　190 proof grain alcohol
½ teaspoon distilled water

1 teaspoon essential oil
To make an ounce of perfume:
　1 tablespoon plus 1 teaspoon
　190 proof grain alcohol
　¾ teaspoon distilled water
　1¼ teaspoons of essential oils

Using vodka: If you can't find 190 proof grain alcohol, use the highest-proof vodka you can find and replace the alcohol and water in the above formulas with it.

Combine ingredients in a glass jar (preferably colored), cap and shake. Use right away or let the perfume sit for a few weeks to allow the scent to fully blend and mature.

Note: Remember that essential oils' odor intensities vary considerably and this will affect how much of them you'll use. For example, sandalwood essential oil is a mild base note that needs to be used in much higher quantities than other essential oils. So in the following Spiced Perfume formula, there is a total of 2 teaspoons of essential oil, a greater quantity than usual because we want the sandalwood aroma to be noticed.

Spiced Perfume for Men

An intriguing, smooth and subtle scent.

1 tablespoon plus ½
　teaspoon 190
　proof grain alcohol
½ teaspoon
　distilled water
1¼ teaspoons sandal-
　wood essential oil

½ teaspoon black pepper essential oil
5 drops cinnamon essential oil
20 drops basil essential oil
15 drops nutmeg essential oil
10 drops cedarwood essential oil

Pour alcohol, water and essential oils into a 1-oz. amber glass jar, cap and shake. It is ready for use, although, as many perfumists suggest, you may want to let the perfume sit for a few weeks to allow the scent to fully blend and mature. Shake bottle and apply a small dab of perfume here and there as desired. It is very concentrated, so use sparingly. Makes 1 oz.

Variations: If you can't find 190 proof grain alcohol, substitute for the alcohol and water with 1 tablespoon plus 1 teaspoon of vodka or brandy. To make the perfume in an oil base, substitute for the alcohol and water with grapeseed oil.

Colognes. As mentioned earlier, colognes are essentially diluted perfumes. They contain more water and less essential oil than perfumes; hence, they can be applied more liberally. However, keep in mind that they still contain a high concentration of essential oils and a significant amount of alcohol, which can be drying and irritating to the skin if applied in too great a quantity. You can either splash on colognes or keep them in a spray mist bottle. Colognes can also be misted into the air and onto upholstered furniture to refresh and scent a room.

Basic Cologne Formula ALL

Use this basic formula to invent your own colognes by employing various essential oils, singly and in different combinations and proportions.

In parts: 7 parts 190 proof grain alcohol
3 parts water
½ part essential oils

In spoon measurements: 2 tablespoons plus 1 teaspoon 190 proof grain alcohol
1 tablespoon distilled water
½ teaspoon essential oil

Combine ingredients in a glass jar (preferably colored), cap and shake. Use as is or let the cologne sit for a few weeks to allow the scent to fully blend and mature.

Exotic Express Cologne ALL

An exotic, woody scent.

7 tablespoons 190 proof grain alcohol
3 tablespoons distilled water
60 drops fir essential oil
60 drops sandalwood essential oil

60 drops black pepper essential oil
18 drops sage essential oil
24 drops cedarwood essential oil
10 drops patchouli essential oil

Combine ingredients in a glass jar (preferably blue or amber) and cap with a tight-fitting lid. Shake well and it is ready to use, although, as many perfumists suggest, you may want to let the cologne sit for a couple of weeks to allow the scent to fully blend and mature. Apply cologne here and there as desired or place in a spray bottle and mist onto body and clothing. The colognes can also be sprayed around the room or onto upholstered furniture to create an exotic ambiance. Makes about 5 oz.

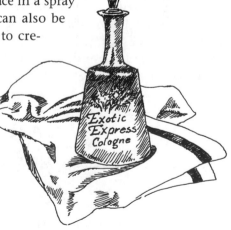

Variation: If you can't find 190 proof grain alcohol, use 10 tablespoons of vodka to replace the alcohol and water.

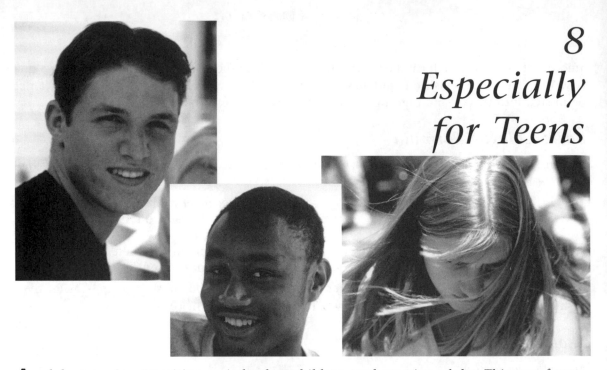

8
Especially for Teens

A dolescence is a transition period, when children are becoming adults. This transformation can be very exciting as new horizons open and new feelings emerge. During this time the body produces hormones to facilitate the passage from childhood into adulthood. In some adolescents these hormonal changes can also cause pimpling and acne. While various topical applications like the ones offered here can help to clear up these conditions, it is extremely important to consider diet and lifestyle changes at this time. Internal herbal support may also be very helpful in dealing with teenaged skin. Below you will find a regimen that provides a natural approach to caring for acne-prone skin. Bear in mind that if adolescent skin is not plagued with acne or breakouts, it does not require special care other than the usual gentle cleansing and nourishing programs found in the first chapter.

The hormonal changes of adolescence can sometimes cause strong body odor. This chapter also offers some natural deodorant formulas designed for teenagers of both sexes. You can also refer to Whole Body Treatments chapter.

CARE OF ACNED SKIN

Breaking Out

Very few teens seem to make it to adulthood without an occasional breakout or pimple attack. When skin breakouts occur, it is important to resist the urge to squeeze or pick. Picking tends to exacerbate the problem, often leading to unsightly and painful localized infections. The next time you suffer a breakout, try one of the following spot treatments just before going to bed. When you wake up in the morning you will find that the pimples have often shrunk considerably or disappeared altogether.

❦ **Vitamin E Treatment:** Squish a vitamin E capsule and squeeze a little onto your index finger. Gently dab the vitamin E directly onto each pimple, covering completely. Leave on overnight.

❦ **Clay Treatment:** Mix a teaspoon of dried clay with just enough water to yield a stiff, pasty consistency. Dab a spot of clay onto each pimple with your index finger, making sure to cover completely. Leave on overnight.

For added benefits, you may also want to try one of the following formulas from this chapter for spot treatments: Echinacea Oat Scrub, Happy Skin Scrub, or Green Goddess Masque.

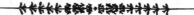

Facial Hot Packs

A facial hot pack offers an excellent way to deeply clean and tone the skin, clearing away dead cells and debris by opening the pores and increasing circulation. A hot pack is one of the best treatments to use for skin affected by pimpling or acne, especially when antimicrobial herbs such as thyme and echinacea are used. This treatment can be done 3 times a week for oily and acne-prone skin. It is most effective to follow up with an appropriate masque or scrub to continue the deep-pore cleansing process. See directions for Facial Hot Packs on p. 7.

You might try an infusion of one of the formulas listed in the Facial Steam section of chapter 1, such as Sweet Fern Citrus Blend, or the Blemish Beautifier Blend found in the section that follows. The formulas given here are also excellent selections.

Pimple Away Pack   ALL/ACNE

32 oz. water   3 drops lavender essential oil
3 drops tea tree essential oil

Follow directions for Facial Hot Pack on p. 7 and drip the essential oils into the water right before applying the pack. Note that the essential oils evaporate quickly, so you may need to add a few more drops of essential oil to the water in the middle of the treatment.

Variation: Replace the tea tree oil with 2 drops of sage essential oil and the lavender with 2 drops of chamomile essential oil.

Sage Rosemary and Thyme   OILY/ACNE

Use the following freshly dried herbs: 32 oz. water
  1 handful sage, ½ handful thyme,   cotton cloth
  ½ handful rosemary

Make herbal infusion with herbs and water and let steep for 8 hours. Follow directions for Facial Hot Packs on p. 7.

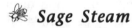

Deep Pore Caress

OILY/ACNE

Use ½ oz. or a palmful of the
following freshly dried herbs:
yarrow, echinacea root (cut),
calendula flowers, chamomile
flowers

32 oz. water
cotton cloth or towel

Make herbal infusion with herbs and water and let steep for 4 hours. Follow directions for Facial Hot Packs on p. 7.

Facial Steams

Steaming is an excellent cleansing technique for acne-prone skin, as it helps open pores and release subdermal toxins. If you have acne or pimply skin you may wish to do a steam 3 times a week. After a steam the pores are wide open, so applying an appropriate masque or scrub is recommended to continue the deep-pore cleansing process.

See Basic Steam Technique on p. 5.

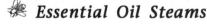

Sage Steam

OILY/ACNE

1 handful sage leaves
16 oz. water

Follow directions for Basic Steam Technique on p. 5. Makes enough for 1 treatment.

Variations: Replace the sage with oregano, yarrow or thyme.

Blemish Beautifier Blend

OILY/ACNE

This exotic-smelling blend contains astringent and antimicrobial herbs to help reduce oil production as it deeply cleanses the pores.

1 handful each of the following dried
herbs: lavender, yarrow, thyme,
calendula blossoms, lemon balm

Combine herbs; use a handful of herbal mixture for each steaming. Follow directions for Basic Steam Technique. Store herbal mixture in a dry, cool place. Makes enough for 5 steams.

Essential Oil Steams

ALL/OILY/ACNE

Some good essential oil choices for acne are lavender, melissa, rosemary, chamomile, lemongrass, tea tree, tangerine and sage.

Place 1–3 drops of essential oil of choice into a bowl that already contains steaming water just before lowering your face over the bowl. Proceed with extra caution when placing your face over the bowl, as the essential oil vapors could irritate your eyes. Note that the steam will carry the essential oils out into the air and dissipate rapidly, so you may need to add a few more drops in the middle of your steam treatment. Follow directions for Basic Steam Technique on p. 5.

Facial Scrubs

These facial scrubs are formulated from dry ingredients that are ground together, moistened and then used to scrub the skin. They contain ingredients that are antimicrobial, astringent and healing to promote a healthy, clear complexion. They gently cleanse and polish, providing excellent exfoliation. Scrubs also help to nourish the skin by stimulating circulation. A scrub is used like a soap-and-water wash, but tends to leave the skin smoother and less stripped of its protective oils. If you generally use soap on your face, you may want to replace it altogether with a scrub, since the latter contains no harsh detergents or artificial scents. Keep in mind that scrubbing too hard can further damage skin that is broken out, so it is important to scrub very gently. Vigorous scrubbing can also make oily skin oilier by stimulating the oil-producing sebaceous glands. Grinding the scrubs to a fine powder will lessen their abrasive and irritating effects. These scrub formulas can also be left on the face and used as facial masques for more sustained cleansing or placed directly on blemishes to clear them up.

The Echinacea Clove Scrub and Rose Blossom Sage Scrub found in the first chapter are excellent formulas for clearing up teenaged skin as well as the following formulas.

Echinacea Oat Scrub   ALL/ACNE

This is a cleansing, healing, soothing scrub for blemished skin.

2 tablespoons dried echinacea root (cut)

1 tablespoon oats (preferably whole oat groat)

1–2 teaspoons water or witch hazel extract

Finely grind the echinacea and oats in a coffee/seed grinder and sift through a fine-mesh strainer, regrinding coarser particles as needed. For a single application, wet 1–2 teaspoons of scrub with water or witch hazel until a pasty consistency is reached and follow the Basic Scrub Technique on p. 9. Or apply directly onto blemishes to help clear them up, leaving on overnight for best results. Makes enough for 3–4 applications.

Variations: You can substitute for the echinacea other herbs such as sage, calendula, yarrow or thyme. And you can replace the oats with rice or other grains.

Happy Skin Scrub   ACNE/OILY

A gentle, healing and cleansing scrub.

½ cup oats
½ cup brown rice
¼ cup comfrey leaf
¼ cup oregano
⅛ cup anise seed
½ cup calendula

¼ cup myrrh
1½ cups clay
1 drops tea tree essential oil
1 drop lavender essential oil
1–2 teaspoons water or witch hazel extract

Using a blender, grind all ingredients except the clay and myrrh into a powder. Sift through a fine-mesh strainer for a uniform consistency and to ensure that all the ingredients have been properly pulverized. Add the clay and myrrh and mix thoroughly. Store in an air-tight container in the refrigerator.

To use scrub place 1–2 teaspoons of the formula into a small bowl and slowly stir in 1–2 teaspoons of witch hazel or water until it reaches a pasty consistency. Add the essential oils, stir in well and follow the Basic Scrub Technique on p. 9. Or apply directly onto blemishes to help clear them up, leaving on overnight for best results. Yields 3 cups.

Variations: You can wet the scrub with equal parts water and tincture of echinacea or goldenseal.

Facial Masques

For pimply or acne-prone skin it is beneficial to use masques 3 times a week. Ideally, masques should be applied following a steam or Facial Hot Pack treatment because the pores are then open, which allows the masque formula to penetrate more deeply.

You may wish to try one of the masques from the first chapter indicated for acne-prone skin, such as the Whole-Wheat Flour Cleansing Masque. The following masques contain ingredients that are antimicrobial, astringent and soothing, making them perfect for broken-out or acne-prone skin. They are meant to provide the skin with gentle, sustained cleansing without causing further irritation. Please refer to p. 13 for Basic Masque Technique.

I Love My Face Honey Masque   ALL/ACNE

This is a gentle, soothing masque for irritated, blemished skin.

> 1 teaspoon honey   1 drop chamomile essential oil
> 1 drop tea tree essential oil

Place honey in palm of hand and stir in the essential oils, apply to face and leave on for 20 minutes, then rinse off with warm water. Makes enough for 1 application.

Variations: Replace the tea tree oil with thuja essential oil and the chamomile with lavender essential oil.

Green Goddess Masque   OILY/ACNE

This formula is good for oily, blemished and wide-pored skin.

> 1–2 tablespoons green clay   1 drop sage or lavender essential oil
> approximately 1–2 tablespoons fresh
>   apple or peach juice (preferred) or
>   water

Mix the clay and juice to create a smooth paste. Add more juice if too thick, more clay if too loose. Add the essential oil. Apply the paste thickly to your face and leave it on for 10–20 minutes. This paste may be used to dry out pimples by applying directly onto blemished area. Makes 1 masque application.

Healing Garden Masque
ALL/DAMAGED/ACNE

This masque gently cleanses and soothes blemished, irritated and damaged skin. The fresh apple juice and lemon juice provide the masque with alpha hydroxy acids that help delicately exfoliate the skin.

1 large handful fresh plantain leaves
1 tablespoon fresh-squeezed apple juice (preferred) or water
a squeeze or ¼ teaspoon fresh citrus juice (from lemon, orange, grapefruit or lime)

1 tablespoon distilled witch hazel
2 tablespoons clay (preferred) or cornstarch

Chop plantain and place in food processor (preferred) or blender and process with liquids, pouring liquid in a little at a time until a thick paste results. Add the clay or cornstarch and continue to blend. If the herbal paste is too loose and won't adhere to your face, sprinkle in small amounts of clay or cornstarch to thicken.

Apply the masque thickly to the face and relax and recline to keep it from dripping off face. You can also place gauze or thin cloth over the masque to keep it in place. Leave on for 20 minutes or longer and then rinse off. This masque will not dry. Makes enough for 1 application.

Variations: Replace the plantain leaves with violet leaves. Replace the apple juice with freshly squeezed carrot juice.

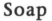

Soap

I don't recommend using soap for the face because it is so effective at removing oil from the skin, which can cause the skin to dry out and become irritated. This oil removal is at times beneficial for very oily skin. However, stripping the skin of its oils with harsh soaps can also cause irritation and further increase oil production. If you are inclined to use soap, try the gentle formula that follows.

Lime Sage Liquid Soap
OILY/ACNE

A gentle but effective cleanser that cuts grease. This soap has a delicious, subtle aroma of lime with a hint of sage.

Use the following dried and crushed herbs: 2 teaspoons comfrey root, 1 teaspoon sage, 1 teaspoon yarrow
1 cup water

3 oz. castile soap
30 drops lime essential oil
20 drops sage essential oil
10 drops tea tree essential oil

Make an infusion with herbs and water, then let steep for 8 hours or overnight and strain. Pour strained infusion and liquid castile soap into jar or squeeze bottle. Add essential oils, cap and shake. It is ready for use. Shake before each use. Store in the refrigerator if not used up within a few weeks. Makes about 9 oz. (See notes and variation on following page.)

Note: For a less drying soap decrease the castile soap and/or add less essential oils, and for a more drying soap increase the castile soap.

Variation: You can use plain water in place of the herbal infusion, although the resulting soap will be less cleansing and toning to the skin.

Astringents and Toners

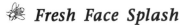

Astringents and toners help remove oily residue while refining and tightening the pores after they have been opened during the cleansing process. In general, they have a drying effect on the skin; the more alcohol or vinegar used to make an astringent or toner, the more astringent and drying it will be. Water-based formulas that include glycerin, aloe or other hydrating substances are less astringent and more moisturizing. Astringents and toners can sometimes be used instead of a cleanser. Those with oily or acne-prone skin may benefit from the use of these products to reduce oiliness. However, keep in mind that overuse can dry out the skin and cause it to produce even more oil. The best way to know how often to use a product is to watch how your skin responds, then tailor the applications accordingly. Start out by applying the following formulas once in the morning and once at night. You can also refer to the first chapter and use the formulas specified for oily and acne-prone skin, such as the Antimicrobial Astringent or the Chamomile Blend Astringent.

Fresh Face Splash

OILY/ACNE

A gentle, refreshing splash that contains alpha hydroxyl acids provided by the citrus juice.

2 teaspoons orange juice (fresh-squeezed preferred)
bowl filled with about 16 ounces cold water

Place bowl in sink and add orange juice. Splash face with water–orange juice solution, catching the solution back in the bowl, and repeat for a minute or so. Makes 1 treatment.

Variations: To increase the astringency and alpha hydroxyl acids add 1 teaspoon of lemon juice or a ½ teaspoon of vinegar to the splash. To increase the antimicrobial action add 1–2 drops of tea tree essential oil.

Grapefruit Mist

OILY/ACNE

A refreshing grapefruit-scented toner with antimicrobial properties.

1 oz. plus 1 tablespoon distilled water
2 teaspoons distilled witch hazel
1 teaspoon 80-100 proof vodka

15 drops grapefruit essential oil
5 drops tea tree essential oil

Pour ingredients into a spray mist bottle (preferred) or jar, add essential oils, cap and shake. Mist or splash on face. Does not require refrigeration. Makes 2 oz.

Chamomile Lavender Delight

OILY/ACNE

This is a soothing, reparative toner for irritated, inflamed, oily and acne-prone skin.

8 drops chamomile essential oil
8 drops lavender essential oil
4 drops thuja essential oil

1 oz. plus 1 tablespoons distilled water
2 teaspoons aloe vera gel
1 teaspoon 80–100 proof vodka

Pour ingredients into a spray mist bottle (preferred) or jar, add essential oils, cap and shake. Does not require refrigeration. Mist or splash on face. Makes 2 oz.

Calendula Comfrey Astringent

OILY/ACNE

This is a soothing, skin-reparative astringent. It contains about 20 percent alcohol, which may be drying for some skin if used undiluted.

Combine the following freshly dried herbs: 1 handful calendula blossoms, 1 tablespoon comfrey root (crushed or powdered)

16 oz. water
8 oz. 80 proof vodka (or other 80 proof liquor)
2 teaspoons aloe vera gel

Make infusion with herbs and water. Let steep for 4 hours. Pour 8 oz. of strained herbal infusion into a 16-oz. jar, then add vodka and aloe. Cap and shake well. It is ready to use. Makes about 16 oz.

Variation: For a less drying effect, dilute ¼–½ teaspoon of astringent with 1 teaspoon of distilled rose water or plain water per application.

Flower Power Astringent

ACNE/INFECTED/OILY

A strong cleansing formula that requires a 6-week period to make, but once made will keep for years outside refrigeration.

Use the following freshly dried herbs: 1 handful yarrow, 1 handful calendula blossoms, 1 handful roses, 1 tablespoon comfrey root (cut)

14 oz. 100 proof vodka

Make tincture with herbs and vodka following Directions for Alcohol Tinctures Using Dried Herbs.

To use as a general facial astringent you may want to dilute tincture before use. For a single treatment dilute ¼–½ teaspoon of tincture in 1 teaspoon of water and apply to face with cotton swab or cloth. To dry out pimples, apply tincture undiluted directly onto affected area as often as needed. This preparation is also excellent for cleaning wounds. Makes about 10 oz.

Variation: Add 1 drop of wintergreen essential oil per treatment for added cleansing.

Moisturizers

In general, people with oily skin do not need moisturizers. However, if a moisturizer is needed, the smallest amount will usually suffice. Keep in mind that a daily moisturizer application may not be necessary and should be applied only on an as-needed basis. It is best to apply moisturizers to a clean face, preferably while the skin is still slightly moist after washing or steaming. In some cases the skin needs moisture and not oil. The best treatment in this case is to increase water consumption to hydrate the skin from the inside. While oil acts as a barrier to help the skin retain moisture, the skin also needs a source of moisture. This is why applying a moisturizer to a damp face is most beneficial. The following formulas offer light, effective moisturizers for oily and blemished skin.

❦ Touch of Grapeseed   Oily

Grapeseed is a light and somewhat drying oil that may be appropriate for oily skin.

> **Several drops grapeseed oil**

Apply oil to fingertips and gently massage into clean and slightly moistened face.

Grapeseed Combination   Acne/Oily

A mixture of essential oils that help soothe and clear-up acne in a light base of grapeseed oil.

> **1 oz. grapeseed oil**   **3 drops lavender essential oil**
> **2 drops chamomile essential oil** **2 drops tea tree essential oil**

Pour oil into a glass jar, add essential oils, cap and shake. It is ready to use. Apply oil to fingertips and gently massage into clean and slightly moistened face. Makes 1 oz.

Rose Water and Grapeseed Oil   Oily/Acne

> **Several drops grapeseed oil**
> **small amount rose water (a few mists if**
> **using spray bottle, or a small palmful**
> **if applying by hand)**

Apply a dab of oil on forehead, chin and cheeks. Then place rose water in a pump spray bottle and mist on face or splash it on face by hand. Massage face, working oil and water into skin. Makes enough for 1 treatment.

Variations: Replace the rose water with an astringent or toner, such as Chamomile Lavender Delight or Grapefruit Mist. Replace the grapeseed oil with other oil of choice, such as calendula-infused oil (see Luscious Lotion p. 29) or the just-given Grapeseed Combination.

Blemish Potions

These are strong cleansing formulas for drying out pimples and should be used with caution, as they could dry and irritate the skin.

Herbal Skin Clear
ACNE/INFECTED

Use for pimples, acne and infected skin. This formula requires a 6-week period to make, but once made will keep for a year or more outside refrigeration.

½ oz. goldenseal root powder
1 oz. echinacea root powder
½ oz. myrrh powder
8 oz. 80–100 proof vodka
1 oz. apple cider vinegar

25 drops of tea tree essential oil
25 drops chamomile essential oil
25 drops wintergreen essential oil
25 drops lavender essential oil

Make tincture with herbs and vodka, following Directions for Alcohol Tinctures Using Dried Herbs. Let steep for 6 weeks and strain. Add vinegar and essential oils.

Apply directly to problem area with cotton swab, and repeat as needed. This preparation is also excellent for cleaning wounds. Makes about 6 oz.

Variation: Wet a teaspoon of clay with Herbal Skin Clear and apply to pimples to dry them out.

Fresh Flower Cleanser
ACNE/INFECTED/OILY

A strong cleansing formula that requires a 6-week period to make, but once made will keep for years outside refrigeration. This formula is made with fresh herbs, and the amount of herb you use will dictate the amount of tincture you end up with.

Use the following fresh herbs in
equal quantities: calendula flowers,
spilanthes flowers, yarrow flowers,
echinacea flowers and plantain leaf

100 proof vodka

Make tincture with herbs and vodka, following Directions for Alcohol Tinctures Using Fresh Herbs.

To dry out pimples, apply tincture undiluted directly onto affected area as often as needed. This preparation is also excellent for cleaning wounds. Yield varies.

DEODORANTS

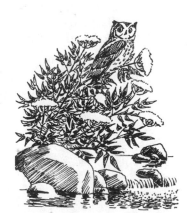

Natural and effective deodorants are easily made with essential oils, witch hazel, vodka, herbs and various other ingredients. You can use the deodorants found in chapter 4: Whole Body Treatments or try one of the following formulas. Teenagers will often enjoy custom blending their own scent for a deodorant, which is easily done by replacing the essential oils in the following formulas with others of your choice.

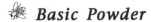 ## Basic Powder   ALL

Sprinkle cornstarch, baking soda, arrowroot powder or clay into underarms to reduce perspiration and gently deodorize.

Variation: Mix a few drops of essential oil of tea tree, rosemary or lavender into powder to increase deodorizing action.

Fresh Scent   ALL

A refreshing, cleansing deodorant for both sexes.

4 oz. distilled witch hazel (available at pharmacies)	4 drops eucalyptus essential oil
	4 drops tea tree essential oil
4 drops lavender essential oil	4 drops lime essential oil

Pour witch hazel into a 4-oz. jar, add essential oils and shake well. It is ready to use. Apply to cotton ball and wipe underarms. Does not require refrigeration. Shake before use. Makes 4 oz.

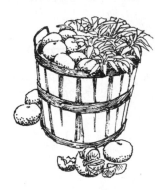 ## Sage Tangerine Deodorant   ALL

Refreshing and deodorizing. An excellent choice for both sexes.

4 oz. distilled witch hazel	10 drops tangerine essential oil
8 drops sage essential oil	2 drops sandalwood essential oil

Place ingredients in a 4 oz. jar and shake well. It is ready to use. Apply to cotton ball and wipe underarms. Does not require refrigeration. Always shake before use. Makes 4 oz.

Calendula Lemongrass Deodorant   ALL

An antimicrobial formula with the exotic and refreshing scent of lemongrass. An excellent choice for both sexes.

4 oz. Calendula Tincture (see p. 100)	20 drops tea tree essential oil
3 oz. distilled water	10 drops rosemary essential oil
½ teaspoon glycerin	20 drops lemongrass essential oil

Pour calendula tincture, water and glycerin into a jar, add essential oils, cap and shake. Apply deodorant onto a cotton swab or cloth and wipe underarms. You can also put the deodorant into a spray bottle and mist into underarms. Does not require refrigeration. Makes 7 oz.

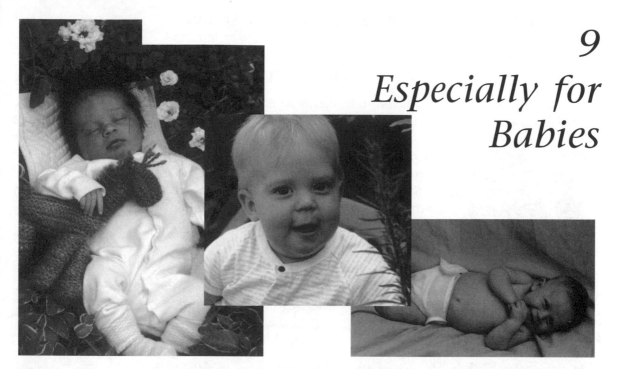

9
Especially for Babies

I am amazed at the number of baby care products available on the commercial market that contain petroleum by-products, artificial dyes and chemical scents. Babies have extremely delicate skin, so the substances we use on them should be very gentle and free of toxins. They should also be very nourishing and protective to the skin, to prevent drying and chapping. Although under certain circumstances a more cleansing antimicrobial action may be needed, in general baby care products should be free of harsh chemicals and detergents, as well as strong scents. A good general rule is that if a formula is too harsh for the sensitive skin around your eyes, it is not suitable for a baby's skin. The oils, herbs and other ingredients used to make baby care products should therefore occupy the gentle end of the skin care spectrum. The most commonly used herbs in natural baby care products, and the ones I rely upon most in the formulas offered in this chapter, are chamomile, lavender, St. Johnswort, calendula, violet, fennel, comfrey and plantain.

The formulas presented in this chapter will help you meet your baby's basic skin care needs. There are emollient baths and after-bath oils and creams to help soothe and protect your baby's skin. There are also some suggestions for gentle herbal baths to help soothe a cranky or colicky baby, and to lull your little one to sleep. You will also find a sampling of healing salves and gentle powders to help prevent and treat diaper rash.

Please note that while the products presented here are specially formulated for baby's tender skin, these — and all skin care products — should be kept out of baby's reach and used according to directions. If your baby has especially delicate skin or is prone to allergies, test a little bit of a given formula, diluted according to any instructions, on a small patch of arm or leg skin before applying it all over. Also, it is a good idea to introduce new products one at a time so that if your baby does develop a reaction, you will be better able to isolate what may have caused it.

BABY BATHS

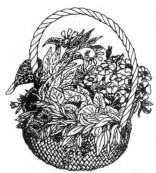

In addition to its cleansing effects, a warm bath is a pleasurable way to soothe a cranky baby. The addition of botanicals and oils can enhance the relaxing effects of your baby's bath. Note that it is not necessary or even advisable to use soap every time you bathe your baby — too frequent baths or too much soap can make the skin dry and flaky. When you do use soap, choose a gentle, natural one that is specially formulated for babies. Adding an emollient to the bathwater can be helpful in keeping your baby's skin from drying out.

Oil in the Baby Bath

Adding oil to the bathwater helps keep your baby's skin nourished and lubricated. This is especially helpful in the winter, when indoor heating dries out the air.

🐝 *Basic Oil Bath*   ALL/DRY

Add a teaspoon of carrier oil, such as almond, jojoba or olive, into the bathwater.

🐝 *Cream Bath*   ALL/DRY

To nourish and protect the skin from drying out. Add a teaspoon of cream into the baby's bath.

Baby Bath Oil   ALL

A rich, soothing and calming oil to add to the bathwater or apply directly onto skin.

1 oz. jojoba oil
1 oz. almond oil
1½ oz. calendula-infused olive oil
   (see Luscious Lotion p. 29)

½ oz. wheat germ oil
5 drops chamomile essential oil

Pour oils, except the chamomile essential oil, into a jar, then add the chamomile essential oil drop by drop, cap and shake well. Add 1 teaspoon of oil into the bathwater just prior to immersing the baby, or massage directly into skin. Makes 3 oz., enough for about 18 baths.

Essential Oils in the Baby Bath

You can add various therapeutic effects to baby's bath with a single drop of essential oil added to the water. The use of essential oils can be especially helpful during stressful times, such as when a baby is teething or recovering from an illness. Remember that essential oils are extremely concentrated and very potent. When using them, please add 1 drop and 1 drop only to the water, as the addition of more can be irritating to baby's delicate skin. Keep an eye on how your baby responds to different essential oils. If you see any sign of skin irritation, avoid using the oil that may have caused it.

Basic Essential Oil Bath ALL

Add 1 drop of essential oil of choice to the bathwater just prior to immersion. Swish the water around with your hand to disperse the oil before placing baby in the bath.

Variations: Add chamomile for relaxing an irritated baby, especially during teething, lavender for a cleansing and calming bath, fennel for a colicky baby and eucalyptus or rosemary for a congested baby.

Herbal Bath for Baby

Herbs, such as chamomile, lavender and calendula, offer gentle cleansing and soothing effects. An herb can be used alone or combined with other herbs to produce an array of bath blends to suit your baby's needs. See the following formulas for some excellent herbal bath choices. You may want to refer to the Botanicals section in the Ingredients chapter for further information and to help you create customized bath blends.

 ### *Basic Herbal Baby Bath* ALL

Use approximately 2 handfuls of dried herb per 32 oz. of water. Note that if you are using powdered herbs, use only about 6 tablespoons. If using herbs that have been cut and sifted, use about ¾ of a cup. If using seeds, use about 2 palmfuls.

Make an herbal infusion with the herbs and water. Strain the infusion and add it to the bathwater. If bathing the baby in a portable basin you can leave the herbs in the infusion if you like, since there is no drain to clog. Either pour the bathwater and herbs directly onto the compost pile afterward, or pour the used water through a sieve and discard the herbs. Be aware that some babies like to pick the herbs out of the bathwater and place them in their mouths. Although the herbs used in the following bath blends are safe for internal consumption, the concern is for a baby who is not old enough to chew and swallow properly, so please keep a watchful eye on your baby during the bath. Makes enough for 1 bath.

Variations: Use plantain leaf to make a healing, soothing bath for itchy, scraped or irritated skin. Use mint for a cooling bath, which is especially nice on a hot summer day. Use chamomile for a calming bath, which can be very effective just prior to sleep. Use fennel seeds to make a bath for a colicky baby.

Hollyhock Flower Baby Bath ALL

This blend of herbs is gentle and healing to the skin, helping soothe minor skin irritations and rashes.

Use 1 large handful or ½ oz. of the following freshly dried herbs: hollyhock flowers, calendula flowers, violet leaf

Use 1 small handful or ½ oz. of freshly dried chamomile flowers

Combine the herbs and store in an airtight jar away from heat and sunlight. To use, take 2 handfuls of herb mixture and 32 oz. of water and make a quart of herbal infusion, letting it steep for 4 hours. Strain and add to the bathwater. If bathing the baby in a portable basin you can leave the herbs in the infusion, as they won't clog the drain, and then throw the bathwater with the herbs into the compost. Makes enough for 2 baths.

Sweet Slumber Baby Bath

ALL

A gentle mixture of herbs used to promote sleep and relaxation.

Use the following dried herbs: 2 large handfuls or 2 oz. chamomile, 2 large handfuls or 1 oz. hops strobiles, 1 large handful or 1 oz. lavender flowers

Combine the herbs and store in an airtight jar away from heat and sunlight. To use, take 2 handfuls of herb mixture and 32 oz. of water and make a quart of herbal inusion. Let steep for 1 to 2 hours. Strain and add to the bathwater. If bathing the baby in a portable basin you can leave the herbs in the infusion, as they won't clog the drain, and then throw the bathwater with the herbs into the compost. Makes enough for 2 to 3 baths.

BABY POWDERS

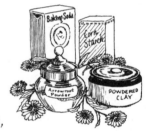

Powders absorb excess moisture on the skin, thus helping to prevent diaper rash. They are also very soothing and deodorizing. I avoid commercial talcum powders because I do not want to expose my child to it. Even though talc is a naturally occurring substance, it can be carcinogenic when inhaled in sufficient quantities. Commercial baby powders, even when made with more neutral ingredients like cornstarch, often contain chemical scents and other harsh ingredients. You can instead use any of the following powders alone or in combination for dusting baby's bottom: cornstarch, arrowroot powder, clay or baking soda. Adding essential oils and herbs to these powders augments their therapeutic properties. You can either use spice shakers or powder canisters for sprinkling on baby powder, or apply it by hand. The following easy-to-make formulas offer an assortment of powders that address various needs.

Orange Cornstarch Baby Powder

ALL

An easy-to-make, sweet-smelling, absorbent and gently disinfecting powder.

1 tablespoon cornstarch
2 drops sweet orange essential oil
1 drop lavender essential oil

Drop the essential oils into the cornstarch and stir them in well. Apply to baby's bottom or wherever needed. Makes enough for 1 or 2 applications, once you've tried it and know you like it, make more by multiplying the ingredients.

Baking Soda Baby Powder

ALL

Baking soda is excellent for acidic skin rashes, such as certain kinds of diaper rashes, and the tea tree oil adds antimicrobial action.

2 teaspoon baking soda
3 drops tea tree essential oil

Drop the tea tree oil into the baking soda and stir well. Makes enough for 1 or 2 applications.

Variation: To make a larger quantity use ½ cup of baking soda and 36 drops of tea tree oil. Place baking soda in a jar, then drop in the tea tree oil while stirring in well. Cap the jar tightly and shake to continue mixing the ingredients. Store in a cool, dark place. Makes ½ cup of powder, enough for 20 or more treatments.

Calendula Lavender Baby Powder

ALL

A refreshing-smelling baby powder to keep skin soothed, dry and deodorized.

1 cup clay
½ cup baking soda
½ cup arrowroot powder
¼ cup freshly dried lavender blossoms
¼ cup freshly dried calendula blossoms
¼ cup slippery elm powder
30 drops lavender essential oil
10 drops tea tree essential oil

Powder herbs, except the slippery elm powder, in a coffee grinder used exclusively for herbs and seeds, then sift powdered herbs through a fine mesh strainer, allowing the fine powder to fall into a bowl under the strainer and regrinding the coarser particles. It is important to grind the herbs as finely as possible so the powder feels soft and silky against the skin. Place powdered herbs, clay, baking soda, arrowroot powder and slippery elm powder into a jar, mix the powders thoroughly, then add the essential oils while stirring them in. Cap and shake jar. Makes about 2½ cups of baby powder.

Bacteria Buster Baby Powder

ALL/IRRITATED/INFECTED

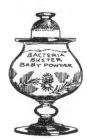

A strong antimicrobial powder for diaper rash and minor skin infections.

1 cup clay
½ cup baking soda
½ cup arrowroot powder
¼ cup goldenseal powder
¼ cup myrrh powder
¼ cup freshly dried calendula blossoms
¼ cup freshly dried yarrow flowers and leaves
¼ cup slippery elm powder
40 drops tea tree essential oil
30 drops lavender essential oil
10 drops melissa essential oil

Process calendula and yarrow in a coffee grinder used exclusively for herbs and seeds into a powder, then sift powdered herbs through a fine mesh strainer, allowing the fine powder to fall into a bowl under the strainer and regrinding the coarser particles. It is important to grind the herbs as finely as possible so the powder feels soft and silky against the skin. Place clay, baking soda, arrowroot powder, slippery elm, goldenseal powder, myrrh powder and the powdered yarrow and calendula into a jar, mix the powders thoroughly and add the essential oils while stirring them in. Cap and shake jar. This powder can also be used as a poultice for diaper rashes. (And it is a good adult foot powder.) Makes about 2½ cups.

BABY EMOLLIENTS

Baby emollients are lubricating substances that gently nourish, soften and soothe the skin. They include baby oils, creams and balms. Some of these emollients are designed for everyday use, and others are specially formulated to address specific conditions such as diaper rash or congestion.

Baby Oils

You can choose from any carrier oil, used alone or in combination, to gently massage and lubricate a baby's skin. These include, but are not limited to, olive, almond, jojoba, coconut and peanut oil (see Ingredients chapter for more information about specific carrier oils). You can also add essential oils to the carrier oil to create a more pleasing and therapeutic formula. However, use caution when preparing an essential oil-enriched preparation for baby, as the essential oils can irritate sensitive skin. Products made for babies should contain proportionately less essential oil than ones prepared for adults — about ⅓ the amount. You can also infuse herbs into a carrier oil to create another kind of gentle oil for your baby with subtle therapeutic effects. Herbal-infused oils such as comfrey root, plantain and St. Johnswort are excellent soothing oils for a baby. They can be used alone or combined with other oils. Here are some choice recipes:

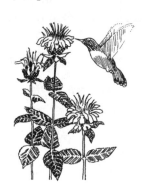

🐝 *Basic Aromatherapy Baby Oil*   ALL

When including essential oils in a baby oil, be sure to properly dilute them, using as little essential oil as possible. Remember that babies' skin is sensitive and easily irritated. These aromatherapy oils can be massaged into the skin or added to the bath.

Up to 5 drops essential oil of choice
1 oz. carrier oil of choice

Pour carrier oil into small-mouth glass jar, add essential oils, tightly cap and shake jar. It is ready for use. Makes 1 oz. *Variations follow:*

Lavender Baby Oil
For calming and soothing the skin.
Use 5 drops lavender essential oil and 1 oz. almond oil.

Winter Night Baby Oil
For warming and decongesting.
Use 1 drop melissa essential oil, 1 drop rosemary essential oil, 2 drops ginger essential oil and 1 oz. sesame oil.

Relaxing Baby Oil

ALL

A refreshing, sweet and soothing body oil. Massage into abdomen for calming colic, stomach cramps and anxious bellies. Good for both babies and adults.

4 oz. Basic Body Oil BLend (see p. 83)
  or 4 oz. almond oil

12 drops fennel essential oil
8 drops lavender essential oil

Place carrier oil into a jar and add the essential oils, drop by drop. Cap jar with a tight-fitting lid and shake well. The oil is ready to use. Makes 4 oz.

Avocado Baby Oil

ALL/DRY

A rich treat for dry, chapped and irritated skin.

2 oz. avocado oil
2 oz. jojoba oil
2 oz. almond oil

½ oz. wheat germ oil
10 drops chamomile
  essential oil

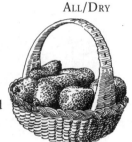

Pour oils into a jar and then drop in the chamomile essential oil. Cap jar and shake. The oil is ready to use. Makes 6½ oz.

Violet Baby Oil

ALL/DRY

This infused oil has healing and nourishing properties. It is a soothing and beneficial oil for skin rashes and irritations, as well as being a wonderful all-purpose baby oil. The recipe must be made weeks ahead of time to allow the herbs to infuse in the oil.

Use the following freshly dried herbs:
  1 oz. violet leaf, 1 oz. calendula

and 1 oz. chamomile
14 oz. cold pressed olive oil

Coarsely grind herbs in mortar and pestle or coffee/seed grinder, and proceed to Directions for Herbal-Infused Oils with Dried Herbs. Makes about 10 oz. infused oil. *Variation follows:*

Light Violet Baby Oil
Dilute the herbal-infused oil with equal amounts of almond or apricot kernel oil. Or substitute almond oil for the olive oil when making the herbal-infused oil.

Antimicrobial Oil

ALL/IRRITATED/INFECTED

A stronger-acting oil for diaper rashes and other minor skin infections. This formula must be made weeks ahead of time to allow the herbs to infuse in the oil.

Use the following freshly dried herbs:
  ½ oz. echinacea angustifolia root
  (small pieces), ½ oz. calendula
  whole blossom, ½ oz. thyme,
  ½ oz. yarrow, ½ oz. myrrh powder

12 oz. cold pressed olive oil
about 24 drops tea tree essential oil
16 drops lavender essential oil

Coarsely grind herbs, except myrrh, in mortar and pestle or coffee/seed grinder. Using myrrh, ground herbs and olive oil, proceed to Directions for Herbal-Infused Oils with Dried Herbs. To every ounce of strained oil add 3 drops of tea tree essential oil and 2 drops of lavender essential oil. Makes about 8 oz.

This herbal-infused oil is used as a main ingredient in other formulas, such as creams and balms. However, the essential oils are omitted from the herbal-infused oil and added at the appropriate time to minimize their evaporation.

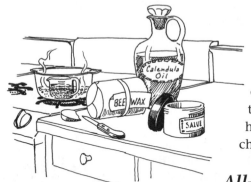

Baby Balms and Salves

Balms and salves are oils thickened with beeswax. The oils used to make balms can be herbal-infused varieties, or plain carrier oils of your choice. You can add essential oils to balms to produce various fragrances and therapeutic effects. The gentle baby preparations offered here are very good for healing diaper rash, cracked or chapped skin, abrasions and other minor skin irritations.

All-Purpose Salve   ALL

All-purpose salve is made with St. Johnswort-, calendula- and plantain-infused oils solidified with beeswax. This is a broad spectrum healing salve useful for minor skin irritations, inflammations, diaper rash, chapped skin, lips and burns. See formula p. 103.

Calendula Salve   ALL

Calendula salve is made with calendula blossoms-infused in cold pressed olive oil and solidified with beeswax. This salve is very popular with mothers. It is gentle but effective in healing minor skin irritations and bacterial problems. See formula p. 105.

Baby Nourish Balm   ALL/DRY

A thick, supernourishing, concentrated balm for protecting, lubricating and healing baby's skin. Good for babies whose skin is chafed and irritated. Note that it is necessary to make the chamomile-infused olive oil weeks ahead of time (if you can't wait, you can use avocado oil instead).

2 oz. chamomile-infused olive oil	1 oz. jojoba oil
(preferred) or avocado oil	1 oz. coconut oil
1 oz. shea butter	1 oz. beeswax

To make chamomile-infused olive oil see Creamy Rose Chamomile Oil pp. 82–83

Pour liquid oils into a heat-proof measuring cup, then add the shea butter and coconut oil, measuring after each addition. Melt, break or grate beeswax into small pieces and add to the oil mixture, enough to bring the level of the measuring cup by 1 oz. Place the measuring cup into a hot-water bath and while stirring well, allow everything to melt and become a uniform liquid free of lumps and clumps. When all the ingredients have melted and thoroughly combined pour the liquid into a wide-mouth jar, let cool undisturbed and cap when solidified. It is now ready to use. Makes 6 oz.

Variation: Replace the chamomile-infused oil with comfrey-infused oil.

Antimicrobial Baby Balm
ALL/IRRITATED/INFECTED

3 oz. Antimicrobial Oil (without
essential oils, see formula pp. 161-162)

1 oz. beeswax
20 drops tea tree essential oil

First make Antimicrobial Oil without the essential oils. Then proceed to Directions for Salves and Balms using Antimicrobial Oil and beeswax. Add the 20 drops of tea tree oil at the end of the salve-making procedure. Apply salve often or as needed. Makes 4 oz.

Baby Creams

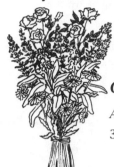

Baby creams are oil and water emulsions that are especially nice to massage into baby's skin after a bath, or whenever a soothing, nourishing and moisturizing effect is needed.

Calendula Cream
ALL

A protective, gentle cream to keep skin moisturized and soothed.

3 oz. calendula-infused
olive oil (see Luscious
Lotion p. 29)
3 oz. almond oil

3 oz. coconut oil
1 oz. beeswax
9 oz. distilled water

Follow Directions for Creams. Apply as often as desired or during diaper changes. Makes 19 oz.

Skin Revival
ALL/DRY

This rich, nourishing cream can be used for children when their skin is dry and chapped. Apply before sleep, after bathing or as needed. When making Skin Revival for infants you may want to omit the essential oils from the recipe, or use ¼ the suggested amount. See formula page 29-30.

Antimicrobial Cream
ALL/IRRITATED/INFECTED

A moisturizer with cleansing and disinfecting properties. May be helpful for dry skin conditions accompanied by minor infections as often seen in diaper rash.

6 oz. Antimicrobial Oil (see pp. 161–162)
without essential oils added
3 oz. coconut oil
1 oz. beeswax

9 oz. distilled water
10 drops lavender
20 drops tea tree oil
5 drops chamomile essential oil

Follow Directions for Creams. Use as needed, and apply frequently if working with active infections. Makes 19 oz.

Herbal Sleep Pillows

These pillows are a wonderful way to help lull a little one to sleep. They are stuffed with herbs that have been used for centuries to promote sleep and relaxation. If you place the pillow next to your child's head, its subtle but effective herbal aromas will help promote sleep. For infants under 6 months of age, I suggest attaching the pillow to the headboard of the crib or placing it under the bedding sheet as a safety measure.

In the Night Kitchen's Herbal Sleep Pillows

The following recipe and instructions will make a 6-by-7-inch herbal sleep pillow.

Herbal Sleep Mixture Formula

Use 1 cup dried lavender flowers, ½ cup dried chamomile flowers, ¼ cup dried linden flowers (crushed), and ¼ cup sage leaves (crushed).

Mix the dried herbs together. Note: Whenever possible use organically grown herbs. Remember to smell the herbs before purchasing them to ensure that they are strongly and sweetly scented. The pillow's sleep-inducing capacity depends on the aroma of the herbs.

For a stronger and longer-lasting scent you can do the following:

Take 1 tablespoon of orris root and place in a glass jar. Put a few drops of essential oil of lavender on the orris root. Close the jar tightly and shake. Place in a closet and leave for 2–4 weeks, shaking the jar once a week. Add to the herb mixture.

Place the herb mixture into the pillow.

Instructions for Making Herbal Pillow

Choose a material that feels soft to the touch — cotton flannel and sand-washed silk are my personal favorites. You can either use the same material for both sides or choose materials of different colors and textures for each. Cut two 8-by-7-pieces of the material. Sew the two pieces together, (along three sides only). Turn inside out and fill with herbal mixture. Fold ¼ inch of the open end inside and sew across to close.

Variations: The size can be adjusted by increasing or decreasing the dimensions of the pillow and the amount of herbal mixture used. For much larger pillows, you can use 100 percent cotton or wool as a filler to add to the herbal mixture. Make sure to use enough herb to retain the feel and aroma of the herbal pillow.

DIAPER RASH REMEDIES

Diaper rash is one of the most common maladies to affect babies. There are a number of gentle and effective ways to prevent and to treat diaper rash. One of the best means of both prevention and treatment is also the simplest: Allow the baby's bottom to be exposed to the air and to moderate amounts of filtered sunlight. You should also change baby's diapers frequently so that wet or soiled diapers are not allowed to linger against the skin for any length of time. Wash the baby's bottom after every diaper change with warm water. If desired, you may also use a very mild soap. Hold baby's bottom under the running faucet for an especially thorough rinsing, but please be very careful to check the temperature of the running water first. Dry with a soft, clean cloth, or allow the bottom to air-dry. Make sure that baby's bottom is completely dry before putting on a new diaper. You may also apply one of the antimicrobial oils, balms or creams, and/or dust baby's bottom with one of the powders just offered. If using cloth diapers be sure to cleanse them properly. To rid diapers of undesirable bacteria, add ½ cup of supermarket-grade white vinegar to the final rinse cycle of the wash and hang them to dry in the sun. For a serious case of diaper rash, try the following:

Bacteria Buster Baby Powder Pack   RASH
    1–2 tablespoons Bacteria Buster Baby Powder (See formula pp. 159–160)
    1–2 tablespoons water

Wet powder with water, adding the water slowly till a smooth and thin paste results. Apply the paste to the baby's bottom and let stay on for a minimum of 20 minutes. Wash off with warm water. Apply Antimicrobial Baby Balm and then dust bottom with a little of the Bacteria Baby Buster Powder. Use this procedure 1–2 times a day and repeat until the rash is gone.

BABY GIFT BASKET

Baby Gift Baskets are useful and beautiful presents filled with heart and soul that both mother and baby will appreciate. Choose from among the formulas in this section, arranging them in a basket decorated with dried flowers, herbs or other appropriate adornments. Please be sure to label the products clearly with ingredients and directions for use. The following is a sample Baby Gift Basket:

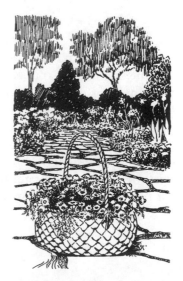

Hollyhock Flower Baby Bath, Avocado Baby Oil, Bacteria Buster Baby Powder and Calendula Cream.

Place the formulas in a basket partially filled with a natural fiber filler (available at craft shops). Arrange dried flowers around them, make a card from handmade or recycled paper, punch a small hole in the card and tie it onto the basket with a natural fiber string.

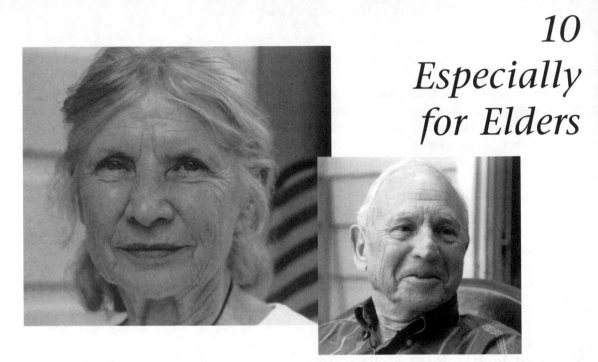

10
Especially for Elders

T he elders are often overlooked in our youth-oriented culture, both in terms of the wisdom we could derive from their experience, and in terms of their special physical, emotional and spiritual needs. In the area of body care, elders generally require gentle cleansing combined with rich nourishing and moisturizing treatments. Besides relaxing and rejuvenating the skin, it is equally important to relax and rejuvenate the spirit. While many of the formulas offered throughout this book can be used by older folks, following are an assortment of pleasurable and effective formulas and treatments created specifically with more mature individuals in mind. Younger folks might consider offering relatives and friends one of the following treatments — a wonderful gift that is sure to be appreciated.

HAND SOAKS

Soaks offer a pleasant and relaxing way to rejuvenate tired, swollen, painful or arthritic hands, conditions often experienced by older people. As we age, our fingernails tend to become drier and more prone to fungal and bacterial growth. These conditions can be addressed easily and pleasurably with soaks. Soaks are especially well suited for elders because they are easy and noninvasive treatments, requiring only that one remain seated for at least 10 minutes. Soaks are especially good for people with poor peripheral circulation, a common problem as we age. Soaks also offer the benefit of affecting the whole body, promoting relaxation and a general sense of well-being. You may refer to the In Your Hands/On Your Feet chapter for hand-soak suggestions, or try some of the following special treatments.

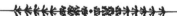

A Gift to Aging Parents, Grandparents and Friends

Remember how much you liked having your elders read to you when you were a child? Consider returning the favor now to the generation who raised you. Set your loved one up with one of the hand soaks offered here, then read a short story or some poetry out loud while he or she relaxes into the treatment. You might even want to read an entire novel in installments. You will both look forward to the relaxation and the time shared over this experience.

BASIC HAND-SOAK TECHNIQUE. Choose a bowl that both your hands fit into comfortably. Fill it with water or herbal infusion, as hot as you can comfortably tolerate. Keep your hands in the water for at least 10 minutes.

 ## Oil and Vinegar Soak ALL

This soak reduces aches and pains while also cleansing unwanted microbes from under the finger-nails. The olive oil provides moisturizing action to prevent the skin from drying out.

2 tablespoons apple cider vinegar
¼ teaspoon olive oil or other oil of choice

optional: **and 3 drops wintergreen essential oil**

Follow the Basic Hand-Soak Technique and add vinegar, oil and optional essential oil to the hand-soak water. Caution: Vinegar may sting raw and open skin.

Variations: To increase the relaxing effects of the soak replace vinegar with chamomile-infused vinegar (see formula p. 97) or mugwort-infused vinegar (see formula p. 97) .

Cleanse and Calm Salt Soak ALL

A strong-cleansing, antifungal hand soak that is calming. The jojoba oil is added to prevent the skin from drying out.

8 drops tea tree essential oil
8 drops lavender essential oil
4 drops chamomile essential oil

2 tablespoons jojoba oil or other rich carrier oil of choice
6 tablespoons sea salt

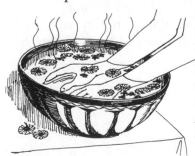

Place salt in a glass jar with a tight fitting nonmetallic lid, add jojoba oil and stir in thoroughly. Add essential oils into the salt a few drops at a time, stirring in thoroughly after each dropping; when done adding the oil, cap tightly so the volatile oils do not evaporate and the salt continues to absorb them. You may use them right away or store them in a cool, dark place. Add 1–2 teaspoon of salts per hand soak. If skin should feel dry after soak apply a moisturizer. Makes enough for 9–18 soaks.

Herbal Rejuvenation Soak

All

This fragrant blend of sweet-smelling herbs is soothing, cleansing and relaxing. Make extra infusion and set aside a cup for drinking as you enjoy your soak. The herbs in this formula have been used traditionally to relieve headaches and other ailments associated with stress.

1 tablespoon lavender flowers	1 tablespoon fennel seeds
1 tablespoon chamomile flowers	16 oz. water

Make herbal infusion with herbs and water. Let steep for a minimum of 1 hour. Pour the unstrained infusion into a pot, gently reheat and pour into bowl. Top off with additional warm water. Makes enough for 1 treatment.

Variations: For a more invigorating soak replace the chamomile with mint. For a more soothing soak replace the fennel with marshmallow root and let the infusion steep for 8 hours.

HAND CREAMS, OILS AND BALMS

As we age our bodies tend to produce less sebum, the protective oily substance that keeps skin moist and lubricated. The following formulas nourish, soothe and lubricate mature skin, keeping it healthy and protected. Aging often brings sluggish circulation, and swollen hands as well. Keep in mind that massage is an excellent way to alleviate these symptoms, and that creams, oils and balms can facilitate the process. You can either massage your own hands or enlist the aid of somebody else for an extra treat. When I visited my grandfather during the last few years of his life, I would bring him a pot of homemade split pea soup and gently massage his hands during our visits. I don't know which he enjoyed more — the massages or the soup. The following formulas offer various therapeutic effects, and are suitable for massage as well as for softening and lubricating the hands.

Happy Hands Oil

All/Dry

This nourishing oil brings relief to dry, sore and irritated hands.

1 oz. almond oil	1 teaspoon wheat germ oil
2 oz. peanut oil	20 drops birch essential oil
1½ tablespoons	20 drops lavender essential oil
avocado oil	7 drops chamomile essential oil

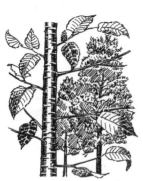

Betula lenta

Pour oils into a small-mouth 4-oz. glass jar (preferably blue or amber), leave ⅛ inch space at the top, add essential oils drop by drop, cap jar and shake well. Apply to slightly moist hands or add 1 teaspoon to hand-soak water. Makes 4 oz.

Recovery Balm
ALL/DRY/DAMAGED

This reparative balm can be used to prevent hands from drying and cracking if applied before and after engaging them in work. It may also be used to soften, soothe and heal already dry and damaged skin. It has a refreshing and calming scent that is pleasing to many older folks.

1 oz. jojoba oil
2 oz. shea butter
2 oz. St. Johnswort-infused olive oil
   (see p. 125) (preferred) or plain
   olive oil

1 oz. beeswax
1 tablespoon wheat germ oil
1 tablespoon cocoa butter
½ teaspoon lavender essential oil
30 drops chamomile essential oil

Place ingredients, except the essential oils, in a heat-proof cup placed in a hot-water bath. Stir until ingredients are thoroughly melted. Remove from heat and stir mixture for a couple of minutes to cool but not thicken; this also helps to evenly distribute the ingredients. Pour into a wide-mouth jar, add essential oils and quickly cap the jar with a tight-fitting lid to prevent the essential oils from evaporating. Allow butter to sit undisturbed for several hours or overnight to completely cool. Massage balm into hands as often as you can; try to do it at least twice a day. Apply it before night slumber for the most reparative action, and if hands are really dry and damaged sleep with gloves. Makes about 7 oz.

Heavenly Hand Cream
ALL/DRY/DAMAGED

A luxurious cream that is excellent for moisturizing dry, irritated and damaged hands.

1 oz. jojoba oil
1 oz. peanut oil
1 oz. comfrey root-infused olive oil
   (see Comfrey Comfort p. 82)
   (preferred) or plain olive oil
2 oz. almond oil
1 oz. avocado oil
1 oz. shea butter

1 oz. cocoa butter
1 oz. coconut oil
1 oz. beeswax
1 teaspoon sandalwood essential oil
½ teaspoon sweet birch essential oil
¼ teaspoon lavender essential oil
2 oz. aloe vera gel
7 oz. distilled water

Follow Directions for Creams. The aloe and water combined make up the water portion. Makes 19 oz. Note that this cream may become slightly granular in cold temperatures.

FOOT SOAKS

Foot soaks are extremely pleasurable treatments that combine thorough foot-cleansing action with relaxation and relief of localized pain. A hot soak will stimulate circulation to the lower extremities, bringing nourishment and relief to cold or numb feet. Foot soaks, like hand soaks, can impart a sense of well-being to the entire body. They are especially well suited for elders, for whom, a full body bath is not always agreeable. To prepare a Foot Soak see p. 106.

🐝 *Foot Marinade*

A an excellent soak for achy, tired and swollen feet.

¼ cup vinegar

1 teaspoon olive oil

1 tablespoon sea salt

4 drops wintergreen essential oil

Prepare Basic Foot Soak and add recipe ingredients to the soak water just before immersing feet.

Variations: For more cleansing action add 2 drops of tea tree essential oil. For a more moisturizing action add another teaspoon of olive oil, and omit the salt.

Fresh Herbal Toes

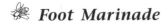

A cleansing and soothing foot soak.

½ oz. comfrey leaf

½ oz. marshmallow

½ oz. yarrow flowers

½ oz. calendula flowers

½ oz. lavender flowers

64 oz. water

Make infusion with herbs and water and let steep for 4 hours. Pour unstrained infusion into the soaking vessel, adding hot water up to the mid-calf level.

FOOT OILS, CREAMS AND BALMS

Oils, balms and creams can the offer the protection and nourishment our skin needs as we age. The formulas offered here are specially formulated for the feet to soften and soothe the skin while offering added benefits such as deodorization and warmth. They are especially good to apply after a soak or bath. Massaging the feet with one of these emollients can be extremely beneficial for improving circulation, and a wonderful gift for an elderly friend or relative. Use the following formulas to enhance the therapeutic effects of massage.

Relax and Rejuvenate Foot Oil

A soothing and nourishing oil for tired, dry and achy feet. This oil mildly deodorizes the feet.

2 oz. chamomile-infused olive oil (preferred)or plain olive oil

10 drops rosemary essential oil

10 drops lavender essential oil

5 drops chamomile essential oil

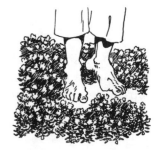

Pour carrier oil into small-mouth glass bottle with a lid, leaving ⅛ inch space at the top, add your essential oils, cap and shake before use. Apply 1–2 teaspoons per foot treatment. For best moisturizing effect, apply to clean and slightly moist feet. Makes 2 oz.

Note: To make chamomile-infused olive oil see Creamy Rose Chamomile Oil pp. 82–83.

Variation: For a more antifungal effect replace the chamomile-infused olive oil with black walnut-infused olive oil (see Antifungal Healing Oil p. 113) and add 10 drops of tea tree essential oil.

Grandpa's Foot Butter   ALL/DRY/DAMAGED

This deluxe and refreshing-smelling butter is excellent for dry, cracked and damaged skin. The essential oils add cleansing and mild deodorizing effects. Grandma will also like it.

3 tablespoons coconut oil
1 tablespoon shea butter
1 tablespoon grated cocoa butter
1 tablespoon plus 1 teaspoon grated
   beeswax
4 tablespoons calendula-infused olive
   oil (preferred) or plain olive oil

30 drops rosemary essential oil
10 drops tea tree essential oil
5 drops lavender essential oil
optional: add an additional teaspoon
   of beeswax to thicken in the warm
   weather

Note: To make calendula-infused olive oil see Luscious Lotion p. 29.

Place ingredients, except essential oils, in a heat-proof cup and put in a hot-water bath. Stir until ingredients are thoroughly melted. Remove from heat and continue to stir for a couple of minutes until mixture is slightly cooled but not thickened; this also helps to evenly distribute the ingredients. Pour into a wide-mouth jar, add essential oils and quickly cap the jar with a tight-fitting lid to prevent the essential oils from evaporating. Allow butter to sit undisturbed for several hours or overnight to completely cool. Massage Grandpa's Foot Butter into problem area as often as you can; try to do it at least twice a day. It is also beneficial to apply generously onto feet before night slumber. Makes about 4½ oz.

Blissful Foot Cream   ALL/DRY/FUNGAL

Use this rich, reparative moisturizer on dry, achy and fungal foot conditions.

3 oz. calendula-infused olive oil
   (preferred) or plain olive oil
3 oz. almond oil
2 oz. coconut oil
1 oz. shea butter
1 oz. beeswax

¼ teaspoon thuja essential oil
40 drops tea tree essential oil
1 teaspoon rosemary essential oil
1 teaspoon wintergreen essential oil
9 oz. distilled water

Note: To make calendula-infused olive oil see Luscious Lotion p. 29.

Follow Directions for Creams. Makes 19 oz.

FOOT POWDERS

Foot powder helps absorb excess moisture to help prevent fungal infections, or to treat them when they do occur. The formulas offered here also have cleansing and deodorizing effects to help eliminate foot odor. Use foot powder as part of a remedial program for fungal conditions in conjunction with other appropriate foot treatments such as antifungal soaks and creams.

Sweet Feet Powder   ALL

A refreshing-smelling powder that is absorbent and deodorizing and provides antifungal action.

Use the following dried herbs:
- 1 tablespoon whole cloves,
- 1 tablespoon coriander seeds,
- 1 tablespoon lavender flowers,
- 1 tablespoon slippery elm powder,
- ¼ cup myrrh powder
- 1 cup clay

- 1 cup cornstarch or arrowroot powder
- 80 drops tea tree essential oil
- 40 drops sage essential oil
- 40 drops lavender essential oil
- 40 drops fir essential oil
- 80 drops rosemary essential oil

Powder herbs, except the myrrh and slippery elm, in a coffee grinder used exclusively for herbs and seeds, then sift powdered herbs through a fine-mesh strainer over a bowl, regrinding the coarser particles as needed. It is important to get the herbs as finely powdered as possible so the foot powder feels soft and silky against the skin. Place powdered herbs, clay, cornstarch and myrrh and slippery elm powders into a jar, mix them thoroughly, then add the essential oils a few drops at a time while stirring them in. Cap and shake jar. To use powder, sprinkle onto feet, and especially between toes. May also be sprinkled into shoes. Store powder in shaker with top or jar with a tight-fitting lid. Makes about 2½ cups.

BODY POWDERS

Body powder can be used to freshen up between baths. Since mature skin tends to dry out easily and frequent baths are often not desirable, these refreshing powders can be enjoyed by older folks for their gently deodorizing effect. The essential oils they contain are also very pleasing to the senses and uplifting to the spirit.

Grandma's Lavender Body Powder   ALL

A sweet-smelling powder that is refreshing and absorbent.

- ½ cup arrowroot powder or cornstarch
- 10 drops lavender essential oil
- 8 drops ylang-ylang essential oil

- 4 drops sweet basil essential oil
- 4 drops sage essential oil

Put arrowroot powder or cornstarch in a small jar, add essential oils and stir them in thoroughly. Cap and shake the jar to continue mixing the ingredients. It is ready to use. To store powder, cap jar with a tight fitting lid. Makes 4 oz.

Variation: Grind and sift 2 tablespoons of dried lavender flowers and add to the powder.

Green God Body Powder ALL

A refreshing-smelling powder to keep dry and deodorized that both grandma and grandpa will enjoy.

1 cup clay
½ cup baking soda
½ cup arrowroot powder
½ cup freshly dried herbs (sage,
   calendula blossoms and thyme
   leaf combined)
2 tablespoons coriander seeds

2 tablespoons slippery elm powder
20 drops cedarwood essential oil
40 drops rosemary essential oil
20 drops sage essential oil
20 drops black pepper essential oil

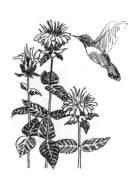

Powder herbs, except the slippery elm, in a coffee grinder used exclusively for herbs and seeds, then sift herbs through a fine-mesh strainer over a bowl, regrinding the coarser particles as needed. It is important to get the herbs as finely powdered as possible so the powder feels soft and silky against the skin. Place all ingredients except the essential oils into a jar, mix the powders thoroughly, then add the essential oils while stirring them in. Cap and shake jar. Makes about 2½ cups.

FACIAL CARE FOR MATURE SKIN

Facial care for mature skin usually means using treatments that are very gentle and nourishing, with mild cleansing and exfoliation properties as needed. As we age our skin tends to become dry, thin and dull. We want to stimulate and increase circulation to the skin to encourage vibrancy and sparkle without causing mechanical or chemical irritation. In the first chapter you will find various preparations that are appropriate for aging skin, or you may want to experiment with the following formulas designed specifically with mature skin in mind. These formulas are very gentle and nourishing. If you find that you want a more astringent and cleansing formula that is less nourishing, please refer to the first chapter and choose among the formulas best suited for your skin type.

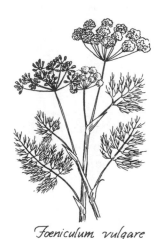

Foeniculum vulgare

Facial Steams

Steams are an excellent way to increase circulation to the skin while deeply cleansing the pores. If you have thread veins or your skin is sensitive to heat, you may not want to use this treatment. Mature skin can often benefit from a weekly or twice-monthly steam.

Lavender Coriander Anise Blend

This is a sweet, refreshing steam for mature skin.

Use the following freshly dried herbs:
2 handfuls lavender flowers, 2 palmfuls
coriander seeds (crushed before use),
2 palmfuls aniseeds (crushed before use)

Combine herbs, use a palmful of herbal mixture for each steaming. Follow directions for Basic Steam Technique see p. 5. Store herbal mixture in a dry, cool place. Makes enough for 6 steams.

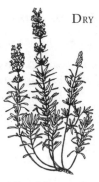

Lavandula angustifolia

Facial Scrubs

Facial scrubs for mature skin should be gentle and nourishing, with minimal but sufficient exfoliating action. Choosing ingredients that are soothing and lubricating, and grinding the ingredients into a fine powder, will make the scrub less abrasive. In the first chapter you will find scrubs that are appropriate for mature skin, such as the Comfrey Fenugreek Scrub. You may also want to try the following formula.

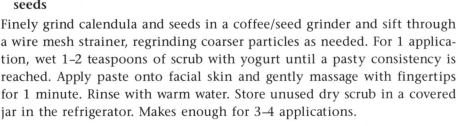

Face Blossom Scrub

ALL/MATURE

A cleansing, soothing scrub for all skin types.

1 tablespoon dried calendula blossom	1 tablespoon sunflower seeds
1 tablespoon fennel seeds	1–2 teaspoons yogurt

Finely grind calendula and seeds in a coffee/seed grinder and sift through a wire mesh strainer, regrinding coarser particles as needed. For 1 application, wet 1–2 teaspoons of scrub with yogurt until a pasty consistency is reached. Apply paste onto facial skin and gently massage with fingertips for 1 minute. Rinse with warm water. Store unused dry scrub in a covered jar in the refrigerator. Makes enough for 3–4 applications.

Helianthus annus

Note: This scrub may also be left on the face for 10–20 minutes and used as a masque.

Facial Masques

Facial masques can be an exhilarating treat for elders. Masques made with nourishing ingredients are best for mature skin. In the first chapter you will find a wide assortment of masques appropriate for mature skin. The following rich masques are also excellent choices.

Glowing Honey Face   ALL/DRY/MATURE

A soothing, moisturizing masque.

½ teaspoon honey
5 drops olive oil, cream or other
    carrier oil of choice

1 squirt fresh lemon juice
1 drop lavender essential oil

Place ingredients into a small bowl and stir until well blended. Massage mixture onto face and apply an even coat on the surface of the skin. Leave on for 20 minute and wash off with warm water. Note: Tie hair back to keep away from honey. Makes enough for 1 masque.

Earthen Beauty   ALL/DRY/MATURE

A rejuvenating, soothing masque.

1 tablespoon clay
1 tablespoon cream

1 drop rosemary essential oil
6 drops vinegar

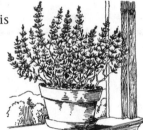

Place ingredients in a small saucer and stir until a pasty consistency is reached. If needed, add more cream to loosen the masque. Massage mixture onto face and apply an even coat on the surface of the skin. Leave on for 20 minute and wash off with warm water. Makes enough for 1 masque.

Hydrating Herbal Toner

These toners are excellent for dry, mature skin, as they are made with reparative herbs, aloe and other skin-restorative ingredients. They are misted on to help moisten, freshen and invigorate the skin.

Rejuvenating Facial Mist   ALL/DRY/MATURE

A gentle, reparative toner that has a sweet floral scent.

2 tablespoons plus 2 teaspoons calen-
    dula infusion (preferred) or
    distilled water
3 teaspoons aloe vera gel

1 teaspoon glycerin
5 drops lavender essential oil
3 drops fennel essential oil
2 drops chamomile essential oil

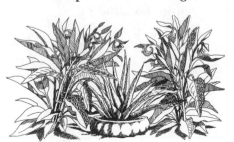

Pour all ingredients into a spray mist bottle, cap and shake well. It is ready to use. Use up within a couple of months; keep refrigerated and check for bacterial contamination periodically. Yields 2 oz.

Note: Make calendula infusion with 1 handful of dried calendula blossoms and 8 oz. of water, let steep for 3 hours and strain.

Far East Facial Mist

All/Dry/Mature

An exotic-smelling restorative toner.

2 tablespoons plus 2 tea-
spoons rose infusion
(preferred) or distilled
water
3 teaspoons aloe vera gel
1 teaspoon glycerin

10 drops sandalwood essential oil
3 drops nutmeg essential oil
2 drops geranium egypt
essential oil
2 drops patchouli essential oil

Pour all ingredients into a spray mist bottle, cap and shake well. It is ready to use.
Use up within a couple of months; keep refrigerated and check for bacterial contamination periodically. Yields 2 oz.

Note: Make rose infusion with 1 handful of dried rose blossoms and 8 oz. of water, let steep for
3 hours and strain.

Moisturizers

Moisturizers are extremely beneficial in rehydrating and lubricating mature skin. In the first
chapter you will find some excellent choices for mature skin, such as Blue Chamomile Face
Cream and Skin Revival. The following formula also serves as an invaluable moisturizer for dry,
mature skin.

Facial Recovery Cream

All/Dry/Damaged

This rich, reparative cream can be used for the body as well as the face.

Liquid oils should total 6 oz.:
3 tablespoons jojoba oil,
2 tablespoons avocado oil,
2 tablespoons peanut oil,
2 tablespoons St. Johnswort-infused
olive oil (see p. 125), 2 tablespoons
wheat germ oil, 1 tablespoon plus 2
teaspoons comfrey root-infused
olive oil (see p. 82), 2 teaspoons
lecithin

Solid oils should total 3 oz.:
3 tablespoons shea butter,
3 tablespoons coconut oil
½ oz. beeswax
9 oz. comfrey root infusion
(preferred) or distilled water
2 teaspoons vegetable glycerin
25 drops lavender essential oil
40 drops sandalwood essential oil
10 drops fennel essential oil

Note: Less beeswax is used in this recipe than in the Basic Cream Formula.
This is because the addition of lecithin helps emulsify creams and therefore
can be used to replace some of the beeswax within a cream formula.

Make comfrey root infusion with 2 tablespoons dried cut comfrey root and
8 oz. water. Let steep for 8 hours and strain.

Follow Directions for Creams on pp. 224–226 instructions. When making Facial Recovery Cream add the lecithin to the liquid oil component and the glycerin to the water component. This cream is very thick and rich and is harder to

pour than other creams, so you will need to scoop it out. The more lecithin you add the thicker the cream, as lecithin is an emulsifier. It's messy, but worth it. Facial Recovery Cream is also one of the most perishable of the creams and so should definitely be refrigerated, especially since its consistency is not compromised by refrigeration. Makes 19 oz.

PAIN RELIEF OILS AND BALMS

Aging often brings with it an assortment of aches and pains. If you exercise regularly, eat properly and get enough rest, the chances of moving into a healthy and virtually pain-free old age is greatly increased. If you are experiencing some minor discomfort you may want to try the formulas in Chapter 4: Whole Body Treatments under the section heading Preparations for Sore Muscles, Bones and Nerves. Some good choices are Fire and Ice Liniment Balm, Arnica Oil, Analgesic Oil and Relaxation Salve.

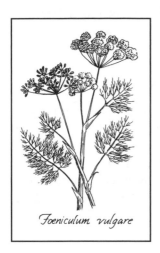

Foeniculum vulgare

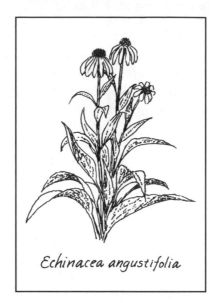

Echinacea angustifolia

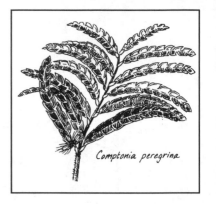

Comptonia peregrina

11
Natural
First Aid

Every now and then your skin may need a little extra protection or remedial action from contact with, or overexposure to, various elements in the environment. An entire book could be written on natural first aid, and I felt it important to at least include a few basic topical treatments, for everything from wounds and burns to poison ivy rashes and sunburn. Since prevention is an important part of natural skin care, I have also included some sunscreen and bug repellent formulas.

SUN PRODUCTS

Sunshine

One of my favorite health and beauty treatments — strange as it may seem — is exposure to fresh air and sunshine. Regular, moderate exposure to the sun can impart a rich, healthy glow to the skin, aid in vitamin D metabolism, support hormonal functioning and general health and even help clear up acne and other skin problems. I advocate an hour or two of exposure on a daily basis, taking care to protect the skin against the sun's damaging ultraviolet (UV) rays when appropriate. In the summer I like to avoid direct exposure to the sun when it is at its greatest intensity, from about 11 A.M. to 3 P.M. In the winter, when the sun's angle is low in the Northeast, where I live, and the light is not as intense, I like to bundle up and bathe my face in the noonday sun. Even if you are sensitive to the sun, you might be able to tolerate direct exposure to the winter sun, then enjoy the summer sun indirectly under the cover of shade or filtered through the leaves of a tree. UV exposure is a definite concern, particularly as air pollution continues to eat away the Earth's protective ozone layer, so please use your good judgment when it comes to sunning yourself. Remember that the sun is always at its greatest intensity from late morning to early afternoon, and that it is still possible to receive a very bad burn on an overcast day. You should also keep in mind that the sun is more intense at high altitudes, and that reflected sunlight from water or snow can intensify your exposure.

The application of nourishing and protective emollients to your skin before and after sun exposure can help prevent the skin from drying out and turning leathery. A number of natural ingredients such as shea butter, PABA (a member of the vitamin B family), sesame oil and St. Johnswort offer varying degrees of protection against UV rays. The following formulas combine various rich emollients with these natural sunscreens, providing nontoxic alternatives to the chemical sunblocks available on the commercial market. I am also of the opinion that eating a healthy diet rich in omega-3 fatty acids — particularly EPA fatty acids — will help provide natural sun protection from the inside. Omega-3 fatty acids are found in especially high concentrations in whole seeds, and cold-water seafood is extremely rich in EPA.

Golden Sun Juice   ALL/NORMAL/DAMAGED

This is a rich, protective, nourishing oil with an SPF-15. It may be used as a general-healing body oil for damaged skin or when protection is needed from sun and wind. (The SPF is based on empirical research and not from laboratory testing.) Notice how your skin responds to the sun with this oil. If it burns, you need a stronger product, or you can increase the SPF by adding additional PABA.

¾ oz. beeswax
2 oz. shea butter
1 oz. wheat germ oil
4 oz. sesame oil
4 oz. St. Johnswort-infused olive oil
  (see Luscious Lotion p. 29)

1 oz. lecithin
3 oz. coconut oil
1 tablespoon PABA
optional: 3 oz. cocoa
  butter, 50 drops essential
  oils of choice

In a 16-oz. heat-proof measuring cup (if adding cocoa butter, use a cup that is 20 oz. or larger) combine all the ingredients except the PABA, lecithin and optional essential oils. Place the measuring cup in a hot-water bath, and while stirring allow the oils and beeswax to melt together and become a uniform liquid free of lumps. In a small cup combine the lecithin and the PABA, stirring and dissolving the PABA into the lecithin. Remove the heat-proof cup from the hot-water bath, add the PABA-lecithin mixture and stir in well. Pour into a squeeze bottle and add essential oils of choice, if desired. Cap and shake bottle to mix in essential oils. If ingredients should separate, shake before using. Makes about 16 oz., if using cocoa butter makes 20 oz.

Dina's Deep Tanning Butter   ALL/DARK OR SUN-RESISTANT SKIN

I developed this butter for myself, as I like to tan and didn't like using the Golden Sun Juice because its high SPF prevented my skin from doing so. This butter allows tanning without drying or wrinkling the skin, keeping it soft, nourished and protected. I approximate it has an SPF-6. When making this butter for myself, I omit the essential oils. However, many of my customers prefer the Deep Tanning Butter made with them.

3 tablespoons jojoba oil
2 tablespoons avocado oil
2 tablespoons peanut oil
2 tablespoons calendula-infused olive oil (see Luscious Lotion p. 29)
2 tablespoons wheat germ oil
1 tablespoon burdock root-infused olive oil

1 tablespoon lecithin
3 tablespoons shea butter
3 tablespoons coconut oil
2 oz. beeswax
optional: 60 drops tangerine essential oil, 30 drops patchouli essential oil, 50 drops lavender essential oil

Note: To make burdock root-infused olive oil use 2 oz. of freshly dried and crushed burdock root and 8 oz. of cold pressed olive oil and follow Directions for Herbal-Infused Oils with Dried Herbs. Yields about 5 oz.

In a 16-oz. heat-proof measuring cup, combine all the ingredients except the essential oils and the lecithin. Place the measuring cup into a hot-water bath, and while stirring allow the ingredients to melt together and become a uniform liquid free of lumps. Remove the cup from heat, add the lecithin and stir in well. Pour mixture into a wide-mouth jar and immediately drop in essential oils, quickly capping jar to prevent them from evaporating. Leave undisturbed to solidify; when solid it is ready for use. If pouring the Deep Tanning Butter into individual 2-oz. jars, add ⅙ the amount of each essential oil into each jar. Makes about 12 oz. or fills six 2-oz. salve jars.

Some people prefer to use creams rather than oils for sun protection because they contain water, which helps to hydrate the skin.

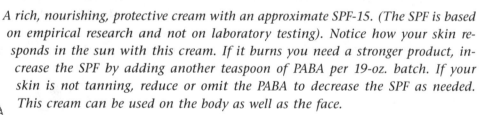

Sun Butter Face Cream   All/Sensitive

A rich, nourishing, protective cream with an approximate SPF-15. (The SPF is based on empirical research and not on laboratory testing). Notice how your skin responds in the sun with this cream. If it burns you need a stronger product, increase the SPF by adding another teaspoon of PABA per 19-oz. batch. If your skin is not tanning, reduce or omit the PABA to decrease the SPF as needed. This cream can be used on the body as well as the face.

See formula p. 31.

REMEDIES FOR BURNS FROM SUN, FIRE AND RADIATION THERAPY

Burns are without a doubt one of the most painful conditions that we can experience. If you have received a first-degree burn — one that causes redness, but that has not penetrated the skin too deeply — there are a number of remedies you can use to alleviate the painful sensation and promote rapid healing. In general, first-degree burns, whether caused by contact with a direct heat source, overexposure to the sun or even radiation therapy, can be alleviated con-

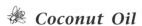

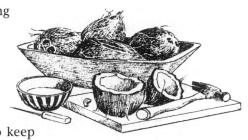

siderably with thick and frequent applications of cooling emollients such as coconut oil or one of the following salve formulas. If you have received a thermal burn from a direct heat source such as a stove, a hot iron or scalding liquid, first apply something cold to the affected area as quickly as possible to draw out the heat; cold water, ice cubes or snow work very well for this purpose. Next apply a thick coat of oil or salve, reapplying it often to keep the affected area covered. Whenever I burn myself on the wood or cooking stove I find that this method soothes the pain, helps prevent blistering and promotes rapid healing. In the case of sunburn, frequent applications of cooling salves can also help prevent your skin from peeling. Keep in mind that the formulas offered here are for first-degree burns, in which the burn has not penetrated too deeply into the body. They may also be used in conjunction with medical treatments for more serious burns. But in such cases, please seek professional medical advice.

Coconut Oil   ALL/DAMAGED

Coconut oil's cooling nature is very helpful in healing burns. After submersing burn in cold water, apply coconut oil generously, and reapply throughout the day to keep burn well coated with the oil.

Lavender Coconut Oil   ALL/DAMAGED

Lavender essential oil is also excellent for burns. By adding rosemary's cleansing action to lavender and coconut oil we have another excellent formula for healing burns. This also makes a great hair treatment.

4 oz. coconut oil   **40 drops rosemary essential oil**
40 drops lavender essential oil

Place the coconut oil in a double boiler or hot-water bath, allow to melt, pour into a wide-mouth jar, drip in essential oils and quickly cap. Let cool and solidify. It is ready to use. Note that in the summer months the consistency of this preparation will be runny and loose, as the coconut oil melts at 76 degrees. After submersing burn in cold water, apply generously and re-apply throughout the day to keep burn well coated with oil. Makes 4 oz.

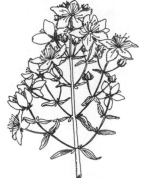

Relaxation Salve   ALL/DAMAGED

This salve contains St. Johnswort and coconut oil, which are both excellent for healing burns. The St. Johnswort helps with inflammation and pain. See formula pp. 92–93

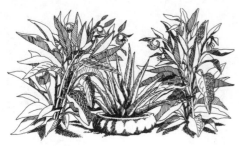

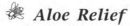 *Aloe Relief* All/Damaged

The gel from the leaf of the aloe plant or bottled gel applied to a burn soothes the pain and speeds the healing process. Apply the inside of the aloe leaf directly on the burn, and tape onto the burn if possible. Or alternatively, apply the gel generously and repeatedly over the burn.

 ## Butter All/Damaged

Dairy butter can be used to soothe the skin and facilitate the healing of a burn where the skin hasn't been broken. Submerse burn in cold water then spread butter over the burn and reapply as needed.

Golden Sun Juice All/Dry/Damaged

Golden Sun Juice, found at the beginning of the chapter, is an excellent oil to apply to sunburned skin. It prevents peeling and blistering while reducing the discomfort of the burn. Generously apply and reapply, keeping the skin well coated.

Superhealing Cream for Radiation Dry/Damaged

I devised this cream for a woman with breast cancer who was receiving radiation treatment. It helped her with healing the burns and scars that resulted from the treatments. She loved to use the cream, as it soothed her wound while the aroma of the lavender was refreshing and uplifting to her spirit.

1 oz. calendula-infused olive oil (see Luscious Lotion p. 29)
1 oz. comfrey-infused olive oil (see Comfrey Salve/Loose Version p. 36)
1 oz. St. Johnswort-infused olive oil (see p. 125)
1 oz. jojoba oil

1 oz. sesame oil
1 oz. wheat germ oil
1 oz. shea butter
2 oz. coconut oil
1 oz. beeswax
2 teaspoons lavender essential oil
9 oz. distilled water

Follow Directions for Creams. Makes 19 oz.

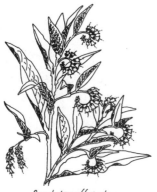

Symphytum officinale

Comfrey Formulations

Comfrey roots and leaves encourage the healing of burns. You can make comfrey poultices from either fresh or dried herb. The following preparations are also used for healing sprains, broken bones and other injuries. In addition, they make excellent, although messy, face and body packs.

Fresh Comfrey Burn Pack   DAMAGED

Large handful fresh comfrey leaves
   and/or roots (chopped)
1–2 tablespoons water

½ teaspoon olive oil
2 drops lavender essential oil
1 drop tea tree essential oil

Place chopped herbs into blender or food processor and puree with water and olive oil until a thick puree results; remove from blender and add the essential oils. Store unused portion in the refrigerator in a covered container.

Apply thickly to burn and cover with a cloth bandage. Leave on for as long as possible and reapply as needed. You may need to double or triple the recipe depending on the size of the burn.

Dried Comfrey Burn Pack   DAMAGED

1 tablespoon comfrey root
1 tablespoon comfrey leaf
3–4 tablespoons water

¼ teaspoon olive oil
2 drops lavender essential oil
1 drop tea tree oil

Grind comfrey into a powder and place in small bowl, pour in water to make a paste, then add olive oil and essential oils. Apply the paste to the affected area. Leave on for as long as possible and reapply as needed. To remove pack, soak area with warm water or apply a warm, wet cloth and gently rinse off. You may need to double or triple the recipe depending on the size of the burn.

Comfrey Salve   DAMAGED

This is another way to prepare comfrey; although not as potent as the preceding preparations, it will often suffice. See formula pp. 102–103.

BUG REPELLENT AND BITE AND STING REMEDIES

Green Bug Juice   ALL

This is an effective bug repellent, based on Julliette de Bairacli Levy's recipe in her book Traveler's Joy. *Its dual action is provided by first extracting the bitter herbs into a carrier oil base and then adding strong-acting essential oils. Apply thoroughly to your skin and reapply as necessary. The effectiveness of the oil depends largely on the bitterness of the wormwood. If you can, taste the wormwood before you buy it. Good-quality wormwood should taste disgustingly bitter and have a strong aroma. Green Bug Juice also makes an excellent after-bite remedy by reducing itching and swelling. And it is excellent for toning pores and softening skin.*

To make with dried herbs use:
- ½ cup wormwood (cut),
- 1 tablespoon rue (cut),
- 1 tablespoon sage (cut),
- 1 tablespoon tansy (cut),
- 1 tablespoon pennyroyal (cut),
- 1 tablespoon southernwood (cut)

8 oz. cold pressed olive oil
1 teaspoon eucalyptus essential oil
45 drops lemongrass essential oil
30 drops spearmint essential oil

Coarsely grind herbs. Proceed to make an herbal-infused oil with the herbs and olive oil by following Directions for Herbal-Infused Oils with Dried Herbs. Pour strained herbal-infused oil into a jar, add the essential oils, cap and shake. It is ready for use. Makes about 5 oz. *Variation follows:*

Green Bug Juice with Fresh Herbs   All

If you are growing these herbs, proceed with stuffing a jar half full with wormwood and then filling the rest of the jar with equal parts of rue, sage, tansy, pennyroyal and southernwood and following Directions for Making Herbal-Infused Oils with Fresh Herbs. For every 2 oz. of strained herbal-infused oil you end up with, add 50 drops of eucalyptus essential oil, 13 drops of lemongrass essential oil and 10 of drops spearmint essential oil.

Easy Bug Juice   All

You can also make a simpler oil with just wormwood infused in olive oil. Add the essential oils as mentioned in the above recipe, if you have them, and apply this oil to the skin to repel bugs.

Artemesia absinthium

Plantain Leaf Poultice   All/Damaged

Fresh plantain leaves, chewed and applied to bug bites, such as bee stings and mosquito bites, effectively reduce swelling, itching and pain. Wrap and tie a cloth over the poultice to keep it in place. See Botanicals section in Ingredients chapter for more information on plantain.

Baking Soda for Bee Stings   All/Damaged

For effective bee sting relief apply a baking soda paste. Bee stings are acid and the alkalinity of the baking soda helps to neutralize them.

1 teaspoon baking soda   1 drop tea tree essential oil
½ teaspoon water

Place baking soda in palm of hand or small vessel and add water, a few drops at a time, until a spreadable paste results. Add the tea tree oil and apply to bee sting. Leave on for as long as needed and reapply new paste if necessary. Makes enough for 1 application.

Vinegar for Wasp Stings   All/Damaged

Wasp stings are alkaline and are neutralized by the acidic qualities of vinegar.

Tissue or cloth (sized to cover the bite)
vinegar

Make a vinegar compress by saturating a cloth or tissue with vinegar and applying it to the wasp bite. Keep cloth on the bite for several minutes or until discomfort is gone. If cloth begins to dry out, add more vinegar. To keep preparation in place, you may want to wrap and tie a bandage around it. Makes enough for 1 application.

Clay Poultice with Tea Tree Oil ALL/DAMAGED

Applying a clay paste with added tea tree oil helps to draw out and disinfect bug bites. Use vinegar to wet the paste if treating a wasp sting.

clay	**tea tree essential oil**
liquid (water, echinacea tincture or vinegar)	

Make a clay paste with equal parts clay and liquid and add 2 drops of tea tree oil per tablespoon of clay paste and apply to bites. Allow to dry and flake off. Rinse off residual paste and reapply as needed.

Black Walnut and Tea Tree Salve ALL

This strong-acting salve for fungal, viral and septic skin conditions is also helpful when applied to a bite to reduce swelling and foster healing. See formula p. 113.

Lavender Sandalwood Cream ALL

A friend reported after his trip to Africa that this cream was a lifesaver at night, when he would be kept awake by irritating bug bites. He applied it to the bites, which soothed and relieved the irritations allowing him to go to sleep. See formula p. 29.

CARE OF CUTS, BRUISES AND SCRAPES

The following remedies have disinfectant, astringent and cell-regenerative properties, making them ideal for minor cuts, scrapes and bruises. Some also have analgesic properties to help alleviate localized pain. Many of these formulas can be used to disinfect and clean wounds before applying a healing salve.

Poultices

Poultices are one of the most ancient methods used to encourage the healing of wounds. They are made by mashing or masticating fresh herbs to release their juices, thereby creating a soft, moist mass that is applied directly to the affected area. If dried herbs are used, they are usually powdered, then moistened with water, herbal infusion, herbal tincture or other suitable liquid to create a paste that is applied to the wound. Once you have applied a poultice, you may wrap it with a cloth or cotton gauze to hold it in place over the wound for more sustained healing effects.

🐝 *Plantain Poultice*   DAMAGED

Fresh plantain leaf chewed and applied to wounds greatly facilitates the healing process.

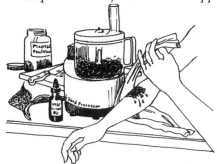

Plantain Poultice (Big Batch)   DAMAGED

If the wound is large you may want to puree plantain leaves in a food processor, as the chewing could get tiring.

Large handful fresh plantain leaves (chopped)
1–2 tablespoons water
2 drops lavender essential oil
1 drop tea tree essential oil

Place chopped herbs into blender or food processor and puree with water until a thick puree results; remove and add the essential oils. Store unused portion in the refrigerator in a covered container.

Apply thickly to wound and cover with a cloth bandage. Leave on for as long as possible, and reapply as needed. You may need to double or triple the recipe depending on the size of the wound. Makes enough for 1 or more applications (again depending on the size of the wound).

Yarrow Poultice   DAMAGED

Yarrow is an excellent first aid herb, offering analgesic, antimicrobial, astringent and styptic effects. Apply fresh-chewed yarrow to wounds. Or powder dried yarrow and sprinkle on affected area to help stop bleeding, reduce pain and minimize bacterial growth. Yarrow tincture may be applied to wounds as well.

First Aid Tinctures

Tinctures made from herbs that have strong cleansing, analgesic and cell-reparative properties can be used directly on injured skin. Keep in mind that the alcohol in tinctures will sting broken skin, you may wish to dilute the tincture with water to minimize this stinging sensation. To dilute the tincture add 1–2 dropperfuls or ¼ teaspoon of tincture into ¼–½ cup of water. Soaking the wound in the diluted tincture solution can help alleviate pain and promote healing. Tinctures are convenient for travel, and make good additions to a first aid kit.

Herbs for Wounds

The following herbs are most appropriate for wound care, and are often found in natural first aid products such as balms, tinctures and washes:

Aloe, arnica, calendula, comfrey, echinacea, garlic, goldenseal, lavender, myrrh, oregano, plantain, sage, spilanthes, St. Johnswort, thyme, witch hazel and yarrow.

Calendula Tincture

DAMAGED

Calendula tincture is often used as a cleansing wash for wounds. You can apply it straight onto the injury; however, if the skin is broken the alcohol will sting. You can dilute the tincture in water to minimize the stinging. Soaking the injured area is also very helpful. Dilute the tincture by adding 1– 2 dropperfuls or ¼ teaspoon of calendula tincture into ¼–½ cup of water. Apply to wounds often to keep them from getting infected while also speeding the healing process.

See formula p. 100.

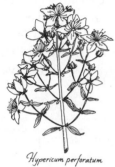

Hypericum perforatum

St. Johnswort Tincture

DAMAGED

St. Johnswort's astringent, anti-inflammatory and pain-relieving properties make it very useful for various kinds of injuries. You can apply it straight onto the injury; however, if the skin is broken the alcohol will sting; you can dilute the tincture in water to minimize the stinging. Soaking the wound in a diluted tincture-and-water solution can be very beneficial. Dilute the tincture by adding 1–2 dropperfuls or ¼ teaspoon of St. Johnswort tincture into ¼–½ cup of water. See formula p. 49.

Defense Formula

DAMAGED

This is a combination of herbs traditionally used for their antimicrobial action. The formula can be used to help clear infections inside and outside the body. You can apply it straight onto the site; however, if the skin is broken the alcohol will sting. You can dilute the tincture in water to minimize the stinging. Soaking the injured area with diluted tincture water solution is also very helpful. Dilute the tincture by adding 1–2 dropperfuls or ¼ teaspoon of tincture into ¼–½ cup of water. See formula pp. 100-101.

Essential Oils for Wounds

Essential oils are by nature strong antimicrobial agents, and are very helpful in dressing wounds. They can be added to water for washing wounds or included in other preparations such as poultices, salves and tinctures.

Essential Oil Wound Wash

DAMAGED

> **Add 3–6 drops of essential oil of choice**
> **a cup of water**

Wash or soak wound with water. Makes enough for 1 application.

Tea Tree Wound Wash

DAMAGED

Tea tree essential oil can be added to water as well as poultices, balms and other preparations for increasing antimicrobial action.

Add 4 drops of tea tree oil to 1 cup of water and use to clean wounds. Makes enough for 1 application.

Variations: Essential oils of lavender, thuja, thyme, rosemary, eucalyptus and sage make excellent wound washes. Check Ingredients chapter for more choices and information on essential oils.

Healing Salves

These salves are made with herbal-infused oils solidified with beeswax. The healing properties of these formulas may also be enhanced by the addition of essential oils. The salves are applied to wounds after they have been cleaned to speed healing and minimize scarring. There are numerous salve and balm formulas mentioned throughout the book that are appropriate for dressing wounds, such as Calendula Salve, Black Walnut and Tea Tree Salve, Relaxation Salve, Comfrey Salve and Skin Soothe Balm.

Do an empirical test on yourself by applying salve to only part of a wound, leaving the other part without. Watch and compare the healing. The part that has been treated with salve should heal faster, with less scarring.

Wound Balm   Damaged

A strong healing balm made with herbs traditionally used for wound care. This formula requires that you first make an herbal-infused oil, which will take about 6 weeks to steep. Once you have made the oil you can use it as is or turn it into a salve with the addition of beeswax. The essential oils are added to increase the cleansing and healing action of the preparation, but can be omitted if desired.

Use herbs that are freshly dried: 1 oz. comfrey root (cut), ½ oz. yarrow, ½ oz. calendula blossoms, 1 oz. myrrh powder, 1 oz. goldenseal roots (cut)
  16 oz. cold pressed olive oil
  4 oz. beeswax
  ¾ teaspoon tea tree essential oil
  1 teaspoon lavender essential oil
  ½ teaspoon thyme essential oil

First make herbal-infused oil by coarsely grinding herbs in mortar and pestle or coffee grinder and placing herbs and olive oil in a glass jar with a tight-fitting lid. Proceed to Directions for Herbal-Infused Oils with Dried Herbs. The strained infused oil is then made into a salve with the addition of beeswax by following Directions for Salves and Balms. Remember when making a salve to add the essential oils at the end of the salve-making procedure as instructed. Makes about 12 oz. of herbal-infused oil or 16 oz. of balm.

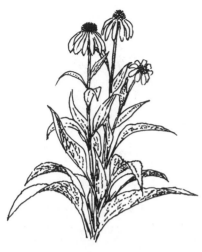

Echinacea angustifolia

All-Purpose Salve ALL/DAMAGED

This salve is made with St. Johnswort-, calendula- and plantain-infused oils solidified with beeswax. This is a broad-spectrum healing salve useful on minor skin irritations, inflammations, diaper rash, chapped skin, lips and burns. Apply salve to wounds after they have been cleaned. See formula p. 103.

Antimicrobial Baby Balm DAMAGED

This balm, found in the Especially for Babies chapter, is made with herbal-infused oils of echinacea, myrrh, calendula, thyme and yarrow and solidified with beeswax. These herbs are strong cleansers and wound healers. Apply after wound has been washed and re-apply throughout the healing process to speed and ease recovery. See formula p. 163.

POISON IVY ANTIDOTES

Although some lucky people are unaffected by contact with poison ivy, others can develop anything from a mild skin rash to an acute systemic reaction. If you know that you have been exposed to poison ivy, the first step you should take is to thoroughly wash any skin that has come into contact with the plant as soon after exposure as possible. You may either want to use a strong cleansing soap to strip the oils off your skin or to try the following baking soda formula, then rinse, rinse, rinse. This will flush away the oils that are responsible for the reaction and prevent them from spreading to other areas of your body. If the offending oils do penetrate the skin and enter the blood and lymph fluids, a rash or systemic reaction may result. The following formulas can help prevent a rash from occurring, alleviate itchiness and discourage the formation of blisters that may lead to spreading the rash. You can also prevent the rash from spreading further by placing the liquid preparations in a spray bottle and misting rather than rubbing them onto the affected areas.

Baking Soda Scrub ITCHY

Baking soda helps neutralize the plant acids.

   baking soda

Gently scrub baking soda on area that has been in contact with poison ivy to prevent rash from occurring. One easy way is to keep a plastic container filled with baking soda in the shower and dip your hand into container and slather baking soda on skin as needed. Rinse well with warm water.

Fresh Jewelweed Poultice

Jewelweed seems to neutralize poison ivy's irritating oils. It will prevent poison ivy from creating a rash if it is applied shortly after contact, or it can be used to minimize the effects of an already established rash.

fresh jewelweed, leaf and stem

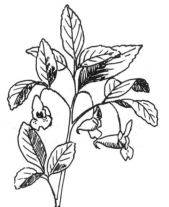

Impatiens capensis

Gather jewelweed and mash it well, till the juices are released. Apply this wet mash to the affected area.

Jewelweed Ice Cubes

If you or a family member are prone to poison ivy rashes you might consider making these jewelweed ice cubes. Stored in the freezer when jewelweed is out of season, they are available year-round and are easy to use once they are made.

fresh jewelweed, leaf and stem
water

Gather jewelweed, chop it up and place it a blender or food processor with just enough water to liquefy the herb. Strain jewelweed puree through a strainer lined with a cloth. Gather up the ends of the cloth and squeeze out all the liquid. Compost the herb and freeze the liquid in ice cube trays. To use, place ice cube over rash and let it melt onto skin. Keep applying as needed. The cold ice cubes along with the jewelweed help soothe the heat and irritation of the rash.

Jewelweed and Friends

Use the following fresh herbs:
  1 handful jewelweed, 1 handful
  wild lettuce (leaf and a little stem),
  1 handful yellow giant hyssop leaves

3–6 tablespoons water

Chop herbs and place in blender or food processor with just enough water to liquefy the herbs. Apply the puree to the affected area or strain through a strainer lined with cloth. Gather up the ends of the cloth and squeeze out all the liquid. Compost the herb and store unused portion in the refrigerator, or freeze the liquid in ice cube trays for future use.

Variation: You can also preserve the liquid by adding an ounce of vodka to every ounce of liquid. Place liquid in a spray bottle and mist on affected area.

Learn about the local wild herbs in your area to find out which ones can be used as antidotes for poison ivy — you will be surprised at how many there are! At the same time you will begin to learn other useful information about the wild foods and healing herbs that grow all around you.

Woodland Essence "Itch Re-leaf"   ITCHY

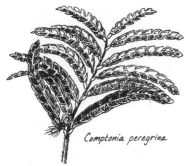

Comptonia peregrina

This formula is used for any inflamed, itching skin reaction such as poison ivy rashes, insect bites and hives. Apply to affected skin as needed. Itch Re-leaf may also be added to clay to create a paste and then applied to the skin to help dry out the rash. Available through Woodland Essence (see Resources).

Gather fresh herbs in equal parts:
     jewelweed (whole plant), plantain leaf and stem,
     comfrey leaf, comfrey root, mugwort leaf,
     witch hazel bark, sweet fern leaf and stem.

Method 1: This makes a tincture using distilled witch hazel and 190 proof alcohol as the menstrum and requires 6 weeks of preparation time.

Cut herbs and roots finely and pack loosely in a glass jar. Add 3 parts witch hazel extract (from drugstore) and 1 part 190 proof grain alcohol to cover the herbs and fill the jar. Cap with a tight-fitting lid. Keep jar away from direct sunlight. Shake daily for 6 weeks and strain and bottle. It is ready for use.

To give approximate amounts: If you use a 16-oz. glass jar and loosely fill it with the herbs, you will need about 5–6 oz. of fresh herbs. The amount of menstrum needed to cover the herbs and fill the jar will be about 10–11 oz. This will consist of 7½–8 oz. of witch hazel extract and 2½–3 oz. of 190 proof grain alcohol. As with all tinctures, the measurements of herb and menstrum depend on the size jar you are using, how tightly the jar is packed with herb and how much moisture the herbs contain.

Method 2: This makes a water-based decoction that is preserved with alcohol. It is a faster method, requiring only 8 hours of steeping.

Place well-chopped herbs in a large nonaluminum pot. Cover herbs with water and simmer on low heat for 1 hour with pan covered. Remove pan from heat and let steep for 8 hours or overnight. Strain. Preserve herbal liquid with 20 percent alcohol by volume. This means that to every 4 oz. of herbal liquid, add 1 oz. of 190 proof grain alcohol.

You may want to place the Itch Re-leaf in a spray bottle; misting a rash feels good and helps prevent further irritation that may result from touching or rubbing the skin.

Ed Smith's Grindelia Sassafras Compound   ITCHY

A specific for allergic contact dermatitis associated with the plants poison oak, poison ivy and poison sumac. Helps relieve the itching and can prevent or lessen the occurrence of blisters. Available through Herbpharm (see Resources).

**1 oz. grindelia tincture made with
     dried flower and leaf**
**1 oz. sassafras tincture made with
     dried root bark**

1¼ teaspoon peppermint essential oil

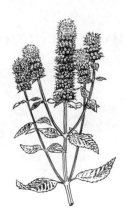

Make tinctures, but use 10 percent glycerin in the menstrum for tincturing the sassafras due to its high tannin content, or purchase them premade. Combine the tinctures and add the peppermint essential oil. Put in a jar with a mist nozzle, and spray on skin or apply with a disposable cotton swab. In severe cases, additional relief can sometimes be gained by internal use of this compound. Take 20–40 drops in water 3–5 times per day.

Note: Herbpharm makes this preparation with menthol crystals instead of the peppermint essential oil. Ed Smith adapted the recipe here for simplicity's sake.

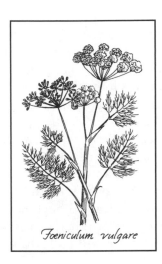

Foeniculum vulgare

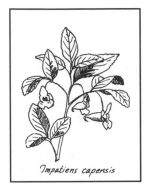

Impatiens capensis

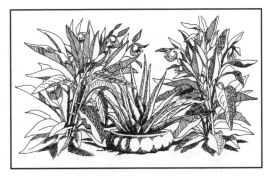

12
Ingredients

When you read the ingredient labels of commercially prepared products for skin, nails and hair, you are often confronted with a long list of chemicals with unpronounce able names, artificial colors, synthetic scents, stabilizers and preservatives. Frequently the labels attempt to seduce you with mystifications like "anti-aging complex" or "amino-en-riched formula" that seem to promise eternal youth and beauty. The sophisticated packaging and alluring ads are often enough to make you believe that if you spend enough money, eternal youth and beauty really can be yours.

Behind the multimillion-dollar, youth-oriented beauty industry is the idea that through "sci-ence" humans can control and improve upon Nature — an idea that springs from a profound sense of alienation from the Earth. Ironically, many of the ingredients that go into the products created by this industry are synthetic versions of naturally occurring substances. The question we should ask ourselves every time we reach for a commercial body care product is whether the synthetic ingredients it contains really are an improvement upon what Nature herself has to offer. From my perspective, the answer is usually a resounding no. If we can accept our-selves as a part of Nature, rather than set ourselves apart from her, then we can begin to accept the simple gifts she has to offer. When we use these gifts to make our own body care products, we are empowered with the knowledge of exactly what we are putting on our bodies, and we can feel reassured by their natural purity. We can also feel satisfied knowing that using these ingredients is generally a more ecologically sustainable choice than using highly processed or synthesized ones.

When choosing ingredients for your body care formulas, keep in mind the principles of sim-plicity and purity. Many of the ingredients called for in the formulas presented here available through health food stores, co-ops or direct mail. When you use agricultural products, try to choose ones that are organically grown. Whenever possible, choose minimally processed ingre-dients that are as fresh and as close to their natural state as possible. For example, if you are making a formula that calls for nuts, you might buy whole nuts and grind them in a blender yourself so that the nutrients are not lost through oxidation. This is also especially important when using seeds and herbs. Avoid ingredients that have unnecessary additives such as artificial scent or color. For example, aloe vera gel is close to colorless in its natural state, but is often tinted bright green when sold commercially. Since many cosmetic dyes are potentially carcinogenic, it is worth the effort to seek out a brand that is free of this unnecessary coloring.

Many of the herbs listed in the Botanicals section that follows can either be gathered wild or cultivated in a garden. Gathering and growing your own herbs can be a very rewarding process. I always feel a great sense of personal satisfaction when the products I make for sale, gifts or home use come from herbs that I have nurtured from seed or gathered from a beautiful meadow or streamside. If you do collect your own herbs, be sure to gather from clean sites located away from roadsides, since the toxic exhaust from automobiles is easily absorbed by plants. And please gather responsibly — never wipe out an entire stand of a wild herb. Always leave enough healthy plants in any given area to ensure regrowth. If you decide to gather your own herbs, it is well worth investing in a good field guide and going on "weed walks" with a qualified herbalist in order to be positive of your plant identifications.

The sampling of ingredients presented in this chapter is enough to get you started on making your own natural body care products. There are many other ingredients you might use, and other books that treat much of the information here in greater depth and detail. I encourage you to use this chapter as a quick reference guide, and to consult the books listed in Resources for further ideas and information.

This chapter is divided into four sections: Oils and Butters, Foodstuffs and Other Natural Ingredients, Botanicals, and Essential Oils. The items within each section are listed alphabetically for ease of reference.

OILS AND BUTTERS

Oils and butters generally function in body care products as carrier or base oils. Carrier or base oils serve as a foundation for skin care products and for essential oils. Carrier oils are generally extracted from fruits, grains, nuts or seeds, such as olive, wheat germ, peanut or sesame. Many of them are the same products that you use for cooking. The various carriers have particular qualities that make them useful in different situations or for different skin types.

I believe it is very important to choose unrefined cold pressed or expeller pressed oils. These grades of oils have been mechanically pressed rather than extracted with petrochemical solvents such as heptane or hexane. Less heat has been used in the production of cold pressed than expeller pressed oils, which keeps them from becoming rancid and retains more of their nutritional value. Also, unrefined oils are more nourishing than refined oils, whether ingested or used topically. Be aware, however, that unrefined oils are stronger in color and scent than refined oils, and that they may have a cloudy appearance.

Keep in mind too that light, heat and oxygen cause rancidity and spoilage in oils. You may want to purchase oils in relatively small quantities and store them in airtight containers in a cool, dark place such as the refrigerator. Oil-based preparations should be stored in the same way. If an oil or oil-based product begins to smell rancid, it is best to discard it or use it for polishing the floor or furniture.

Almond Oil, pressed from almond kernels, enjoys a lot of popularity in the natural skin care arena. It is a light and nearly odorless oil with a great deal of nutritional value. I find it to be somewhat on the dry side, and often combine it with richer, heavier oils such as peanut or olive. Although cold pressed almond oil is available, the solvent extracted type is much more common. Please read the label to be sure, since the solvents used in the latter are not good for the skin.

Apricot Kernel Oil is made from the inner kernels of the apricot. It possesses properties similar to almond oil, being light, odorless and somewhat drying. Like almond oil it can be used in most skin care preparations, but may also need to be enriched with more emollient oils.

Avocado Oil is a wonderfully rich oil made from the pulp of the avocado fruit. A heavy but penetrating oil that is rich in nutritive and therapeutic components, it is an excellent oil for dry, damaged skin.

Canola Oil is a new hybridized oil from the seeds of the rape plant, a mustard family member used as a forage crop for livestock that was created by the Canadian government for its low erucic acid content. Expeller pressed canola oil is now widely available. It has a neutral and light quality that is good for most skin types and useful in creams and massage oils. Canola oil does not contain many nourishing components, and may be combined with richer oils to increase the nutritive value.

Cocoa Butter, made from the cocoa bean, is solid at room temperature but melts when applied to the skin. It has a delicious chocolate scent that can enhance a product's aroma. It is used as an emulsifier and stiffener in creams. Cocoa butter can also be added to body oils to thicken them. It is highly protective because it stays on the surface of the skin, which helps prevent dehydration. It also has water-repellent properties, which is helpful in swimming situations and with sunscreen products. However, cocoa butter may feel too heavy for some skin types, and a few people are allergic to it.

Coconut Oil is made from the fruit of the coconut palm. It is solid at room temperature, but liquefies when temperatures exceed 76 degrees F. Thus, it tends to loosen and liquefy during the summer months. Coconut oil has a cooling property, which lends itself to sun products and burn remedies. It is used in creams to help emulsify and stiffen them. Coconut oil has long been used by tropical peoples for hair care. I enjoy using it as a hair conditioner, and often include it in the hair products I make.

Flaxseed Oil, pressed from the seeds of the flax (linen) plant, has gained a lot of popularity in the natural health movement due to its high concentration of omega-3 essential fatty acids. Products made from this oil must be kept refrigerated, since its superpolyunsaturated nature is very unstable and goes rancid easily. It also has a strong odor. It may be used alone or added to oils and creams for eczema, psoriasis and other skin conditions.

Grapeseed Oil, made from the seeds of grapes, is the lightest of the oils and virtually odorless. It is also very drying, which should be kept in mind when making products for dry-skin problems. I have not been able to find cold or expeller pressed grapeseed oil, it all seems to be produced with chemical solvents. However, because the oil is so light and odorless, it is favored as the carrier oil by aromatherapists. It serves as an excellent base for perfume blending.

Jojoba Oil is pressed from the seeds of a small desert shrub with leathery leaves. It is technically not an oil, but a liquid wax ester that resembles human sebum, the natural coating that protects our skin and keeps it supple. Jojoba oil can act as a second skin, providing protection and emolliency while still allowing the skin to breathe. It is used extensively in products for dry, aged and damaged skin and hair. I like to use it in sun protection products as well.

Olive Oil is made from the fruit of the olive tree. Virgin-grade olive oil is the first cold pressing of the olive and the most nutritious of olive oils. I find it to be the most stable oil and the least likely to go rancid, so it is a good choice for making herbal-infused oils. Olive oil contains many beneficial substances and can be used alone or in combination in various preparations. Keep in mind that olive oil is a heavy oil with a strong aroma, which should be considered when creating a product. It is absorbed by the skin, but may take a bit longer than other oils. You may choose to combine it with another lighter oil, such as almond, for massage products.

Peanut Oil is rich, heavy and strongly scented. I find that it penetrates the skin well. It is especially appropriate for skin products for dry, malnourished skin. Peanut oil can be used in skin preparations to increase the product's overall nutritive value. It was recommended especially by Edgar Cayce because he thought it resembled human oil and was easily accepted by the skin. However, due to the peanut's susceptibility to fungus, peanut oil can contain undesirable contaminants.

Sesame Oil, made from sesame seeds, is widely available in cold pressed form. It contains natural antioxidants that make it a rather stable oil. It contains natural sunscreen properties, so I like to use it in the sun products I make. It has a very strong odor, and has a warming and drying effect. I often combine sesame oil with more lubricating oils like peanut to create a less drying product. In the Ayurvedic tradition, sesame oil is very popular as a warming substance, and is used for poor circulation and nervous skin problems. While in India I saw many women with long, beautiful black hair coated with sesame oil, which is an excellent conditioner.

Shea Butter comes from the shea tree (Butyrospermum parkii), which grows in West and Central Africa. Its seeds are harvested to make shea butter for food, skin and hair products. Since the French colonized West and Central Africa, it has been used in French cosmetics under the name of karite butter. Shea butter is solid at room temperature and may be used in creams to help emulsify and stiffen them, or in body oils as a thickener. It can make a cream or balm slightly grainy, but this will not alter the effectiveness of a product. Shea butter is extremely therapeutic, helping to heal cracked, aged or damaged skin. It contains some ultraviolet protection, approximately SPF-6, and is therefore useful in sun products. It also contains chemical constituents that help to heal bruising and soreness. It is a very heavy butter that penetrates the skin, leaving it soft and smooth; some people find it too heavy for normal use. Shea butter can be quite expensive and difficult to find, but I have listed some sources of it in the Resources section.

Wheat Germ Oil, pressed from the germ of the wheat berry, is extremely nourishing, and contains significant amounts of vitamin E. It can be added to skin care preparations to increase their therapeutic benefits. However, the odor of cold pressed, unrefined wheat germ oil is very strong and nutty, which should be considered when creating a product. You only need to add a little wheat germ oil to skin care products, as it is extremely concentrated.

FOODSTUFFS AND OTHER NATURAL INGREDIENTS

Alcohol functions as a solvent and a preservative in skin care products. When applied to the skin it is cleansing, astringent and cooling. It can also be very drying for some skin types, which should be taken into consideration when creating formulas. Diluted alcohol can serve as a menstrum for tincturing herbs, and is used as an ingredient in facial astringents, deodorants, mouth rinses and body splashes. To figure out the alcohol content of a liquor, simply divide the proof in half. Thus, 80 proof alcohol contains 40 percent alcohol and 60 percent water; 100 proof alcohol contains 50 percent alcohol and 50 percent water. To use as a preservative, such as in a facial astringent, you will need 1 part pure alcohol to 4 parts other liquid. This means that if you are using 80 proof brandy, for instance, which is 40 percent alcohol, you will need an ounce of brandy for every ounce of other liquid. Brandy, vodka and other 80–100 proof liquors contain high enough alcohol-to-water ratios to use straight for tincturing. Occasionally 190 proof alcohol is used in a recipe to optimally extract the chemical constituents of an herb, such as St. Johnswort or resinous herbs like vanilla bean and myrrh. These high-proof extracts are usually diluted before use. Wines may be used in skin preparations, but they contain less alcohol than brandy or vodka. Wines are only about 15–20 proof, and may also have a strong color and odor, which you may or may not find desirable. Because of wine's low alcohol content, it has less preservative action than distilled liquor. If you are tincturing with wine you will also end up with less alcohol-soluble constituents in your product. Warning: Whenever alcohol is indicated in a recipe here, I am referring to food-grade liquor, not rubbing alcohol, which is poisonous when ingested.

Arrowroot powder is made from the refined powdered root of the Maranta arudinacea plant. It is a thickening agent with excellent absorbent properties, and can be added to pastes and facial masques to thicken and make them adhere better to the skin. Arrowroot is also used as a main ingredient in body powders, giving a smooth, silky feeling to the skin and helping to absorb moisture. Arrowroot powder is widely available in health food stores.

Baking Soda, also known as sodium bicarbonate, cleans and deodorizes while providing alkalinity. It can be used in body powders, teeth cleansers, baths and hand and foot soaks.

Beeswax is an important ingredient used to emulsify creams and thicken salves. It should be bought in as unadulterated a form as possible, unbleached and minimally purified. It has a sweet smell that I find especially pleasing. I get my wax from a local beekeeper because the quality is high and his prices are the lowest I have found. If you can't find a beekeeper near you, look in the Resources section for beeswax. Please do not try to substitute paraffin (a petroleum product) for beeswax. When using beeswax to harden oils for making salves and balms, I generally use 1 oz. of beeswax to 2½ oz. of oil for a hard salve. Use 1 oz. beeswax to 3 oz. of oil for a looser salve. Some herbalists I know use 1 oz of beeswax to harden 8 oz. of oil. This will make a very loose balm with the consistency of petroleum jelly; if the temperature rises above 70 degrees F. it will usually melt into a thickened liquid oil. Modify the amount of wax you use depending on what you are making, where on the body it will be applied and the temperature conditions in which it will be used.

Borax — sodium borate or sodium tetraborate — is a naturally occurring mineral composed of sodium, boron, oxygen and water. It is most commonly used as an alkaline water softener and cleansing agent, which makes it useful in mineral bath blends. It also serves as an excellent emulsifier for creams, because it helps water and oil blend together.

Clays are absorbent, drawing, cleansing, thickening and tightening agents, which makes them useful in facial masques, body powders, deodorants and creams. Clays are available in a variety of colors, a function of their place of collection and mineral composition. White kaolin clay has more neutral effects and is less drawing. Green clay, derived from volcanic deposits, is richer in mineral composition and is also more drawing and drying than kaolin clay. You can use any clay accessible to you — just be sure that it is clean and that it has been collected from an un-contaminated source. Make sure when purchasing clays that their color is a reflection of their natural mineral composition and not added for effect, making them appear to contain miner-als they don't. When clay is moistened with an equal amount of water or other liquid and made into a paste, is can be used for masques and poultices.

Cornstarch is made from whole corn that has been softened with a "weak acid," then fur-ther processed to remove the germ and hull, leaving behind the starch. This residue is then filtered, washed and dried. Cornstarch may be used in the same way as arrowroot powder. It is widely used as a thickening agent and has excellent absorbent properties.

Distilled Water is made by evaporating water, then recondensing it for the purpose of re-moving minerals, bacteria and other substances. It is frequently used when making body care products, especially creams, to minimize bacterial contamination. You can use plain water, but bear in mind that it will usually cause a product to spoil more rapidly.

Glycerin is a sweet, sticky, soothing humectant that is a chemical component of oil and fats. It also has preservative qualities. It is preferable to use nonsynthetic vegetable glycerin made without petroleum by-products. The humectant properties of glycerin are useful in moisturiz-ing and soothing dry, parched skin. The addition of glycerin is useful in creams, facial astrin-gents and body splashes. It is added to the menstrum when extracting tannin-rich herbs to help liberate their medicinal properties while neutralizing the tannins. The menstrum should be 10 percent glycerin to 90 percent diluted alcohol. Herbs tinctured in glycerin diluted with water are called glycerites. For a short-term preservative (perhaps a few months), you will need to use at least 25 percent glycerin to 75 percent water or other perishable liquid. For a stable preserva-tive you might need to use at least 60–75 percent glycerin to 25–40 percent water. However, note that even 25 percent glycerin in a product can make the skin feel too sticky.

Grains and Beans are used in scrubs and masques for the face and body. They provide vita-mins, minerals and other nourishing substances while exfoliating skin and absorbing dirt and oil. Different grains and beans affect the skin differently. Some are more astringent and drying, while others are more soothing and emollient. The emollient and soothing grains — such as barley and oats — tend to have more gluten. The astringent and drying grains include rice, corn, millet and most beans.

Grapefruit Seed Extract is used as a preservative in creams and other body care products. It is considered to be a nontoxic, broad-spectrum antimicrobial with no known side effects for the body or the environment. Unfortunately, the manufacturing process is kept secret, as I discovered while doing research for this book. I did learn that grapefruit seeds and pulp are used to manufacture the extract, but various other chemical processes are also involved that completely transform the organic structure of the raw materials. For this reason, I wonder whether the extract can be considered a truly "natural" product. However, many people are using the extract with good results for various antimicrobial body care preparations. All of the extracts I have seen available on the market are diluted with 60 percent glycerin. Still, the manufacturers always recommend diluting grapefruit seed extract further to prevent it from irritating the skin. This means using anywhere from 2–20 drops diluted in liquid, depending on the quantity and purpose of the formula you are making. I called a manufacturer of the extract to inquire about its preservative properties. I was informed that 1 drop of extract added to 16 oz. of water will purify the water, similar to chlorination. In addition, 1½ oz. of grapefruit seed extract added to 1 gallon of water will preserve it for a period of 3 months or longer. To bring the measurements down to scale, I approximate that 1 teaspoon of grapefruit seed extract will preserve 14 oz. of perishable liquid. The figures given are approximations only, but can be used as a starting point.

Lanolin is secreted from the sebaceous glands of sheep into their wool, and is often referred to as wool fat. It is highly emollient, soothing and softening. It may be used in creams, salves and hair products. Note that some people are allergic to lanolin, and that unrefined lanolin can have a very strong odor.

Lecithin is a thick, orange-yellow viscous liquid derived from egg yolks, soybeans or corn. It makes oil and other skin care products spread well over the skin's surface and has a softening and soothing effect. It is also a very good emulsifier. Be sparing in the addition of lecithin to creams, as it will make them very thick. I like to use ½ tablespoon of lecithin for an 19 oz. batch of cream.

PABA (para-aminobenzoic acid) is a member of the vitamin B family that is used topically to increase the skin's resistance to burning and damage from harmful ultraviolet rays. People who have experienced allergic reactions to PABA in commercial products may find that they are not allergic to naturally occurring PABA, or that the product which caused an allergic reaction may have contained other irritating substances. Food-grade PABA is available as a white crystalline powder that is water-soluble. It may therefore be difficult to keep it evenly dispersed in an oil unless the oil is shaken prior to use in order to redistribute the PABA. When creating a sun protection product it is important to use other skin-protective and -restorative substances like shea butter or jojoba oil in conjunction with the PABA; this augments the product's effectiveness. The amount of PABA added to a product will depend on how easily you burn and what other ingredients you combine it with. For example, I use only ¾ oz. of PABA (a heaping tablespoon) in a 32-fluid-oz. batch of my Golden Sun Juice. This formula contains only approximately 2½ percent PABA, but its protective qualities are enhanced by the other naturally occurring sun protection ingredients. It provides a sunscreen with an approximate SPF-15, which is not a sunblock. (This SPF is based on empirical research and not from laboratory testing.) Notice how your skin responds in the sun while using a particular formula. If it burns you need a stronger product, so increase the SPF by adding another teaspoon of PABA per 19-oz. batch. If your skin is not tanning, reduce or omit the PABA to decrease the SPF. Experiment with the formula, starting with a little and adding more or less PABA as needed.

Sea Salt is drying, cleansing, abrasive and drawing. It is useful for tooth cleansers, body scrubs, baths and hand and foot soaks. Use the purest, crudest salt available. The less refined the salt, the more therapeutic it will be, since unprocessed salt contains more of the minerals from the ocean and fewer of the chemicals used during the refining process. Eating unprocessed sea salt also provides the body with numerous minerals and trace elements, along with the sodium chloride found in regular table salt. If the cost of unrefined salt is too high for you to justify using it in baths or scrubs, then reserve it for ingestion.

Seeds such as sunflower, sesame, green pumpkin (often referred to as pepitas) and flax provide excellent nourishment for the skin when either ingested or applied topically. You should always start with fresh, raw, whole seeds, and preferably ones that are organic. Using whole seeds and grinding them immediately prior to use is essential for keeping their oils from oxidizing and becoming rancid. I store my whole seeds in the freezer to keep them from spoiling. Seeds contain appreciable amounts of essential fatty acids, vitamin E, zinc, iron and other nutritive substances. They should be included in the daily diet and can be incorporated into face and body scrubs and masques. Flaxseeds are very slimy due to their mucilage content, and may be applied topically to soothe inflamed or irritated skin. However, the addition of too much flax in a masque or face scrub can make the formula too slippery to adhere to the face.

Vinegar has astringent, deodorizing and antifungal properties, and can also function as a menstrum for extracting herbs, although not as effectively as diluted alcohol. Vinegar is especially useful in facial astringents and hair rinses. I use organic, nonfiltered apple cider vinegar that still contains the "mother," a by-product of enzymatic activity that has congealing properties which can give your liquid product a cloudy appearance. This enzyme-rich substance is highly beneficial both when eaten and applied topically. However, this kind of vinegar has a strong smell, and the cloudy appearance bothers some people. So you may want to use an organic white vinegar, or perhaps a more refined, filtered apple cider vinegar. When making products for the skin, especially for the face, I discourage the use of supermarket-grade vinegars, since they tend to be more caustic and irritating. Reserve supermarket-grade vinegars for housecleaning and perhaps foot soaks. Note that vinegar tends to be drying, and its acid content can sting open skin and delicate tissues.

BOTANICALS

Alkanet (*Alkanna tinctoria*) is used in the food and cosmetics industry as a nontoxic coloring agent. The roots of the plant are used to impart a red color. This is a good herb for coloring lip balms and rouges, or for giving oil a red hue. Although not commonly used therapeutically, alkanet root is astringent and contains antimicrobial and wound-healing properties.

Aloe Vera Gel (*Aloe barbadensis*) is an extremely soothing, cooling and healing substance that comes from the swordlike leaf of this succulent tropical plant, which is often kept as a houseplant. It is useful in regenerative creams, soothing and softening astringents, sun products and other reparative skin preparations. The fresh gel scooped from the inside of the aloe leaf and applied directly to a burn will help cool down the skin and prevent it from blistering, as well as aiding in the skin-regeneration process. In the tropics it is applied to freshly washed hair, allowed to dry in the sun, then rinsed out to add softness and luster. Be sure to use pure aloe vera gel from your own houseplants, or packaged aloe vera gel that is pure and minimally processed. Avoid commercially prepared aloe vera gel that has artificial additives. Unfortunately, fresh aloe vera gel from houseplants doesn't blend well with other ingredients when making products such as creams and astringents; I find it necessary to use bottled aloe gel for these purposes.

Aniseed (*Pimpinella anisum*) is a common culinary spice. It is sweet and smells like fennel. It can be added to face scrubs and steams for both its pleasing aroma and the cleansing qualities of its volatile oils. Aniseed added to tea blends adds sweetness, and is helpful in clearing oily skin as well as for alleviating indigestion and other complaints.

Arnica Flowers (*Arnica montana*) are used to heal bruised and painful skin and muscles. The flowers are infused in an oil or liniment base and applied topically for injury and trauma relief. Arnica is a beneficial addition to massage oils. It is toxic when ingested, and should not be taken internally except in homeopathic preparations.

Ocimum basilicum
(Basil)

Basil (*Ocimum basilicum*), a favored culinary herb, also has merit in skin care as a cleansing and invigorating ingredient. It can be used in facial steams, scrubs, masques, astringents and massage oils. This mint family member is an easy-to-grow annual that is well worth the effort, since freshly harvested or freshly dried basil is significantly more potent than commercial-grade basil. As with all mints and herbs that contain strong volatile oils, the effectiveness of the herb is directly connected to the strength of the oils. The integrity of the oils depends on how the herb is harvested, dried and stored. Pick basil when the flowers are about to open and hang the plants to dry without touching each other in a dark, well-ventilated space. When they are thoroughly dry, store them in airtight containers away from heat and light.

Bay Laurel Leaves (*Laurus nobilis*), another well-known culinary herb, can be used to add a spicy, warming quality to steams, oils, astringents and bath mixtures.

Berry Leaves of strawberry, raspberry or blackberry plants, whether wild or cultivated, may be used for their highly astringent and skin-toning properties. All are excellent for oily, large-pored, "dirty" skin. There is often an abundance of berry leaves growing wild in fields, wood edges and meadows. Put them up fresh in vinegar or tincture or dry them. They may be used during their growing season for fresh face masques, and are wonderful additions to facial astringents or face scrubs. They can also be used to make delicious, high-calcium vinegar for salads and sauces.

Calendula (*Calendula officinalis*) is an annual garden flower that is easy to grow from seed.

It will reseed itself in subsequent years if some of the flowers are allowed to mature and drop their seeds. Pick the blossoms at the flower base and place them with the petals facedown on a screen for drying, or use them fresh to make infused oils, tinctures and facial astringents. The flowers may also be broken up and their petals sprinkled into a salad, adding beauty and nourishment to the meal. Calendula contains carotenoids that nourish the skin either when ingested or applied topically. The flower has healing, antimicrobial, antifungal and life force-enhancing properties. Calendula is used in various preparations, from lip balms to wound washes. If you need to purchase it, be sure that it is a vibrant yellow or orange color and that it has been dried whole and not cut and sifted (commonly labeled as c/s in herb catalogues). The commercial herb market generally offers very poor-quality calendula with broken and pale flowers. The higher-quality calendula that is available is generally sold out by early winter. So it pays to grow your own if you can. Healing Spirits and Pacific Botanicals, both listed in the Resources section, offer exceptionally high-quality calendula.

Catnip (*Nepeta cataria*) is a perennial herb with spreading roots, like many of its cousins in the mint family and like other mints, it is very easy to grow. Catnip loses a lot of its value with age, and should be used either fresh or freshly dried. It's invigorating and cleansing properties can be used in facial steams, bath mixtures, astringents, masques and scrubs. Catnip tea is helpful with anxiety-related stomach disorders, flus, colds and general stress.

Cayenne Pepper (*Capsicum frutescens, C. annuum*) is a very hot spice used to warm the body and increase circulation. It is a rubefacient, meaning that it brings blood to the surface of the skin. Cayenne can be added to baths, balms, liniments and oils for muscle pain and stiffness, rheumatic aches and unbroken chilblains. But add just a little of it to your preparations, as too much can burn your skin.

Matricaria chamomilla

Chamomile (*Matricaria recutita)* an annual, and *Anthemis nobilis*, a perennial) is an excellent herb for relaxing and healing nervous and inflamed skin conditions. It can be made into an oil, cream, salve, tincture, infusion or astringent, or used in facial scrubs, masques and steams, as well as in baths. Its gentle and effective healing attributes make it suitable for baby products. It is easy to grow, though it takes a considerable amount of time to pick enough of the tiny blossoms for a preparation. Good-quality chamomile is abundantly available on the commercial herb market, but be sure it has been organically grown.

Cinnamon (*Cinnamomum zeylanicum, C. cassia*) is a circulatory stimulant. This warming spice is added to formulas to increase blood flow, and may be used in cold-weather products like warming body oils and bath blends. Its circulatory aspect can also be useful in liniments and balms for arthritic, rheumatic conditions. When using cinnamon in your preparations proceed with caution, as the volatile oils are very strong and can burn the skin. The cassia cinnamon has more heat than the zeylanicum species.

Citrus Peels of lemon, orange, grapefruit, lime and tangerine are both aromatic and therapeutic. Buy organic citrus, save the peels and add them to your skin care preparations for their astringent and cleansing properties. Put fresh peels into facial astringents and dry ones into facial scrubs.

Comfrey (*Symphytum oficinale*) is a handsome garden perennial with aggressively spreading roots that often escape to the wild. Plant away from the garden and allow it to create a nice patch of its own. Comfrey is one of the most well-known herbs for helping to heal skin. Both its leaves and its roots are used to heal wounds, burns, cuts and breaks in bone and skin. One of its common names is knit-bone, because it helps to repair damaged tissue. Allantoin, a chemical constituent of comfrey, is said to be responsible for cell proliferation. For deeper wounds, comfrey should be used on the second or third day of healing, as its cell-proliferative action may cause the skin to close over too quickly, causing the outer skin to heal before the inner wound is ready. When comfrey is used in the later phase of wound healing, it helps to prevent scar formations. The roots are very rich in mucilage, which offers relief to dry and irritated skin. The leaves are rich in chlorophyll and minerals, and also contain some mucilage. This cooling, soothing, healing ally is used to make infused oil, salves, creams, facial astringents and other preparations. When making comfrey-infused oil, follow the procedure for wet plants that are high in protein, as discussed in the Techniques and Definitions chapter.

Echinacea (*Echinacea angustifolia* and *E. purpurea* are the most commonly used species) is the herb of choice for antimicrobial action. It is ideal for wound and infected-skin preparations. The root of the plant is the most highly prized and most stable part of the plant, and the only part to use if you are buying market-dried echinacea, since the other parts of the plant lose much of their potency upon drying. When purchasing echinacea augustifolia you can judge its strength by placing a small piece of the root on your tongue; the more your tongue tingles and vibrates, the more potent the echinacea. If you grow your own, you can incorporate the flowers, leaves and seeds into your products. Echinacea purpurea

Echinacea angustifolia

is a popular perennial with bold purple flowers. In the garden trade it is referred to as purple cone flower, and I find it worth growing for its beauty alone. Once established in the garden, it is easy to grow and will often reseed itself. Echinacea angustifolia is a Midwestern wildflower that is currently being overharvested. I have found this variety difficult to cultivate in my garden, but herb farmers are starting to grow it and to offer it on the market. I think the angustifolia root is stronger than the purpurea, even though experts say they may be used interchangeably. Echinacea can be both ingested and applied topically where acne and other puslike activity is occurring, as it cleans and supports the lymph and immune systems. Make a tincture for internal and external immune support. Use in masques, creams, wound washes and soaks.

Elder (*Sambucus canadensis*) is a shrub that grows wild in rich soil along riverbanks and woods. The flowers and leaves are used in wound and reparative skin preparations. Elder aids sprained, bruised, cut or damaged skin. Fresh elder flowers yield the most potent oils, tinctures and vinegars for use in creams, salves, massage oils, facial astringents and liniments. Elder flowers are also useful when dried to make infusions for

Sambucus nigra

bathing and drinking. Taken internally as an infusion or tincture, elder flowers can be included in a detoxification program for acne-prone and blemished skin. When purchased, elder flowers should be off-white and sweet-smelling. If they are brown and odorless they have lost their potency. When gathering your own flowers, pick them at the base of the umbel and place them to dry on finely meshed screens. Spread them apart rather than piling them on top of each other in order to prevent molding and browning.

Evergreens — pine, hemlock and spruce — are available fresh year-round for steams, baths and beverages. In the spring the green tree tips are at their peak potency, and are collected for tincturing and oil infusions. The evergreen's invigorating, immune-enhancing, cleansing and astringent properties can be used in face and body splashes, body oils and balms. The needles of the evergreens can be chewed as a fresh winter source of vitamin C.

Fennel Seed (*Foeniculum vulgare*) is a popular culinary spice added to facial scrubs and steams for its sweet, cleansing, hydrating and stimulating effects. Fennel, added to tea blends for sweetness and flavor, makes the tea more palatable while also helping to alleviate indigestion.

Fenugreek Seed (*Trigonella foenum-graecum*) is soothing when added to scrubs and poultices, helping to heal irritated, inflamed skin.

Garlic (*Allium sativum*) is a strong antimicrobial useful in augmenting the body's immune response during infectious states. Use for eardrops and make garlic honey for infected skin.

Ginger Rhizome (*Zingiber officinale*) is a spicy, heating herb that is used to warm the body and increase circulation. It is excellent in foot and body baths, as well as in massage oils and balms. It also makes a nice winter tea when the body is chilled.

Goldenseal Root (*Hydrastis canadensis*) is a strong antimicrobial used in wound preparations and acne products. It is an endangered wildflower that grows in rich woods, and so should be

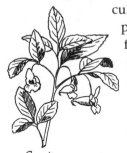

cultivated. Although cultivation can be difficult, it is worth the effort for the preservation of this extraordinary plant. If you choose to buy, please look for sources of cultivated and not wild-harvested goldenseal to purchase. The difficulty of cultivation and the endangered status of goldenseal is reflected in its extremely high price.

Jewelweed (*Impatiens capensis, I. pallida, I. biflora*), a wild plant that grows in rich soil, is best known as the poison ivy antidote. However, it can be used in other products for rashes, irritations, inflammations, burns, bruises, warts and ringworm. This plant must be used fresh when making preparations, and wilts quickly upon harvesting. Harvest the plant at the stem and

Impatiens capensis

use both leaf and stem in your preparations. It is so abundant in the wild that it is not worth growing.

Lavender (*Lavandula vera, L. angustifolia* and other *L.* species) is a strongly fragrant herb with cleansing, astringent and skin-reparative properties. It is used extensively in skin care products such as scrubs, steams, astringents, bath blends, body oils, creams and balms. Lavender's scent is helpful in relaxing and uplifting the spirits. I love growing this attractive plant in the garden, but because the flowers hold their strength when dried and are abundantly available commercially, growing your own is not essential. Put up fresh or dried flowers in oil, vinegar or vodka.

Lemon Balm (*Melissa officinalis*) is a strong, lemon-scented perennial of the mint family. It is very easy to grow and should be used fresh, since the volatile oils responsible for its aroma and healing attributes are largely lost in the drying process. Lemon balm can maintain its potency for a 6-month period if harvested when the flowers are about to open, hung to dry in a dark, well-ventilated space and stored in a cool, dry place away from light. However, the fresh plant is decidedly better for making tinctures, astringents, vinegars and oils. Its astringent, cleansing and gently invigorating properties are useful in steams, splashes, baths and scrubs. It is also delicious to add small, fresh pieces to salads or to use for herbal-infused vinegar, honey or tea. Lemon balm is reputed to have antidepressant and anxiety-relieving properties.

Licorice Root (*Glycyrrhiza glabra*) is used to soothe inflamed skin and can be added to facial masques and scrubs, creams and hair rinses. The sweetness of licorice is 50 times that of sugar, and it can be added to tea blends to add this quality. It is widely available and not necessary to grow especially since the roots maintain their properties when dried and properly stored.

Marshmallow (*Althaea officinalis*) roots, leaves and flowers are useful for their soothing and drawing qualities when used either topically or internally. The root contains significant amounts of mucilage, and was once used to make the confection of the same name. The high mucilage content makes the herb (but not the confection!) great for use in masques and scrubs for irritated or inflamed skin. It may be added to a formula to balance out acidic or caustic ingredients. The leaves can be eaten for the significant amount of calcium they contain, and the flowers are especially nice in a salad. This handsome and hardy perennial is easy to grow, and was once a popular member of cottage gardens both for its beauty and its medicinal and culinary virtues. You can purchase good-quality dried marshmallow root for your preparations, so is not necessary to grow your own. Other mallows contain similar properties and can be used similarly, although I find marshmallow root to contain more mucilage than the other species.

Althaea officinalis

Mint (*Mentha spicata, M. viridis, M. X piperita*) adds a refreshing, stimulating quality to skin care preparations. Use in scrubs, steams, masques, baths, body splashes and hair rinses. Put up fresh mint in vinegar, vodka or oil and dry some for teas, to add to dry scrub formulas and for winter use when fresh mint is unavailable. Mints are very easy-to-grow perennials that tend to propagate through spreading roots. Plant mint away from the garden to create a healthy patch of its own. Harvest mint stem and leaf just as flowers begin to open.

Mugwort (*Artemisia vulgaris*) leaves and flowers are used to cleanse and increase circulation in bath and steam preparations. It is a very aromatic weed found growing in depleted, marginal lands all around us, especially in abandoned city lots. Put some fresh mugwort up in vinegar for salad dressings, astringents and foot soaks, and put some up in oil for massage and salve products. Mugwort is also used in acupuncture for moxibustion and in smudging, and to make dream pillows; it has a long history of "magical" uses. It is best to harvest your own in order to ensure potency or to check sources carefully for good dried mugwort. I have come across dried mugwort on the commercial herb market that is odorless and unrecognizable and therefore useless.

Myrrh (*Commiphora myrrha*) is a tree that grows in northeast Africa and southwest Asia. The exuded oleo gum resin of this tree has antiseptic and antimicrobial properties, making it useful for various wound and teeth preparations. The powdered resin, as opposed to the resin chunks, is the easiest form of myrrh to work with in making preparations.

Nettle (*Urtica dioica*) leaves, roots and seeds are used for skin and hair health. This weed likes to grow in rich soil at the edge of woods. Nettle leaves contain generous amounts of minerals, chlorophyll and other beneficial chemical constituents that provide a nourishing skin-rejuvenative tea. Put up fresh nettle in vinegar or vodka. The freshly dried herb should be used for making oils, since the fresh herb contains a lot of moisture and protein that can make the oil go rancid. Nettle's antifungal properties can be used in hair and scalp products. I use the roots and seeds for controlling dandruff and scalp funk. Nettle is a stimulant that is traditionally used to encourage hair growth. Nettle's rubefacient properties make it ideal for arthritic and rheumatic liniments, balms and oils. Gather nettle for tea before flowers appear, and always gather any part of the nettle with gloves and long sleeves to prevent being stung by the nettle hairs, which contain formic acid.

Oak Bark (*Quercus alba, Q. rubra*) is used for its astringent and antiseptic properties. Put it up in vodka or vinegar, or use the dried and powdered bark for its wound-healing capacities. Its astringency is partly due to its high tannin content, which once made it useful in the hide-tanning industry. Oak bark can be add to preparations for oily and porous skin, such as scrubs, steams and splashes.

Oregano (*Origanum vulgare*) is a familiar, strongly aromatic kitchen herb that is stimulating and antiseptic. It can be used in steams or baths to open and cleanse the pores as well as the upper respiratory tract. It may be added to scrubs, astringents and wound washes. Fresh oregano put up in vinegar is a powerful facial astringent and delicious in a salad dressing. Infuse oregano in oil and use it to make wound balms or tasty sauces. Oregano's antiseptic properties are directly linked to the strength of its volatile oils, which are reflected in its odor. If oregano has a strong odor, it will have strong cleansing properties.

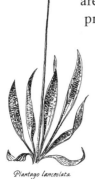

Plantago lanceolata.

Plantain (*Plantago major, P. lanceolata*), a common weed that grows abundantly in disturbed soil, is an astringent, soothing, antimicrobial agent used in wound preparations. A wad of freshly chewed leaf can be applied as a poultice for wounds and bug bites or stings. The ability of such a poultice to draw out and neutralize bites and stings is very impressive. On one occasion a carpenter who was installing new insulation in my attic disturbed a wasp nest and was stung. I quickly took him outside, plucked a leaf of plantain and told him to chew it up, spit it out and apply it to the wasp sting. Within a few minutes the swelling and pain had lessened considerably, and after a few more minutes the sting was completely neutralized. The carpenter was amazed at the effectiveness of this common, lowly weed. Plantain is best used when fresh. Harvest fresh leaves in the growing season and put them up in oil, vinegar and vodka to make salves, liniments, astringents, creams and wound washes.

Rose Flowers (*Rosa spp.*) are used extensively in skin care preparations for their astringent and skin-toning properties. Use organically grown or wild roses, never ones that have been sprayed with pesticides. Pick fresh flowers as they begin to open and put them up in vinegar, oil or vodka for use in facial astringents, massage oils, creams and bath preparations. Dry rose flowers to use in face and body scrubs. Add fresh rose petals to your salad. Excellent-quality dried roses are available on the commercial herb market, which you can use for all of your preparations. Still, I much prefer fresh roses when making vinegars and tinctures.

Sage (*Salvia officinalis*) is a popular, aromatic culinary herb with strong astringent and cleansing properties. This hardy perennial member of the mint family contains potent volatile oils. To capture the strongest potency, the leaf and flowers should be picked just as the flowers are opening and continue to harvest leaves throughout the growing season. Cut at the stem and hang to dry in a dark, well-ventilated space. Sage retains its properties well if harvested, dried and stored properly. I prefer to make my tinctures and astringents with fresh sage, reserving dried sage for face and body scrubs. Its strong antimicrobial action lends itself to wound washes, bug bite antidotes and acne remedies. Use sage in steams, bath blends, tooth powders, mouthwashes, hair products and deodorants.

St. Johnswort (*Hypericum perforatum*) is a summer solstice-blooming yellow wildflower found growing in fields, ditches and roadsides. It is used in nerve-related skin problems such as shingles and nervous skin rashes. It is excellent in massage products, since it helps to release spinal pain and nerve tension transdermally. Its astringent and anti-inflammatory properties make it appropriate for wound, burn and sunburn products. It also contains natural ultraviolet protection, which makes it useful in sunscreen lotions. This plant must be harvested fresh to reap its healing attributes, so commit to hunting for it around

Hypericum perforatum

June 21 in the Northeast; it can still be found blooming well into July. The unopened flower buds and flowers contain the highest concentration of hypericin, the chemical component responsible for many of St. Johnswort's healing attributes. Hypericin is red, and if you squeeze an unopened flower bud between your fingers it will bleed red. These unopened flower buds yield the richest red tinctures and oils. The unopened flower buds should not be mistaken with the seed capsules, which appear throughout the flowering season. Do the squeeze test to be sure, since the seed capsules don't exude the red juice. If the picking of flowers and buds proves to be too time consuming, you can simply clip the upper portion of the flowering tops for a reasonably potent preparation.

Seaweeds are a wonderful category of weeds that grow wild in the ocean. They have many health benefits, whether ingested or applied topically. They contain large amounts of minerals and trace elements not found in land foods. Seaweeds are also very high in mucilage, providing a soothing and protective effect on irritated and inflamed surfaces both inside and on the body. Seaweeds make excellent face and body scrubs and masks. For skin, nail and hair health, I suggest eating half an ounce of seaweed daily. Two of my favorite seaweeds are dulse and kelp. Choose whole strips and pieces (see Resources section), available through mail order rather than the powdered variety. Seaweed can be eaten raw, a handful at a time, making it convenient and easy for daily consumption. Some individuals may find it difficult to digest raw seaweeds, and will benefit from cooking it for a couple of hours to break down the long-chain complex sugars. They make an excellent addition to soups and stir-fries.

Slippery Elm Bark (*Ulmus rubra, U. fulva*) contains large amounts of mucilage, which is useful for soothing inflamed, irritated skin. Dried, powdered bark is added to body scrubs, bath blends, powders and poultices. I suggest purchasing already powdered bark, as I have found it very difficult to powder at home with a blender or seed/coffee grinder. The addition of too much slippery elm powder in masques, scrubs and body packs can make them so slippery that they won't adhere well to the skin. It is thus advisable to add slippery elm in small quantities.

Spilanthes (*Spilanthes acmella, S. spp.*) is a low-growing South American plant used for toothaches; hence its popular name, toothache plant. It is a strong antimicrobial and analgesic that can be added to wound preparations. Spilanthes is used in acne and infected-skin conditions, and can either be taken internally or applied topically. I also add it to mouth-cleansing products. It is easy to propragate but has a long growth period, so in the colder climates it should be started in the greenhouse in April. Its peculiar yellow, conical brown-eyed flowers are harvested and put up in vodka or dried throughout the growing season; then the entire plant is harvested prior to frost and tinctured or dried. Seeds are available in the United States (see Resources).

Comptonia peregrina

Sweet Fern (*Comptonia peregrina*) is a strongly aromatic shrub that grows in dry soils. Its astringent properties are used in poison ivy washes and wound preparations. The sweetly scented leaves make a delicious vinegar for eating and facial splashes. The leaves are also useful in steam and bath blends. Sweet fern is not commonly available on the commercial herb market, so you may need to find a wild patch and harvest your own supply.

Thyme (*Thymus vulgaris, T. spp.*), another popular culinary herb, has strong antiseptic properties due to its thymol content. It is useful in wound washes, facial steams, body scrubs and baths. Thyme is harvested at the stem when its flowers are opening. The leaves and just-opened flowers are put up in vodka, vinegar, oil or honey, and can also be dried. Fresh and freshly dried thyme is far superior to the commercial-grade variety and it is easy to grow your own supply. If purchasing dried thyme, be sure that it has a strong scent; the strength of the aroma reflects the potency of the herb. Thyme can be added to formulas for acne-prone, oily and infected skin. It is commonly used as a culinary herb, and thyme vinegar and honey are wonderful in food preparations. Thyme-infused honey makes an excellent facial masque, and is also delicious on toast or as a sweetener for tea.

Violets (*Viola odorata, V. spp.*) should always be gathered fresh when making preparations. Violets grow abundantly in the wild. If you can't find a wild patch, it is very easy to grow in the garden. The flowers come out early in the spring before the leaves are really developed. The leaves stay with us for most of the summer, are larger than the flowers and contain more reparative properties, so most of the preparations will be made with them. Violets have soothing, anti-inflammatory properties useful for eczema and irritated skin. They are put up fresh in vodka, vinegar or oil for making body splashes, creams, facial astringents and body oils. Fresh violets can also be made into pastes and poultices. When making violet-infused oil, follow instructions for making oil with high-water-content plants. Violet leaves and flowers are beneficial additions to salads and soups, offering significant amounts of vitamins C and A. The violet's mucilage content soothes the inside (the mucous membranes) and the outside surfaces of the body. The flowers add considerable beauty to a salad and can be used as a garnish to dress up any dish.

Wild Lettuce (*Lactuca canadensis, L. spp.*), a wild cousin of the common lettuce, is a biennial that grows from 3–6 feet tall. It can be added to poison ivy washes and other preparations for skin irritations. Tincture the fresh leaf and stem in vinegar or vodka. You can also press fresh juice from the leaf and stem for topical use. The fresh latex from wild lettuce is used to remove warts.

Witch Hazel (*Hamamelis virginiana*) is a common wild shrub found in woods. Harvest the leaf buds and green tips in early spring, and prune out unnecessary branches and peel off the bark for making oils, tinctures and vinegars. You can also dry the bark. Witch hazel's astringent and soothing actions are useful for oozy, flaccid or porous skin conditions. It is used to make facial astringents, hemorrhoid preparations, poison ivy washes and pimple and acne antidotes.

Yarrow (*Achillea millefolium*), a perennial wildflower easily grown in the garden, is a powerful wound healer. The white variety is used for medicinal purposes, and its leaves and flowers are harvested when the flower is almost in full bloom. If the leaves are the only part available at the time of need, then use them. Yarrow is an effective styptic (it stops bleeding) and has strong antiseptic, analgesic and astringent properties. It can be made into a tincture or infused oil, or dried for use in wound and hemorrhoid preparations, facial astringents and salves. Yarrow is invigorating and cleansing in steams and baths. It is an excellent first aid remedy in the wild. Chew up a bit of the fresh plant to make a poultice for cuts and wounds. To clean your teeth with yarrow, simply rub a fresh leaf or flower into the teeth and gums. The analgesic and antiseptic properties are useful for gum and tooth problems: Just rub and pack the fresh plant onto the problem area.

Yellow Giant Hyssop (*Agastache nepetoides*) is a perennial wildflower that grows to 6 feet or more. I have not seen it growing wild

Achillea millefolium

where I live in the Catskill Mountains of New York, but it is easy to grow in the garden and makes a nice spectacle. I use the fresh leaves and flowers to make poison ivy washes.

ESSENTIAL OILS

Essential oils are concentrated, volatile plant extracts obtained from various flowers, roots, barks and peels, usually by a steam-distillation process. Essential oils should not be confused with herbally infused oils, which are produced by infusing plant materials into a carrier or base oil that are then allowed to steep for a period of time. Essential oils enhance preparations with their scent, and can add therapeutic value. Aromatherapy uses essential oils for their subtle influence on mental, emotional, spiritual and physical well-being. Essential oils are also generally strong antimicrobials, and can thus function as natural preservatives. They can be added to creams, salves, oils, baths, scrubs and almost any skin or hair preparation. These plant essences are very volatile, meaning that they evaporate into the air, so they must be stored in a dark, cool, dry place with their lids tightly capped. When using essential oils it is necessary to dilute them, since they are so concentrated; using them "neat" (undiluted) can irritate and burn the skin. Be sure to store essential oils out of the reach of children. I would not suggest ingesting essential oils without qualified supervision.

There are literally thousands of essential oils from which to choose. I have provided only a brief list, which nonetheless offers a broad scent and therapeutic spectrum with which to work. There are many excellent books that focus entirely on essential oils, some of which are listed in the Resources. Certain essential oils have a stronger odor intensity than others, meaning that a drop of one oil may have a more concentrated aroma and potency than a drop of another. In the list of essential oils that follows I note odor intensities; if this is not mentioned, the oil has an average odor intensity. This is important information for the successful blending of oils and creation of products.

Learning About Aromas and How to Blend Them

When making scented body care products, it is important to familiarize oneself with the various essential oil scents, learning the aroma of each one individually before combining them. To smell an essential oil simply open the bottle, hold it a few inches from your nose and sniff. Another way to smell an oil is to dip a wooden toothpick into the oil, then hold it a few inches away from your nose. When teaching classes I pass around one essential oil at a time for students to sample, asking them to write down their preferences and dislikes as well as their personal response to each scent.

It is perfectly acceptable to make a product using only one essential oil. You can also make intriguing scent combinations with two or more oils. It is always a good idea to smell a scent combination before going on to make a product with it. One way to experience combined scents is to hold the open bottles of the different essential oils together and pass them quickly and repeatedly under your nose. Change the position of the bottles, recessing the ones that are intended to be more subtle and lifting the ones closer to your nose that are to be stronger. Although this technique will not produce the exact aroma of the combination, it will provide you with an idea of how the scents will work together. I've used this technique with great success when blending aromas for various products, and have found it extremely helpful in teaching.

When creating an aroma blend, it is important to remember that different essential oils have different odor intensities. For example, 1 drop of peppermint essential oil will completely overpower 1 drop of sandalwood essential oil. This information is largely learned through experience. I share this knowledge in the list of essential oils that follows. If the odor intensity is not mentioned, the oil is average in that category.

Keep in mind that when essential oils are mixed together, then left to age and mature over time, subtle changes occur in the aroma. The different ingredients used to make a product will also affect the final aroma. Also bear in mind that once they are applied, scents interact with an individual's own body heat and chemistry, altering the aroma slightly.

A Word of Caution: Essential oils should only be smelled in a well-ventilated area, preferably outdoors. You may want to restrict yourself to sampling only a few at a time so as not to overwhelm your sense of smell. In addition, headaches and nausea can result from overindulgence. Some people have a much higher tolerance level and can smell dozens of oils without ill effect, while others can only smell a few before feeling discomfort.

These procedures and principles provide some simple initial guidelines for aroma blending. Of course, as you continue experimenting with and using the oils, you will learn more about them.

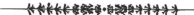

Anise (*Pimpinella anisum*) oil is a sweet, traditional flavoring agent added to produce a pleasant licoricelike aroma in products. It can be used when a nonfloral scent is desired. Anise oil has a weak odor intensity, so a lot needs to be added to a product to yield a sufficient scent. When mixed with other essential oils the anise aroma may be lost due to this low odor intensity.

Basil (*Ocimum basilicum*) oil has a sweet, floral, spicy, refreshing odor that is often used in uplifting aromatherapy blends. Add it to bath, body oil or other skin care products to lighten, sweeten and enhance their aroma.

Bay (*Laurus nobilis*) oil is a spicy, warm oil often added to products for men. It is also added to liniments for sprains and bruises. It contains some antiseptic properties.

Black Pepper (*Piper nigrum*) oil is a pleasant, spicy, warm oil used in products to heat the body and increase blood flow. It is added to oils, balms and other preparations for rheumatic and arthritic conditions. Black pepper oil is often used to scent products for men.

Cedarwood (*Juniperus virginiana*) oil has a deep, woody scent similar to that of the wood from which it is derived. Its odor intensity is very strong and will need to be highly diluted to keep it from irritating the skin and overpowering other scents in a blend. It has a base note, like other wood-derived oils, that blends well with high floral notes like ylang-ylang. It is also a good fixative for stabilizing a perfume. Cedar oil's antiseptic and astringent properties are used in helping oily and acne-prone skin. It has a calming effect that is useful for nervous or irritated-skin conditions. It is also known for its bug-repellent properties.

Chamomile (*Matricaria chamomilla*) oil, also referred to as blue chamomile oil, contains azulene, which gives the oil its blue color and its anti-inflammatory properties. Chamomile oil is used in creams, washes and oils for eczema and psoriasis. Its skin-healing attributes are used for burns, sunburn and skin irritations and inflammations. Its calming effects are added to baby care products and aromatherapy oil blends. Although expensive, it is a very concentrated oil that can be used highly diluted and still maintain its effectiveness.

Cinnamon or Cassia (*Cinnamomum cassia*) oil is a hot, spicy, sweet oil with antimicrobial properties. Add cinnamon oil to circulatory preparations; be cautious, though, because if added in too high a concentration it can burn and irritate the skin. Cinnamon oil is drying and should be added only in small doses to any moisturizing formula. Its drying qualities make it useful for oily scalp and skin conditions. It is also used in dental preparations as a cleansing, stimulating and flavoring agent.

Eucalyptus (*Eucalyptus globulus*) oil has strong antimicrobial and expectorant properties. It is used in inhalation therapy for upper respiratory ailments. Its cooling, refreshing and stimulating nature makes it ideal for balms, creams, body powders and body oils. It can be added to foot and underarm preparations for its deodorant properties. Eucalyptus is also effective as a bug repellent.

Fennel (*Foeniculum vulgare*) oil has a sweet, spicy and invigorating scent similar to that of anise oil. It serves well in massage oils for colicky or cramping abdomens, and is thus a desirable addition to baby oils.

Fir (*Abies canadensis, A. siberiensis*) oil smells like the forest and is considered a masculine aroma. It has disinfectant properties and can be added to cleansing creams and body scrubs. It has a strong odor intensity that requires using less of it than you might other oils. Its scent is low and deep.

Geranium Egypt (*Pelargonium graveolens*) oil has a mid to high, sweet and deep roselike scent, with a very strong odor intensity that easily overpowers other aromas. Use ¼–½ the amount of geranium egypt as other oils. For example, when making 1 oz. of scented body oil, 20 drops of essential oil are generally used; when using geranium egypt essential oil, you will only need to use 5–10 drops. geranium egypt is used extensively in skin care products for its refreshing, astringent, cleansing and skin-reparative properties. Add it to creams, oils, scrubs, body powders, splashes and hair rinses.

Ginger (*Zingiber officinale*) oil is warm and spicy, and is used in preparations to increase circulation. Add it to bath blends, body oils, balms and liniments for sprains or achy, cold and rheumatic muscles and bones. Ginger mixed with other oils adds an exotic tone to the aroma blend. When adding ginger oil proceed with caution: Ginger's heat can redden and irritate the skin if used in excess.

Lavender (*Lavandula officinalis*) oil has a strong, clean, refreshing, sweet, floral fragrance with a mid to high note. It is highly regarded for its therapeutic properties, and can be added to most skin preparations. Add to baths, oils, creams, splashes, scrubs, balms, steams, hair products and body powders for its antimicrobial, anti-inflammatory, analgesic and skin-regenerative properties. It is a normalizing oil that stimulates while relaxing.

Lemongrass (*Cymbopogon citratus*) oil has antiseptic, astringent, deodorizing and stimulating properties that can be added to creams, salves, oils, scrubs, hair products and body powders. It has a lemony aroma with an exotic, sweet tone. Lemongrass oil has a strong odor intensity, so use less of it than you would other oils. It is also added to bug repellents.

Melissa (*Melissa officinalis*) oil, also known as lemon balm oil, has calming, antiseptic and antidepressant properties, and is often used in aromatherapy. It has a lemonlike scent and a strong odor intensity that easily dominates a fragrance blend, so use less of it than you would other oils.

Nutmeg (*Myristica fragrans*) oil has a sweet, warm, spicy aroma that adds a nice note to fragrance blends. The oil is antiseptic and effective in preparations for muscular and rheumatic pains. It is excellent in body oils.

Sweet orange (*Citrus aurantium*) oil is a refreshing, sweet, orange-smelling oil with very drying effects on the skin. Use highly diluted in products that are intended to be moisturizing. It can be added to formulas for oily and acne-prone skin. It is a solvent and degreaser, and has antiseptic properties.

Patchouli (*Pogostemon cablin*) oil has a deep, rich, musty, woody, spicy scent that adds a base note to aroma blends. It is used as a fixative for stabilizing fragrances. It has antiseptic, astringent properties and can be added to various skin care preparations for both its aroma and its therapeutic properties. It is experienced by some as an aphrodisiac, but repels others. Patchouli has a strong odor intensity that can easily dominate a fragrance blend, so you may want to use it sparingly.

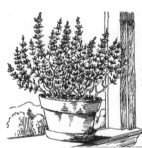

Peppermint (*Mentha piperita*) oil is a stimulating, cleansing, cooling and refreshing oil used to add an invigorating, sweet and minty aroma to creams, foot preparations, baths, splashes, scrubs, body oils, mouth cleansers and lip balms. It has a strong odor intensity that dominates other fragrances, so use less of it than you would other oils. It is effective in preparations to counteract fatigue and muscle aches.

Rosemary (*Rosmarinus officinalis*) oil is a stimulating, astringent and antiseptic oil that is excellent on hair, scalp and skin. Use to cleanse the scalp and skin by adding it to hair rinses, body oils, scrubs, steams and baths. Add rosemary essential oil to massage balms and oils for muscular and rheumatic complaints. It has a refreshing, invigorating, camphorlike odor that adds an uplifting quality to a product.

Sage (*Salvia officinalis*) oil has cleansing, astringent and invigorating properties, and a fresh, stimulating, camphorlike, mildly medicinal aroma. Use sage oil in skin splashes, hair products, acne and infected-skin preparations and massage balms and oils.

Sandalwood (*Santalum album*) oil has an exotic, woody, sweet and subtle aroma. It has a weak odor intensity and it's aroma is easily dominated by other scents, so you may need to add more of it in blends to create the desired scent. Sandalwood oil is used as a fixative for fragrances. It has hydrating, anti-inflammatory and antiseptic effects, and can be added with great benefit to body oils, creams, balms, body powders and hair products.

Spearmint (*Mentha spicata*) oil, like other mint essential oils, has invigorating, cooling, antiseptic, refreshing and stimulating properties that can enhance mouth preparations, body oils, baths, steams, scrubs, creams and foot powders. Its odor is true to the spearmint herb, and it is used widely as a food-flavoring agent.

Tangerine (*Citrus reticulata*) oil has the delightful aroma of the fruit itself. Like all citrus oils, it is drying, so use it diluted in products intended to be moisturizing. Add to bath and body oils for its muscle-relaxant properties. Use tangerine oil in preparations for acne and oily skin.

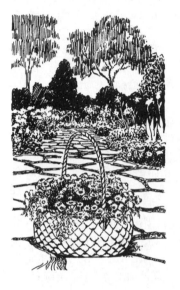

Tea Tree (*Melaleuca alternifolia)* oil, a strong antifungal and antiseptic, is added to wound washes and foot and nail preparations designed for fungal problems. It is also useful in acne and infected-skin preparations. It is added to creams, salves, powders, scrubs, baths and mouth and hair products. It has a clean, spicy yet medicinal aroma.

Thuja (*Thuja occidentalis*) oil is a strong antiseptic, antiviral oil. Add it to cleansing creams, foot products and preparations for acne and infected skin. Thuja oil should be added to products in small doses, as the oil can be irritating to the skin. It is also useful in muscle-relaxing preparations. Thuja oil can be applied directly to warts to remove them.

White Pine (*Pinus strobus*) oil is a strong disinfectant with a very medicinal smell that is not always appealing. Yet its cleansing and muscle-relaxant properties make it a valuable addition to certain formulas. It has a strong odor intensity, so use it sparingly. White pine oil can be combined with other oils to create a pleasing fragrance blend.

Wintergreen (*Gaultheria procumbens*) oil is used as an analgesic in balms and oils for sore muscles and bones. It has a cool, refreshing aroma, and can be added to creams, baths, lip balms, facial astringents and body powders.

Ylang-Ylang (*Canangium odoratum*) oil has a high, sweet, exotic, floral scent traditionally used in aphrodisiac and euphoric aromatherapy blends. Ylang-ylang's appealing aroma can be added to creams, body oils, baths, deodorants, perfumes and body powders. It has moderate antiseptic properties, and can be used for oily-skin problems. It has a strong odor and should be used sparingly so as not to be overpowering or to dominate other oils.

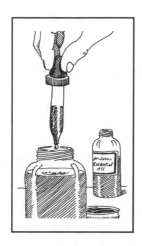
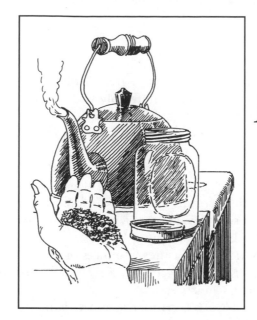

13
Basic
Equipment

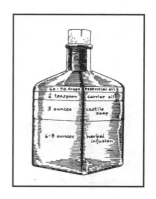

2-quart cooking pot to use for hot-water baths when melting ingredients.

Blender and/or food processor (preferably with whipping cream attachment), or **mixer** for whipping creams. You can use the blender and the food processor interchangeably, although I prefer the food processor for making purees. You can also use either a blender or food processor for grinding large quantities of herbs, nuts and seeds.

Bowls of various sizes.

Chopsticks for stirring. You can also use a spoon, knife or other implement.

Containers for making and storing formulas and ingredients, preferably made of glass. Save your jars! You will need various sizes: Wide- and narrow-mouth with tight-fitting lids, bottles, salt and spice shakers, lip balm jars, etc. Mason jars with lids in 8-, 16-, 32-, 64- and 128-oz. sizes are useful for making herbal infusions, tinctures, infused oils and vinegars. Nonglass containers such as squeeze-type bottles, fine spray mist bottles and tins with tight-fitting lids also come in handy. If you can't meet your jar needs through recycling, the Resources chapter lists companies that offer excellent jar choices at very reasonable prices.

Poly/cotton cloth, such as old sheets and pillowcases, cut into 12-by-12-inch squares for lining colanders and strainers during the decanting process.

Pure cotton cloth for cleaning the face. I save old pieces of good-quality fabric (such as old flannel sheets), cut them into small pieces as needed and use them as washcloths or as an improved and reusable replacement for store-bought cotton pads.

Cutting board

Glass eye droppers for dispensing essential oils, found in pharmacies and by direct mail. It is good to have a dozen or so droppers to use when a recipe calls for many essential oils. To clean them, wipe off essential oil and soak the glass part in alcohol for several minutes, then allow to air-dry.

Grater

Knife

Measuring spoons and cups. Pyrex or other heat proof measuring cup in 8-oz., 16-oz., and 32-oz. sizes, preferably with spouts for pouring. Try to get measuring cups that measure in 1-oz. or ½-oz. gradations.

Rags made from old socks and clothing do a much better job than paper towels when cleaning oily residue from jars, spoons, blenders, etc. Rags are the preferred choice environmentally as well. You will save time and hassle if you thoroughly wipe off equipment used for any recipe containing oil or beeswax, such as creams and salves, before washing it with soap and hot water.

Rubber spatulas for removing creams and other products from blenders, bowls, jars and cups.

Scale that measures in ounces or less than 1-oz. gradations. Although not absolutely necessary, a scale can make the preparation of certain formulas much easier.

Seed/Coffee grinder or mortar and pestle for grinding seeds, nuts and herbs in small quantities.

Wire mesh strainers of varying mesh size for sifting powders and straining infusions and tinctures.

Techniques and Definitions

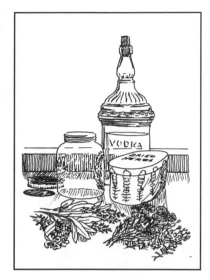
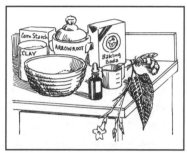
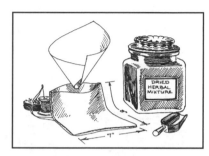

For many of the students who attend my classes, one of the biggest surprises comes from learning how easy it is to make body care preparations with herbs and other natural ingredients. No special equipment is needed beyond the tools found in most kitchens, and most of the techniques are easily mastered. With the exception of creams, which demand careful measurement and mixing, most preparations also leave ample leeway for trial-and-error experimentation and improvisation. Once you've tried the basic techniques described in this chapter a few times, you'll probably begin to develop an intuitive feel for how to mix and transform separate ingredients into finished products. Because certain terms that appear here may be unfamiliar to those who are new to the herbal and natural skin care arena, I've also included a Short List of Definitions at the end of this chapter.

Labeling Your Creations

Be sure to label your creations with a name, the date of manufacture, the list of ingredients and their proportions and directions for use. The date is important in terms of tracking the shelf life. Writing the recipe on the labels reminds you of exactly what went into a given formula and provides an accurate reference for making a new batch. It is especially important to label formulas that are refrigerated so that they are not mistaken for foodstuffs. Use permanent markers or cover the label with clear tape to prevent fading or obliteration of the information.

HERBAL INFUSIONS

The simplest herbal preparation is an infusion, which uses water as a menstrum to extract the active chemical constituents of the herbs. The best-known herbal infusion is herb tea. Be aware that the herbal infusions indicated throughout this book are made with a greater quantity of herb and steeped for a much longer period than the common cup of tea, which makes them much stronger and more concentrated. These strong herbal infusions are used as ingredients in baths, creams, hand and foot soaks, deodorants, facial toners, shampoos, hair conditioners, mouth rinses and more.

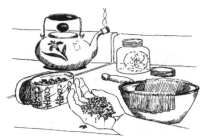

Directions for Herbal Infusions

In general use 1 pint of water per handful of whole dried herb, which is equivalent to approximately 1 oz. of herb by weight. Note that barks, roots, seeds and berries weigh more than leaves and flowers, so adjust your handfuls or volume measures accordingly. For example, a large handful of calendula flowers is equal in weight to a palmful of fennel seeds. When using powdered herbs, use about 3 tablespoons per pint of water. If using herbs that have been cut and sifted, often referred to in herb catalogues as c/s, use about 6 tablespoons per pint. When a recipe calls for a quart or gallon of herbal infusion, just multiply the proportions accordingly. It is important to remember that some loss of liquid through absorption will occur when making infusions with dried herbs — expect about a 20–30 percent loss. In some cases, such as in baths and soaks this loss is not important. However, in creams and other formulas this loss must be compensated for with more infusion, as you will notice in various recipes. If you are employing fresh herbs, use about 4 times the amount that you would the dried herb. No loss of liquid should occur. Keep in mind that dry herbs release their chemical constituents into water more effectively than fresh herbs, since their cell walls have been broken through dehydration.

The amount of herbs you use for an infusion does not need to be exact. The proportions provided here are a guideline. The potency of the herbs — which will vary according to how old they are, how they were grown, dried, and stored and how concentrated the herb is — can alter how much of it is necessary for attaining the desired therapeutic results.

Place the herbs in a jar with a tight-fitting lid and pour boiling water over them. To prevent the jar from cracking you can either place a metal object such as a spoon in it or initially pour only an ounce of the boiling water over the herb, allowing it to sit for a minute before pouring in the rest. Place the lid on the jar and let the herb steep for a minimum of 1 hour. I like to steep most herbs for 8 hours. The longer you steep an herb, the stronger your infusion will be. Bear in mind that roots, barks and berries are denser than flowers and leaves and thus may take longer to release their properties into the water.

After the herbs have steeped for the desired amount of time, strain the infusion through a colander or strainer lined with a thin cloth that is not too absorbent. I like to save old cotton/ poly sheets and cut them into 12-by-12-inch squares for lining the strainer. Tightly woven cheesecloth is also very good, though sometimes difficult to come by. Place the cloth-lined strainer over a bowl that is large enough to catch the liquid and pour the contents of the jar into it, allowing the liquid to seep through. If you are making a gallon of infusion for a bath, you may need to use a bucket or to strain the infusion in two parts. Squeeze out the remaining liquid left in the herbs by gathering up the ends of the cloth and twisting them together. Note that for certain preparations, you don't have to strain the infusion. When I prepare a footbath, I like to leave the herbs in the infusion.

TINCTURES

Tinctures are highly concentrated herbal infusions in which the menstrum can be a combination of water and alcohol, vinegar or glycerin. Tinctures are most often used internally for medicinal purposes. They can also be used topically, in such preparations as antimicrobial wound washes, mouthwashes, facial astringents, deodorant preparations and many other formulas. Tincturing with alcohol and water allows more active constituents to be extracted from an herb than does a water-based infusion. Tinctures are easy to use, and have the advantage of long shelf lives. They provide an optimal way to preserve an herb's volatile properties. Some herbs, such as St. Johnswort, are medicinally potent only when tinctured fresh. Other herbs can be tinctured dried, especially roots, bark and seeds. However, I generally make my tinctures from fresh herbs, since this seems to yield the strongest tinctures. When the herb is fresh its life force is stronger than it is when dried. The Ingredients chapter indicates which herbs are best tinctured fresh to obtain their healing attributes. Following are instructions for the basic tincturing techniques.

Simple Tinctures are made using a single herb tinctured alone.

Compound Tinctures are made with two or more herbs tinctured together. The total herbal quantity used will remain the same, but it is made up of a combination rather than just a single herb.

Directions for Alcohol Tinctures Using Dried Herbs

In general, use 1 part herb to 4 parts menstrum. Place 1 oz. of freshly crushed or powdered herb by weight into a 6 oz. glass jar with a tight-fitting lid. Pour 4-oz. of 80–100 proof liquor, such as vodka or brandy, over the herbs in the jar. Stir the alcohol into the herbs until they are thoroughly saturated, then cap tightly. Bear in mind that if the herbs being tinctured are particularly fluffy and voluminous, such as flowers like chamomile, calendula or yarrow, you may need to use 1 part herb to 5 or 6 parts menstrum. So for every 1 oz. of chamomile flower by weight you will use 5 or 6 oz. of menstrum by liquid measure. Because commercial drinking alcohol contains a certain percentage of water, you need not add extra water to the solution (please refer to the Alcohol section in the Ingredients chapter for a further explanation). In a few of the formulas, 190 proof alcohol is used to make a tincture with resinous herbs such as vanilla, but for the most part tinctures in this book are made with 80–100 proof alcohol. Label the jar with the date and contents, and keep it in a dark place away from direct light or heat; a cupboard is a good place. Try to shake the jar daily — the agitation maximizes the release of the herbal properties into the liquid — but even if you don't shake the jar you will have a potent tincture. Let the herbs steep in the liquid for a minimum of 3 weeks. (I like to let my tinctures steep for 6 weeks or longer.) After steeping, strain the tincture by placing a strainer lined with a thin cloth over a bowl and pour the entire contents of the jar into the cloth-lined strainer. Allow the liquid to seep into the bowl, then gather the ends of the cloth together and squeeze out any remaining liquid. The more you squeeze or press, the more tincture you end up with. However, you can expect a loss of about 20–30 percent even after thoroughly squeezing and pressing, since the dried herbs absorb a portion of the menstrum. Note that the tincture can also be stored unstrained until needed.

Directions for Alcohol Tinctures Using Fresh Herbs

Use a glass jar with a well-fitting lid and pack it tightly with fresh herbs of choice. Pour 80–100 proof liquor such as vodka or brandy over the herbs and let it filter down through them. Keep pouring in liquor until the herbs are completely covered by the menstrum, then cap jar tightly. Label the jar with the date and contents, and keep it in a dark place, such as a cupboard, away from direct light or heat. Let the herbs steep in the liquid for a minimum of 3 weeks. (I like to let my tinctures steep for 6 weeks or longer.) After steeping, strain the tincture by placing a strainer lined with a thin cloth over a bowl and pour the entire contents of the jar into the cloth-lined strainer. Allow the liquid to seep into the bowl, then gather the ends of the cloth together and squeeze out any remaining liquid. The more you squeeze or press, the more tincture you end up with. Note that the tincture can also be stored unstrained until needed.

The fresh herb tincture procedure uses approximately 1 part fresh herb by weight to 2 parts menstrum by liquid measure. This herb-to-menstrum ratio will vary depending on how tightly you pack the jar with herb and how much water the herb you are tincturing contains. Obviously the more tightly you pack the jar with herb, the greater the herbal portion and the less the menstrum portion will be. Fresh roots usually contain a lot of water, and these can be chopped or pureed and tinctured in a ratio of 1 part herb to 1 part menstrum. So for every 1 oz. of fresh root by weight, you can use 1 oz. of menstrum by liquid measure. Although it is not necessary to know the weights and measures when preparing a fresh herb tincture, this information can be helpful for planning ahead, obtaining necessary ingredients and using as a reference point regarding the strength of your tincture.

It's important to remember that fresh herb tinctures require more herb than do dry, since dry herbs are equal to 4 or more times the amount of fresh ones. Remember, too, that while drying herbs concentrates them, it can also decrease their potency.

Unlike tinctures made with dried herb, where a loss of menstrum through absorption occurs in the final product, there will be no loss of menstrum in the fresh herb tinctures. There may even be a slight gain in liquid, supplied from the water content of the fresh herb. The amount of liquid gained will depend on how much water the herb you are tincturing contains and how well you squeeze or press the tincture during the straining process.

STORAGE OF TINCTURES. Store tinctures in amber glass bottles, away from direct light or heat. Amber glass bottles (with or without eye-dropper caps) are available through mail order (see Resources).

Purchasing Herbal Tinctures

When purchasing herbal tinctures read the labels to see how much herb was actually used to make the tincture. If the label indicates a 1:10 ratio of fresh herb to menstrum, you know that only 1 oz. of herb was used to 10 oz. of menstrum, and you can assume that this is not going to be as strong as a tincture with a 1:2 ratio.

Directions for Herbal-Infused Vinegars

To make herbal-infused vinegar (also known as a vinegar tincture), follow the instructions for tincturing with alcohol, using vinegar as the menstrum. When making herbal-infused vinegars I prefer to use organic raw apple cider vinegar. It is important to a use a jar with a plastic or other nonmetallic lid, since vinegar corrodes metal. Because of its acidity, vinegar has the ability to extract calcium and other minerals from herbs, which is ideal for making calcium-rich edible vinegars for mineral supplementation. Vinegar tinctures are used as an ingredient in facial astringents and hair rinses, and are beneficial additions to baths and foot or hand soaks. They are also often delicious and nutritious to eat.

ABBREVIATED DIRECTIONS FOR HERBAL-INFUSED VINEGARS WITH DRIED HERBS. Place freshly crushed or powdered herb into a glass jar with a tightly fitting plastic lid. Pour vinegar over the herbs; stir the vinegar into the herb until thoroughly saturated, then cap tightly. Label the jar with the date and contents, and keep in a dark place. Shake daily and let steep for 3 weeks or longer. Strain vinegar when needed.

ABBREVIATED DIRECTIONS FOR HERBAL-INFUSED VINEGARS WITH FRESH HERBS. Use a glass jar with a plastic well-fitting lid and pack it tightly with fresh herbs of choice. Pour vinegar over the herbs and let it filter down through them. Keep pouring in vinegar until the herbs are completely covered by the vinegar, then cap tightly. Label the jar with the date and contents, and keep in a dark place. Let steep for 3 weeks or longer and strain when needed.

HERBAL-INFUSED OILS

These are oils in which herbs have been steeped so as to extract the healing properties of the herbs, along with their subtle color and scent. They are used topically in massage oils, salves, lip balms and creams. Please note that herbal-infused oils are not the same as essential oils and cannot be used interchangeably. Please see the Essential Oils section in the Ingredients chapter for further explanation. Herbal-infused oils can be made with dry or fresh herbs, with or without the use of heat. The different techniques and methods are described below. When infusing herbs in oil it is best to use a stable oil that will not go rancid quickly, such as cold pressed olive or sesame oil. When infusing with a less stable oil, such as canola or almond, you will need to use it up more quickly.

Directions for Herbal-Infused Oils with Dried Herbs

Making an herbal-infused oil with dried herbs is similar to making an alcohol tincture with dried herbs, except that oil is used as the menstrum. Use 1 oz. of herb by weight to 4 oz. of oil by liquid measure. Place 1 oz. of freshly crushed or powdered herb by weight into a 6-oz. glass jar with a tightly fitting lid. Pour 4 oz. of cold pressed olive oil or other carrier oil of choice over the herbs in the jar. Stir the oil into them until they are thoroughly saturated, then cap tightly. Bear in mind that if the herbs being infused are particularly fluffy and voluminous, such as flowers like chamomile, calendula or yarrow, you may need to use 1 part herb to 5 or 6 parts menstrum. So for every ounce of chamomile flower by weight you will use 5 or 6 oz. of oil by liquid measure. Label the jar with the date and contents. Place it on a wooden cutting board or in a shallow bowl to prevent the oil from dripping onto unwanted places. Try to shake the jar daily — the agitation maximizes the release of the herbal properties into the liquid — but even if you don't shake the jar you will have a potent oil. Let the herbs steep in the oil for a minimum of 3 weeks. I like to let my oils steep for 6 weeks or longer. I often place herb-and-oil-filled jars on a jelly roll pan in the oven — with the pilot light on, as the warmth helps to encourage the extraction process. After steeping, strain oil by placing a strainer lined with a thin cloth over a bowl, and pour the entire contents of the jar into the cloth-lined strainer. Allow the oil to seep into the bowl, then gather the ends of the cloth together and squeeze out any remaining oil. The more you squeeze or press, the more oil you will end up with. However, you can expect a loss of about 20–30 percent even after thoroughly squeezing and pressing, since the dried herbs absorb a portion of the oil.

About Herbal-Infused Oils with Fresh Herbs

The process of making Herbal-Infused Oils with Fresh Herbs is similar to that of making tinctures with fresh herbs. However, more care is needed when making infused oil with fresh herbs, since these are prone to mold and unwanted bacterial growth due to their moisture content, and the sterile environment provided by alcohol tinctures is lacking. This can cause the infused oil to go bad, indicated by an unmistakably rotten smell. If this happens, you should discard the entire contents of the jar and start over. In the event that an oil grows mold but still smells good, you can save it by scooping off the mold and adding more oil to keep the herbs submerged. In my earlier years of making comfrey leaf oil, I always made it with fresh leaf, and the oil would always end up smelling like blue cheese. Nobody would use the products I made with it because of the horrendous smell. It became a running joke at the local natural foods store that my comfrey oil formulas were the worst-smelling products in the shop. I have had enough oils go bad that I now prefer to use freshly dried herbs to make herbal-infused oil. An exception to this is St. Johnswort, which must be prepared when the herb is fresh. In general, if the herb contains a lot of moisture or is high in protein — such as comfrey leaf and root, chickweed, burdock root, nettle leaf, jewelweed, marshmallow root and violet leaf — you are better off drying it for a few days before using it for an infused oil. Or you may want to try out the following heat method. On the other hand, there are many herbalists who are very successful in making these oils. The following directions should get you started on the right track.

Directions for Herbal-Infused Oils with Fresh Herbs

Use a glass jar with a well-fitting lid and pack it somewhat loosely with fresh herbs of choice (more loosely than when making a tincture). Make sure the jar is absolutely dry; moisture can ruin the batch. Pour cold pressed olive oil or other carrier oil of choice over the herbs and let it filter down through the herbs. Keep pouring in oil until the herbs are completely covered by it. Make sure the herbs are submerged in the oil so that no plant matter is exposed to the air. (Marbles and rocks can be used to weigh them down.) Cap and label the jar with the date and contents. Place a bowl under your oil jar as it steeps, since a little oil usually seeps out from beneath the lid, running down the side of the jar and creating an oily mess. By keeping the lids off the jars you can avoid some of the mess, and this also provides an aerobic environment that can help to prevent the growth of mold. I often place herb-and-oil-filled jars on a jelly roll pan in the oven — with the pilot light on, as the warmth helps to encourage the extraction process. After steeping, strain the oil by placing a strainer lined with a thin cloth over a bowl and pouring the entire contents of the jar into the cloth-lined strainer. Allow the oil to seep into the bowl, then gather the ends of the cloth together and squeeze out any remaining oil. Allow the strained oil to sit for a couple of days, which allows the water from the fresh herbs to collect at the bottom of the jar. Next pour or siphon off the oil and discard the liquid that has collected at the bottom. If you don't separate out the water, the oil may spoil. Store oils in a cool, dark, dry place.

HERBAL-INFUSED OILS WITH HEAT. This method is excellent for fresh herbs that contain a lot of moisture or protein. It can also be used with dried herbs to speed the infusion process, and sometimes yields a more potent oil. Heat helps to evaporate water from the fresh herbs, which discourages the growth of mold and prevents the oil from rotting. The addition of heat also speeds up the infusion process, making the herbal-infused oil ready in about 10 days. Place your herb-and-oil-filled jar uncovered on a heat source that does not exceed 125 degrees. You may want to place the mixture in a wide pot so that more surface area is exposed to the air, promoting the evaporation of water. The heat source can be a radiator, warming tray, warmer shelf of a woodstove or whatever else in your home will offer this kind of consistent, gentle heat. You can also place the mixture into an electric cooking pot or turkey roaster, with the lid on but the vent open, set on low. With an electric cooking pot, the lowest setting is above 125 degrees, so you will need to turn it on and off throughout the day to adjust the temperature. Keep infusing the herb-and-oil-mixture for 10 days, then proceed to strain and separate the oil as described above. Note: If you don't have a thermometer, use your skin as a guide and feel the oil to make sure it is not too hot. Oil at 125 degrees is still cool enough to touch without burning yourself, although if you continue to touch the oil for a few seconds it should feel a little too hot for comfort.

SALVES AND BALMS

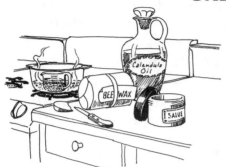

Salves or balms are effective and convenient preparations for soothing and healing skin. One very popular salve is lip balm. These preparations are very easy and satisfying to make. Any herbal-infused oil or carrier oil can be turned into a salve with the simple addition of beeswax, which solidifies the oil. The hardness or softness of the salve depends on how much beeswax you use. In general, I like to make balms on the harder side because they are then more stable and don't ooze out of the jar and into my bag on a hot day. The addition of beeswax slows down the oil's oxidation process, delaying rancidity and prolonging shelf life. The formulas in this book have varying beeswax-and-oil ratios, resulting in softer or harder consistencies depending on the purpose of the salve.

Directions for Salves and Balms

In general use 3 oz. of oil to 1 oz. of beeswax (liquid measures, in both cases).

Put a pot filled 4 inches high with water on the stove over medium heat. Fill a heat-proof measuring cup with liquid oil to the 3-oz. mark, then grate or cut small pieces of beeswax and add it to the oil up to the 4-oz. mark. Place the measuring cup in a hot-water bath and heat until the beeswax has thoroughly melted into the oil, stirring it well with a chopstick or spoon. Pour the preparation into a dry, wide-mouth, 4-oz. glass jar and watch it solidify as it cools. If you are going to add essential oils to your salve you should do so right after pouring the mixture into the jar and cap the jar immediately to prevent the volatile essential oils from evaporating. Leave the salve undisturbed while it is cooling. Some people use a separate double boiler for melting the beeswax adding it in liquid form to your already heated oil. This method reduces the amount of time the oil is heated. If you choose this method, the oil has to be hot enough to accept the beeswax or it will clump up. If this happens, just continue heating the mixture and stirring until the wax is thoroughly melted.

To test salve consistency, drip a small amount of melted salve onto a saucer and place it in the freezer for 1 minute. You may choose to experiment and change the oil-to-beeswax ratio if you prefer either a harder or softer salve.

Store salves tightly capped away from heat and direct light.

SUMMER SALVES. During the summer months use more beeswax for a thicker and more stable salve, since the ambient heat can turn a salve into a thick liquid and also may cause the oil to go rancid. Use 1 oz. of beeswax, 2 oz. of oil and a 3 oz. glass jar, proceeding as above.

CREAMS

Creams are luscious preparations applied to the skin that are highly nutritive, moisturizing and emollient. They are largely made of water and oil, which hydrate and lubricate the skin, respectively. Oils can range from somewhat drying to highly lubricating. The type of oil combined with the other ingredients you choose will help to determine the properties of your final product (see Ingredients chapter).

Creams are probably the trickiest preparation in this book to make, but once you have mastered the technique you will be able to turn out a perfect batch every time. It is important to follow the instructions very closely, measuring the ingredients as accurately as possible. Creams are prone to bacterial contamination and should be made with distilled water, if water is used, along with very clean equipment and hands.

Basic Cream Formula

Use 6 oz. liquid oil, 3 oz. solid oil, 1 oz. beeswax and 9 oz. water.

This basic recipe makes approximately 19 oz. of cream.

The liquid oil portion can be made from carrier oils such as peanut, jojoba, olive or apricot kernel, and/or herbal-infused oils (see Ingredients chapter). If you include lecithin or other fat-soluble ingredients, these should be added to the liquid oil and included in the total liquid oil measurement.

The solid oil portion refers to oils that are solid at room temperature, such as coconut oil, shea butter or cocoa butter.

The water portion can be made from distilled water, floral waters, distilled witch hazel, herbal infusion or fruit or vegetable juice. Aloe gel, herbal tinctures, glycerin and other water-soluble ingredients should be added to the water portion and included in the total water measurement.

Keep in mind that plain water, herbal infusions and juices will cause a cream to spoil more rapidly. So use them up quickly or add a natural preservative such as grapefruit seed extract. Also note that when alcohol is used as part of the water portion, the cream will often change texture, become less smooth and begin to separate after a few weeks. Cold temperatures seem to make creams made with alcohol separate more quickly. This can be a detriment when making cream for sale, since people like their creams to look smooth and creamy. However, when making creams for yourself, you may not be bothered by the cream's appearance, since it does not hamper the effectiveness of the formula.

Optional ingredients include essential oils, PABA for sun protection and natural preservatives such as grapefruit seed extract or vitamins A, C or E.

Essential oils also act as preservatives due to their antimicrobial properties. However, you need to use a lot of essential oil to preserve creams. For example, the Lavender Sandalwood Cream in the Whole Body Treatments chapter is extremely stable and very resistant to bacterial contamination. The recipe calls for 3 teaspoons of essential oil per 19 oz. batch.

Directions for Creams

Begin by pouring 6 oz. of liquid oil into a 16-oz. heat-proof measuring cup. Add pieces of solid oil to the liquid oil until the total volume reaches the 9-oz. mark on the measuring cup; this will give you an exact 3-oz. measurement of solid oil. Next add pieces of beeswax to the cup until it reaches the 10-oz. mark; this will give you an exact 1-oz. measurement of beeswax. Put the cup containing the oils and beeswax into a pot partially filled with water, place over medium heat and stir with a chopstick or spoon until the oils and beeswax melt and dissolve into a single uniform liquid.

Remove the cup from the hot water and allow the mixture to cool to body temperature. I check the temperature by simply touching the cup to my skin. As it cools, the mixture will become thick and opaque. Stir it as it cools to keep the consistency smooth and uniform. If it becomes cooler than body temperature, just reheat the mixture.

While the oils are cooling, pour 9 oz. of distilled water into a measuring cup and heat to body temperature by placing it into the hot-water bath after the oil mixture has been removed from the heat. Test the temperature with a clean finger.

When the oil mixture and the water have both reached body temperature, pour the water into a blender, food processor (preferably using a whipping cream attachment) or mixing bowl and add optional water-soluble ingredients such as vitamin C, grapefruit seed extract or PABA. Process at high speed. If using a high-power blender such as a Vita mixer, set it on low. Slowly add the oil mixture by pouring a thin drizzle into the whirling water. It will begin to thicken and sputter. Continue to process until the oil and water have blended together into a thick, creamy liquid. This may take 5–10 minutes in a blender or food processor. If using a high-power blender, generally you will only need to blend for 20–30 seconds. If using an electric mixer, beat at the highest speed for about 15 minutes. I get the best results with the Vita mixer set on low speed, where an emulsion occurs in 20–30 seconds. This process of emulsification, whereby water and oil merge into one liquid, is the secret to creams.

Scoop the cream into a 32-oz. measuring cup with a spout for easy pouring. If you are going to add essential oils to the cream, do so at this point, making sure to stir them in well. Pour the cream into very clean, dry jars, filling them to the top and leaving as little airspace as possible. Cap with tight-fitting lids. Leave undisturbed overnight so that the cream will set thoroughly. Store the cream out of direct heat and sunlight. Use up quickly or refrigerate for longer storage. Unfortunately, cold temperatures often alter the consistency of a cream, causing the water to bead out and the solid oils to turn slightly granular. But this is only a visual problem and will not change the effectiveness of the cream. If the cream should separate after a period of time, stir vigorously to whip it back together. Try adding a pinch of borax while slightly warming the cream as you stir to help reemulsify it.

In applying cream, make sure that your fingers are very clean when you scoop the cream out of the jar, in order to minimize bacterial contact. Because truly natural creams are so perishable, they are hard to come by on the commercial market. In the Resources section I've included a number of wonderful, mostly small companies that make excellent natural creams.

AROMATHERAPY OILS

These are strongly scented oils whose therapeutic properties are largely attributed to their scent, although they are beneficial in other ways as well. They are made with pure essential oils diluted in a nut or seed oil known as a carrier oil. The essential oils provide the aroma as well as such actions as cleansing, toning and stimulating. The carrier oil offers lubrication, protection and emolliency. The essential oils can be added alone or in combination to create a unique scent with various effects. It is important to understand that aromatherapy oils are not the same as herbal-infused oils. You can use an herbal-infused oil as part or all of your carrier oil when making an aromatherapy oil. You can make aromatic oils for bath and massage, face oils, and other therapeutic products using the following guidelines.

Directions for Aromatherapy Oils

AROMATHERAPY OILS FOR BODY. Dilute 15–30 drops of pure essential oil with 1 oz. of carrier oil.

AROMATHERAPY OILS FOR FACE. Use a more diluted ratio of 5 drops of pure essential oil to 1 oz. of carrier oil.

Begin by filling a small-mouth 1-oz. jar with the carrier oil of your choice, leaving an 1/8-inch space at the top. Add the essential oils drop by drop, then cap the jar and shake well. Be sure to label the ingredients and their proportions, and your oil is ready for use.

Although the basic ratios just given are useful as general guidelines, the amount of essential oil you use will vary considerably depending on the odor intensity of the essential oil you choose and how you intend to use the formula. You may also prefer a stronger or lighter scent. Consult the Ingredients chapter to find out the odor intensity of the various essential oils.

It is advisable to store products containing essential oil in amber glass with well-fitting lids, since light and air degrade the oil.

POWDERS

Powders are made by combining and pulverizing different ingredients such as herbs, grains, nuts and seeds, then adding absorbent powders such as clay, cornstarch, baking soda or arrowroot. The powdering process is very simple, and often necessary when making face and body scrubs, foot, baby and deodorant powders and a variety of other products.

Directions for Powders

To make a powder, grind all the unpowdered ingredients in a coffee/seed grinder that you do not use for grinding coffee. Sift the ground ingredients through a mesh strainer into a large bowl. The finer the strainer, the smoother the powder will be. If you have partially ground particles remaining in the strainer, simply regrind and strain them again, repeating the process as many times as necessary until all the ingredients are ground to the desired consistency. Depending on the quantity of product, you may have to do the grinding in batches. A food processor or blender can be used to grind larger quantities of ingredients.

For formulas that call for clay, arrowroot powder, cornstarch and/or other powdered ingredients, add these ingredients after grinding the other ingredients, then mix thoroughly. If using essential oils, add them at this point, a few drops at a time, stirring well after each addition. Store in an airtight container. Save used powder canisters and salt and spice shakers, or purchase powder cylinders (see Resources) for powders that will be sprinkled on the skin.

Refrigerate the powder if it contains nuts or seeds and will not be used within a month. The nuts and seeds, once ground, are vulnerable to oxidation, which can make the powder go rancid.

Warning: Powders, even those made from natural herbal ingredients, should not be inhaled. When making powders prevent inhalation by handling them gently so they don't blow into the air. If necessary, wear a handkerchief around your nose and mouth or make the formula outdoors.

CLEANUP

You will save time and hassle if you wipe oils and waxy residues from your equipment before washing it with soap and hot water. This is important to do after making oils, salves and creams. Cotton rags from old shirts, socks, sheets and the like work best for this purpose — much better than paper towels. Once you have wiped the surfaces clean, proceed to wash with very hot water and soap.

A SHORT LIST OF DEFINITIONS

Antimicrobial. A substance, such as tea tree oil, that is antifungal, antiviral or antibacterial and that helps to clean and disinfect.

Aromatherapy. The use of aromas to influence one's sense of well-being. Essential oils are typically used to provide the therapeutic aroma.

Base Oil. These oils are generally extracted from fruits, grains, nuts or seeds, and serve as a foundation for skin care products and essential oils. Some of the more commonly used base oils are almond, peanut, olive, corn, grapeseed and jojoba. See Ingredients chapter for more information.

Carrier Oil. See Base Oil.

Compress. Also referred to as a fomentation, it is a cloth dipped in liquid — such as an herbal infusion — and then wrung out and applied to the skin for therapeutic purposes.

Decant. To separate solids or plant materials from a liquid, such as when making a tincture, herbal oil or infusion.

Emollient. A substance that soothes, softens and protects the skin, such as an oil, salve or cream.

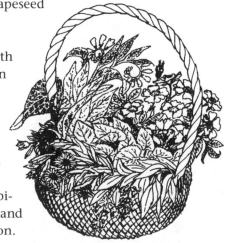

Emulsion. The mixing of a couple of liquids that are typically incompatible, such as water and oil, in making creams and other products. Mayonnaise is a commonly known emulsion.

Hot-Water Bath (or Bain Marie). This is an improvised double boiler made by placing a heat-proof vessel into a pot partially filled with simmering water. The ingredients in the vessel are gently and indirectly exposed to heat, thereby removing the danger of overheating.

Humectant. A substance, such as honey, glycerin and sorbitol, that encourages the retention of moisture. When applied to the skin it promotes hydration.

Hydrate. To provide water and moisture.

Infuse. To steep or soak herbs in a liquid, such as water, to extract their soluble constituents.

Maceration. The process of extracting herbal properties into a liquid by soaking or steeping them, such as when making a tincture.

Menstrum. A solvent, such as water, alcohol or vinegar, that is used to extract the medicinal properties of an herb.

Poultice. A soft, moist quantity of herb, meal or other therapeutic substance that is applied directly to the skin for healing purposes. Poultices have been used since ancient times to encourage the healing of wounds. They are made by mashing up fresh herbs or foodstuffs until the juices are flowing to create a soft, moist mass, which is then applied directly to the affected area. When dry ingredients are used, they are usually powdered and then moistened with a liquid such as water or an herbal tincture to create a paste that is applied to the skin. A cloth is often wrapped over the soft, moist mass or paste to bind it to the skin.

Sebum. An oily secretion of the sebaceous glands that mixes with other skin secretions to lubricate and moisturize the skin and hair, keeping them soft, flexible and water-resistant.

Table of Measures

Measurements by volume

1 teaspoon = ⅓ tablespoon = 5 milliliters
1½ teaspoons = ½ tablespoon = 7.5 milliliters
2 tablespoons = ⅛ cup (1 oz.) = 30 milliliters
4 tablespoons = ¼ cup (2 oz.) = 59 milliliters
5⅓ tablespoons = ⅓ cup = 79 milliliters
8 tablespoons = ½ cup (4 oz.) = 118.4 milliliters
16 tablelspoons = 1 cup (8 oz.) = 236.8 milliliters
1 cup = 8 fluid oz. = .2366 liters (approx. ¼ liter)
2 cups = 1 pint (16 oz.) = .4732 liters (approx. ½ liter)
4 cups or 2 pints = 1 quart = .9463 liters (approx. 1 liter)
4 quarts = 1 gallon (128 oz.) = 3.79 liters

❦ *Resources* ❦

Suppliers of Herbal and Natural Body Care Products, Ingredients and Packaging

Boston Jojoba Company, P.O. Box 771, Middleton, MA 01949, 800-2JOJOBA. Excellent and affordable jojoba oil. www.bostonjojoba.com.

Dancing Willow Herbs, 960 Main Ave., Durango, CO 81301, 888-247-1654. Debra Reuben, practicing herbalist, runs an herbal apothecary and mail order business offering excellent-quality tinctures, herbal-infused oils, liniments and more.

Essential Oil Company, 1719 SE Umatilla St., Portland, OR 97202, 800-729-5912. Offers a complete line of essential oils, carrier oils and other cosmetics ingredients.

Falcon Formulations, 468 County Route 2, Dept.EB4, Accord, NY 12404, 845-687-8938. This is the line of natural body care products and medicinal tinctures I make. Many of the formulas in this book originate from this line. I make these products in small batches and often customize them to order.

Green Terrestrial, 1449 Warm Brook Rd., Arlington, VT 05250, 802-375-8087. Founded by Pam Montgomery, owned by Brenda Nicholson, wise woman herbalist, offers a line of organically grown and wild-crafted herbal products, tinctures, infused oils, salves, etc.

Healing Spirits, 9198 State Route 415, Avoca, NY 14809, 607-566-2701, A small, family-run business offering excellent-quality organically grown and wild-crafted dried herbs, beeswax and other herbal products. HealingSpirits@juno.com.

Heartsong Farm Healing Herbs, RFD 1 Box 275, Groveton, NH 03582, 603-636-2286. Small family-run business offering excellent quality organically grown and wild-crafted dried and fresh herbs, healing preparations and more. mphil@together.net.

Herb Pharm, P.O. Box 116, Williams, OR., 97544, 800-348-4372. Offers the most extensive line of exceptional quality herbal tinctures, compounds, salves, liniments and more.

Island Herbs, c/o Ryan Drum, Waldron Island, WA 98297. Send SASE for a list of dried bulk herbs and seaweeds. Exceptional quality, but be patient.

Janca's Jojoba, 465 East Juanita Ave., #7, Mesa, AZ, 480-497-9494. Offers a complete line of carrier oils, essential oils, shea butter, PABA, jars, beeswax, cosmetic ingredients and more.

Jean's Greens, 119 Sulphur Springs Rd., Newport, NY 12147, 888-845-TEAS. This small business, run by Jean Argus, offers a complete line of exceptional herbal products plus all the materials to make your own body care products at very reasonable prices. An extensive list of herbs, essential oils, jars, tinctures, salves, books, beeswax, infused oils and more. Jean carries several of my products, including the Earthly Extracts line of medicinal tinctures that I make.

Larch Hanson, Seaweed Supplier, P.O. Box 57, Steuben, ME 04680, 207-546-2875. A small, conscientious business offering excellent-quality sea vegetables and garden fertilizer at reasonable prices.

Liberty Natural Products, Inc., 8120 SE Stark St., Portland, OR 97215, 800-289-8427, Wholesale supplier of high quality botanical ingredients, $50 minimum. www.libertynatural.com.

Mountain Rose Herbs, 85472 Dilley Lane, Eugene, OR 97405, 800-879-3337. Offers a complete line of herbs, essential oils, beeswax, carrier oils, jars and containers, herbal body care products, face creams and hair products, books and more. All items available in small quantities. www.mountainRoseHerbs.com.

Pacific Botanicals, 4350 Fish Hatchery Rd., Grants Pass, OR 97527, 541-479-7777. Excellent-quality dried and fresh herbs, organically grown and wild crafted. Available in bulk only.

Sage Mountain Herb Products, P.O. Box 6091, Holliston, MA 01746, 508-429-8627. A small, family-run business offering tinctures, salves, creams, etc., all formulated by Rosemary Gladstar and made from organically grown and wild-crafted herbs. www.sagemtnherbproducts.com.

7Song Botanicals, P.O. Box 6626, Ithaca, NY 14851, 607-564-1023. An extensive and eclectic line of herbal remedies as well as classes on herbalism.

Starwest Botanicals Inc., 11253 Trade Center Drive, Rancho Cordova, CA 95742, 800-800-HERB. Offers oils, essential oils, herbs and more.

Wolf Howl Herbals, Earthwings Farm, 208 Bisson Rd., Orange, VT 05641, 802-479-1034. Sage Blue offers handcrafted body care products, infused oils, Breast Balm, salves, tinctures and teas from organic and wildcrafted herbs.

Woodland Essence, 392 Tea Cup St., Cold Brook, NY 13324, 315-845-1515. Kate Gilday and family prepare herbal products, including the "Itch Re-leaf." This small, family-based business also makes flower essences from the forest and their gardens.

Wood Song Cottage Gardens, 207 River Rd., N. New Portland, ME 04961, 207-628-2542. "Preserving the Cottage Tradition in Herbal Industry," offering excellent quality certified organic and wild-crafted medicinal herbs.

Zack Woods Herb Farm, 278 Mead Rd., Hyde Park, VT 05655, 802-888-7278. Offers over 40 varieties of organically certified or ethically wild-crafted dried and fresh medicinal herbs. zackwoods@PShift.com.

Herbal Seed Resources

Abundant Life Seed Foundation, P O Box 772, Port Townsend, WA 98368, 360-385-5660.

Fedco Seeds, P.O. Box 520, Waterville, ME 04903.

Flowery Branch, P.O. Box 1330, Flowery Branch, GA 30542.

J. L. Hudson, Seedsman, Star Route 2, Box 387, La Honda, CA 94020.

Books

NUTRITION AND COOKING

Diet and Nutrition: A Holistic Approach, by Rudolph Ballantine, MD. Honesdale, PA: Himalayan International Institute, 1978.

Fats that Heal and Fats that Kill, by Udo Erasmus. Burnaby British Canada Canada: Alive Books, 1993.

Food and Healing, by Anne Marie Colbin. New York: Balantine Books, 1986.

Native Nutrition, by Ron Schmid, N.D. Rochester Vermont: Healing Arts Press, 1994.

Nourishing Traditions: The Cookbook that Challenges Politically Correct Nutrition and the Diet Dictocrats, by Sally Fallon with Mary G. Enig, Ph.D. Washington, DC: New Trends Publishing, 1999. Available from Falcon Formulations, 845-687-8938 or Price Pottenger Nutrition Foundation (see below).

Nutrition and Physical Degeneration: A Comparison of Primitive and Modern Diets and Their Effects, by Weston A. Price, D.D.S. 2000. Available through the Price Pottenger Nutrition Foundation, P.O. Box 2614, La Mesa, CA 91943, 619-462-7600. www.pricepottenger.org.

HERBALS

The Family Herbal, by Barbara and Peter Theiss. Rochester, VT: Healing Arts Press, 1989.

Herbal Healing for Women, by Rosemary Gladstar. New York: Simon & Schuster, 1993.

The Herbal Medicine Maker's Handbook, by James Green. Forestville, CA: Simplers Botanical Co., 1990, 707-887-2012.

Herbal Renaissance: Growing, Using and Understanding Herbs in the Modern World, by Steven Foster. Salt Lake City: Gibbs Smith, Publisher, 1993.

The Herbs of Life, by Leslie Tierra. Freedom, CA: Crossing Press, 1992.

The Holistic Herbal, by David Hoffman. Scotland: Findhorn Press, 1983.

The Male Herbal, by James Green. Freedom, CA: The Crossing Press, 1991.

Menopausal Years: The Wise Women Way, by Susun Weed. Woodstock, NY: Ash Tree Publishing, 1992.

Menopause, by Amanda McQuade Crawford. Freedom, CA: Crossing Press, 1996.

Natural Medicine for Children, by Julian Scott. New York: Avon Books, 1990.

Nutritional Herbology, by Mark Pedersen. Bountiful, UT: Pedersen Publishing, 1987.

Planetary Herbology: An Integration of Western Herbs into the Traditional Chinese and Ayurvedic Systems, by Michael Tierra. Santa Fe, NM: Lotus Press, 1988.

Potter's New Cyclopaedia of Botanical Drugs and Preparations, by R. C. Wren. Essex, England: The C.W. Daniel Co. Limited, 1988.

The Roots of Healing: A Woman's Book of Herbs, by Deb Soule. New York: Carol Publishing Group, 1995.

Sage Healing Ways Series, by Rosemary Gladstar. P.O. Box 420, East Barre, VT: Sage Mountain Herbs.

The Wise Woman Herbal for the Childbearing Years, by Susun Weed. Woodstock, NY: Ash Tree Publishing, 1986.

Witches Heal, by Billie Potts. Ann Arbor, MI: DuReve Publications, 1988.

NATURAL HERBAL BODY CARE AND BEAUTY; AROMATHERAPY

The Art of Aromatherapy: The Healing and Beautifying Properties of the Essential Oils of Flowers and Herbs, by Robert B. Tisserand. New York: Inner Traditions International, 1977.

The Complete Book of Essential Oils and Aromatherapy, by Valerie A. Worwood. San Rafael, CA: New World Library Press, 1991.

The Complete Book of Natural Cosmetics: An Authoratative Guide to Natural Beauty Aids that Can Be Prepared in the Buyer's Own Kitchen, by Beatrice Travern. New York: Simon & Schuster, 1974.

The Herbal Body Book, by Stephanie Tourles. Pownal, VT: Storey Publishing, 1994.

Jeanne Rose's Herbal Body Book, by Jeanne Rose. New York: Putnam Publishing Group, 1976.

Natural Beauty at Home, by Janice Cox. New York, NY: Henry Holt and Co., 1995.

Natural Organic Hair and Skin Care, by Aubrey Hampton. Tampa, FL: Organica Press, 1987.

The Natural Soap Book: Making Herbal and Vegetable-Based Soaps, by Susan Miller Cavitch. Pownal, VT: Storey Publishing, 1995.

FIELD GUIDES

A Field Guide to Wildflowers of Northeastern and North-central North America, by Roger Tory Peterson and Margaret McKenny. Boston: Houghton Mifflin Co., 1968.

Identifying and Harvesting Edible and Medicinal Plants In wild (and Not So Wild) Places, by "Wildman" Steve Brill, with Evelyn Dean. New York: Hearst Books, 1994.

Peterson Field Guides: Eastern/Central Medicinal Plants, by Steven Foster and James Duke. Boston: Houghton Mifflin Co., 1990.

Peterson Field Guides: Edible Wild Plants, by Lee Allen Peterson. Boston: Houghton Mifflin Co., 1977.

Herbal Organizations

Northeast Herbal Association, P.O. Box 103, Manchang, MA 01526. A networking and educational organization that publishes an excellent newsletter and directory.

United Plant Savers, P.O. Box 77, Guysville, OH 45735. A nonprofit organization for replanting and protecting endangered plants. www.plantsavers.org.

ℑ *Subject Index* 𝕎

❧ Ingredient Index ☙

❧ *Ceres Press Order Form* 🌿

Clean & Green: *The Complete Guide to Nontoxic and Environmentally Safe Housekeeping* by Annie Berthold-Bond. 485 ways to clean, polish, disinfect, deodorize, launder, remove stains — even wash your car, without harming yourself or the environment. Recipes based on harmless, non-polluting, renewable ingredients. 100,000 in print. *(160 pages/Paper/$9.95)* .... $ _____

American Wholefoods Cuisine: *Over 1300 Meatless, Wholesome Recipes from Short Order to Gourmet* by Nikki & David Goldbeck. Considered "the new *Joy of Cooking*" by authorities from *Food & Wine* to *Vegetarian Times*, this major cookbook introduces a contemporary cuisine that "tastes great and happens to be healthy." 1300 recipes, plus 300 pages of valuable kitchen information. Over 250,000 in print. *(580 pages/Paper/$25.00)* .... $ _____

The Good Breakfast Book: *Making Breakfast Special* by Nikki & David Goldbeck. 450 vegetarian recipes from elegant brunches to quick workday and schoolday "getaways." Attention to high fiber, complex carbohydrates and fat control. Recipes for vegans, as well as people with wheat, dairy and egg sensitivities. *(206 pages/Paper/$9.95)* .... $ _____

The Healthiest Diet in the World: *A Cookbook & Mentor* by Nikki & David Goldbeck. This groundbreaking work blends the science and art of cooking and nutrition with the authors' 25 years of experience. Includes the Goldbecks' "Eight Golden Guidelines" and 300 exciting recipes that reach a new level of health and enjoyment. Nikki's "Dialogue Boxes" are like having a nutritionist in the kitchen. *(561 pages/Paper $18.00)* .... $ _____

NEW **Healthy Highways:** *The Traveler's Guide to Heathy Eating* by Nikki & David Goldbeck. Eat well away from home with this guide to 1,900 healthy eateries and natural food stores in the U.S. Maps and local directions guide the way. Belongs in every glove compartment. Free updates and more at HealthyHighways.com. *(420 pages/Paper/$18.95)* .... $ _____

NEW **EAT WELL The YoChee Way:** *The Easy and Delicious Way to Cut Fat and Calories with Natural YoChee [Yogurt Cheese]* by Nikki & David Goldbeck. Improve your diet without forgoing your favorite dishes with low calorie, low fat, calcium rich YoChee. A great substitute for cream cheese, sour cream, mayonnaise. Guide and 275 recipes with nutritional analysis. If you can use a spoon, you can make YoChee. YoChee makers available online. *(310 pages/Paper/$18.95)* .... $ _____

___ **Earthly Bodies & Heavenly Hair** by Dina Falconi *(Paper/$17.95)* .... $ _____

MERCHANDISE TOTAL .... $ _____

SHIPPING: First item $4.75, additional items $1.75 each; Canada $7.25, plus $3.25 additional items ..... $ _____

NY SALES TAX (NY residents must add local sales tax to both merchandise AND shipping.) .... $ _____

TOTAL ENCLOSED .... $ _____

Charge VISA/Mastercard/AmEx/Discover (please circle one)

Card# _____ Expires _____

Signature _____ Phone _____

Name_____ Email _____

Address _____

City/State _____ Zip/Postal Code _____

* All orders must be accompanied by payment in U.S. funds or charged to Visa/MC. Sorry, no CODs.

CERES PRESS • PO Box 87 EB5 • Woodstock, NY 12498 • Ph/FAX 845-679-5573 or 888-804-8848

Please visit our website at www.HealthyHighways.com